HEALTH OBSERVATION OF SCHOOL CHILDREN

Health Observation
of School Children

A GUIDE FOR HELPING TEACHERS
AND OTHERS TO OBSERVE AND
UNDERSTAND THE SCHOOL CHILD
IN HEALTH AND ILLNESS

GEORGE M. WHEATLEY, M.D., M.P.H.
*Third Vice-President and Medical Director, Health and
Welfare, Metropolitan Life Insurance Company*

GRACE T. HALLOCK
*Coauthor of Health for Better Living Series, Health for
Life, Health Heroes Series, and other health books*

Third Edition

The Blakiston Division

McGRAW-HILL BOOK COMPANY

New York   London   Sydney   Toronto   1965

PREFACE

The first edition of this book appeared in 1951. The primary purpose in writing it was to furnish teachers in training and teachers in service with information that would aid them in making the most of their unique opportunities for identifying children with health problems and for educating and guiding all students in the ways of health.

With the passing years there has been no change in purpose. But there has been steady progress in the sciences that supply a large part of the knowledge upon which the text is based. Consequently there was much material to be brought up to date in preparing this edition. Also many suggestions for improvement of the book have been made by those who have used the previous two editions as teaching aids in courses for future teachers and school nurses. These suggestions have led to very extensive reorganization of, additions to, subtractions from, and in some cases simplification of, the text.

MAJOR VENTURES IN REORGANIZATION

The setting up as chapters in their own right of certain subdivisions of several of the original chapters represents the major change in reorganization. The school health program has been given a whole chapter to itself in order to emphasize the constantly increasing opportunities it offers to teachers for the health observation, health education, and health guidance of their students. The chapter originally entitled *The Growing Child* has become three separate chapters, each one devoted to one of the three main aspects of growth and development—the physical, the social and emotional, and the intellectual. The chapter in previous editions in which descriptions of the nervous and endocrine systems were combined with descriptions of the defense reactions and organic and functional disturbances associated with them have been broken down into four separate chapters.

Everything that has to do with the food requirements of the body and what happens when they are not met now occupies a chapter of its own. The same is true of the first station on the alimentary route—the mouth —which in this edition is dealt with separately in order to point up the importance of measures taken to control one of the major health problems among school-age children—the problem of dental caries.

Information about the structure, functions, and disorders of the eyes and ears and descriptions of the screening tests for vision and hearing which were originally combined in one chapter are now presented in two chapters. This was done so as to emphasize the very valuable part played by teacher observation in detecting children in need of professional eye and ear examinations.

As a result of these major ventures in reorganization, the third edition contains 18 chapters as compared with the 9 chapters in previous editions. This does not mean that the amount of text has been doubled—only that in the authors' opinion the book's readability and its usefulness as a text for study and reference have been increased.

MAJOR ADDITIONS AND REVISIONS

With the aim of bringing the text up to date, new material has been added or old material revised to reflect the more recent advances in physiology, medicine, and public health and to report the more significant changes that have occurred in the statistical picture illustrating the chief health problems of childhood and youth. All statistical charts and tables giving mortality or morbidity figures have been revised according to the latest information available. The immunization timetable and all other tabulated information on communicable diseases which are presented in this edition as appendices have been carefully revised according to the most recent recommendations of the American Academy of Pediatrics and the American Public Health Association. Great care has been taken to bring up to date all reference materials—books, pamphlets, and visual aids—as well as the list of organizations that have available educational material on subjects related to health and safety.

New or greatly expanded material to be found in the third edition is outlined in the following summary:

1. Expansion of the text on heredity (Chap. 1) and the addition of information on inherited mental defectiveness (Chap. 8) made available by recent research in genetics.

2. A review of the characteristics and needs of school children by age groups (Chap. 4).

3. A more detailed and comprehensive account of the educational problems that teachers encounter as a result of differences in intellectual ability exhibited by the slow learners, the gifted, and the mentally handicapped (Chap. 5).

4. Considerable expansion of the material on the identification and treatment of emotionally disturbed children and youth (Chap. 9) together with a discussion of several social problems of increasing concern to the schools—smoking, delinquency, venereal disease, teenage pregnancies, teenage drug addiction, and teenage drinking, so often associated with motor vehicle accidents.

5. Expansion of the material on heart trouble in children (Chap. 10)

so as to include (a) a review of the more common congenital heart-blood vessel defects and the great progress being made in their surgical correction; and (b) a discussion of the ways in which teachers, in co-operation with school health-service personnel, can assist in the identification and guidance of children with heart and circulation problems.

6. An account of the recent research on the thymus gland which has succeeded in throwing light on the hitherto unknown functions of that gland (Chap. 10).

7. Additional material on the subject of nutrition and malnutrition relating to dietary problems of increasing public interest and concern and to the many valuable learning experiences in nutrition education available to the students in most schools (Chap. 12).

8. Expansion of the text on vision (Chap. 16) so as to include new material on screening tests, classroom lighting, and the provision of adequate assistance for partially seeing children.

9. Addition of a section on physical fitness in the chapter on body mechanics (Chap. 18) with particular emphasis on the value of exercise in attaining and maintaining it.

10. Thorough revision or complete rewriting of all parts of the text wherever located which deal with infectious disease so as to acquaint teachers with the latest developments in immunization, chemotherapy, and other means of prevention and treatment now available to the medical profession.

MAJOR OMISSIONS

Several omissions or radical reductions have been made in the text on various subjects largely as a result of recommendations by users of previous editions. The more important changes in this category are as follows:

1. Omission or reduction of descriptions of first-aid procedures except for measures that must be taken immediately in order to save life. Those retained include the latest recommended method of giving artificial respiration—rescue breathing—and measures for dealing with severe external bleeding and traumatic shock.

2. Reduction of the text dealing with body measurements other than for weight and height and omission of the graphs and tabulated information on measurements of skeletal, muscular, and subcutaneous tissue (Chap. 3). In the table giving selected percentiles for weight and height for ages 6 to 18 years, the measurements for height are recorded in inches rather than in centimeters for easier reference.

3. Omission of the section on suggested activities included at the end of each chapter in previous editions because experience in using the book with college classes had shown that there was not time for the students to carry out most of the activities suggested. The tests have been re-

tained, however, because as one teacher put it, "They serve as a good review for each chapter."

Although the third edition is a greatly altered version of the first two editions, there has been no change in the main lines of approach. In general these lines have two major objectives.

BASIC SCIENTIFIC INFORMATION

The first major objective is to supply the knowledge drawn from physiology, psychology, bacteriology, medicine, and public health which is needed to place health observation on a firm and broad scientific basis.

A large part of the knowledge that has to do with appraising, conserving, promoting, and restoring health can be acquired and used only after undergoing years of education and training in the science and art of medicine and its allied disciplines. Another part, however, is made up of facts about the body and mind and the things that affect them for good or ill which laymen can learn and apply both in their own lives and in their dealings with others. It is this knowledge that the authors believe that teachers, school nurses, and all others working with children should possess in order to understand the physiological and psychological basis of observable deviations from good health in individual students and to make good health meaningful and worth working for to all students and their parents.

Their own health is rightly of no less concern to teachers than that of their students. They will be better equipped to take care of it if they have some understanding of the ways in which the body takes care of itself and of what it needs from its owner to operate most efficiently. Also there is much to be said for the conviction of many physiologists that no one can consider himself to be well educated and still remain ignorant of the structure and functions of his own body. As Dr. Walter B. Cannon put it in his autobiography:[1]

> As a physiologist I am especially impressed by the common ignorance of bodily organs and their functions. It seems to me now, as it seemed to Robert Boyle nearly three hundred years ago, that it is "highly dishonorable for a Reasonable Soul to live in so Divinely built a Mansion as the Body she resides in, altogether unacquainted with the exquisite structure of it."

INFORMATION ABOUT SCHOOL-AGE HEALTH PROBLEMS

The second major objective of this book is to acquaint teachers and other lay readers with the principal disorders and defects that are most commonly encountered in the school ages and to report what is currently known about their prevention, detection, and treatment. In giving this

---

[1] Walter B. Cannon, M.D., *The Way of An Investigator*, W. W. Norton & Company, Inc., New York, 1945, p. 171.

information the authors in no case intend to furnish grounds for diagnosis. The teacher's responsibility as a lay observer ends with the reporting of observations to the proper person in the school-health-service setup. There is no end, however, to a teacher's responsibility for each child's welfare. The information given in this book is, in the authors' opinion, only that which any intelligent layman who has a responsibility for children would wish to have.

Knowledge of the health status of each child is bound to contribute to success in teaching as measured by the teacher's ability to help the child to realize his potentialities for good health in the broadest sense of this term. If any physical or mental or emotional condition is interfering with the child's progress toward this goal, it often happens that the task of convincing parents of the need for taking the action recommended by the physician falls on the teacher or nurse or on both working together. Knowing something about a disease or defect, if medical diagnosis indicates that a child has it, will be helpful in interpreting the physician's findings and recommendations to the parents and sometimes to the child himself. The teacher who has this knowledge will be able to cooperate intelligently with the physician and the parents in any follow-up procedures required, and in the supervision of the child in school.

We trust that the extensive changes made in the original version of this book will serve to enlarge its usefulness as a text in courses for teachers and school nurses in training. We hope, too, that we have succeeded in increasing its value for those teachers and nurses already serving in the schools who will use it to gain keener insight into, and deeper understanding of the health problems of, their students.

ACKNOWLEDGMENTS

It is with pleasure and gratitude that we acknowledge our indebtedness to colleagues and friends who gave us invaluable assistance in preparing the third edition of this book.

We wish especially to thank the following reviewers of the second edition for their general recommendations for improvement and their specific critical comments: Dr. Warren H. Southworth, Professor of Health Education, University of Wisconsin; Miss Elizabeth C. Stobo, Professor of Nursing Education, Teachers College, Columbia University; Miss Julia M. Pratt, Associate Professor, Health and Education, Adelphi College, New York; and Miss Lena A. Hovey, Nursing Consultant, National Society for the Prevention of Blindness, New York.

We wish also to thank the following persons who gave us the benefit of their specialized knowledge in reviewing those portions of the manuscript for the third edition which deal with subjects in their particular areas of interest: Miss Marjorie L. Craig, Program Coordinator, Health and Welfare Division, Metropolitan Life Insurance Company; Dr. C. Glen

King, President, The Nutrition Foundation, Inc., New York; Dr. John W. Ferree, Executive Director, National Society for the Prevention of Blindness, New York; and Dr. Herbert G. Birch, Research Professor of Pediatrics, Albert Einstein College of Medicine, New York.

Finally, we owe a special debt of gratitude to friends in the Metropolitan Life Insurance Company who took an active part in preparing the manuscript for this edition: to Miss Dorothy McGovern for her patient typing of the manuscript over and over again; to Mrs. Emily Hammond for help in revising the references; to Mr. William Holland for assistance in revising the statistical charts and tables; and to Mrs. Sophia C. Dertz who acted as our editorial and research assistant at every stage of this book's three-year journey to and through the press.

Acknowledgments for illustrative material that apply to all three editions of this book were recapitulated in the second edition. Here we wish to acknowledge once again the courtesy of the Metropolitan Life Insurance Company for permitting us to reproduce the colored photographs (Plates 1–16) that were taken by the late Dr. Lewis Henry Koplik in the children's clinic of the New York Hospital–Cornell Medical Center, and at the Hunter College Elementary School in New York City. These photographs were used to produce the Metropolitan sound filmstrip entitled "Teacher Observaton of School Children." Later with further explanatory text they were reproduced in the Metropolitan booklet "What Teachers See." The enthusiasm with which these materials were received by the schools, together with impressions gained through conversation and correspondence that a more comprehensive approach would be welcomed, led to the writing of this book.

George M. Wheatley, M.D., M.P.H.
Grace T. Hallock

CONTENTS

Chapter 1   HEALTH OBSERVATION

IN ACTION

Health Observation: Its Historical Background
The Art of Observing Children
The Child as a Whole

It is no new thing for American schools to be interested in the health of children. Early in the life of our democracy free public education was strongly advocated, and somewhat later all children were not only guaranteed the opportunity to go to school but also were required by law to take advantage of that opportunity. The traditional barriers to universal public education—sex, social class, economic status, intellectual potential —were let down. One still remains, however, that cannot be legislated out of existence. A child cannot go to school if he is physically or mentally ill or if he has some infectious condition that threatens the health of other children. If for no other reason than this, and there are many others, the health of its school children is of vital concern to a nation that believes so strongly in the value of education for all its citizens.

HEALTH OBSERVATION: ITS HISTORICAL BACKGROUND

In point of time, the observation of pupils for signs of infection came first in the development of the school's concern for child health. Natural population growth and the flood of immigration in the last quarter of the 1800s led to great increases in the number of children of school age, especially in the larger cities. With the base of exposure to infection broadened, the American ideal of education for all children was threatened by the rising prevalence of infections and other conditions that can keep children out of school. As late as the 1890s eye infections, notably trachoma; debilitating diseases, such as malaria and hookworm; nutritional deficiencies, such as pellagra and scurvy, were interfering with many children's capacity to learn. Epidemics of diphtheria and scarlet fever periodically decimated the schools, even in rural districts, all too often leaving children who escaped death with permanent defects. The blight of tuberculosis kept thousands of boys and girls in their teens from going on with their schooling and deprived many a classroom of its young teacher.

Relief was in sight, however. With the progress in medicine and public health made possible by the bacteriological discoveries of the latter part

1

of the nineteenth century, educational and public health authorities were able to take intelligent action to control the spread of infections that interrupted the schooling of so many children.

The Rise of School Health Services

The first step taken marked the beginning of what we know today as school health services. This measure was the setting up in the schools of several large cities of a system of daily medical inspection for the purpose of detecting early signs of infection. Right from the beginning teachers took an active part in this enterprise. Following epidemics of diphtheria and scarlet fever in Boston in 1894, school physicians appointed by the city commissioner of health visited the schools daily and examined all children *thought by their teachers* to be ailing. In New York City, in 1897, the department of health assigned medical inspectors to call at three or four different schools every day, to ask the teachers whether any of their children seemed ill and to inspect those whom the teachers reported for signs of communicable disease. As it worked out, many inspectors did not go to the schools at all but questioned the teachers over the telephone. When an obviously infected child was found, the only measure taken was to exclude him from school. Infectious eye and skin diseases were found in so many thousands of children that the schools in many sections of the city became practically deserted. Lillian Wald's suggestion in 1902 that public health nurses working with the school medical inspectors might help to clear up some of these conditions led eventually to the establishment of the public health nurse as an invaluable member of the school-health-service team.

As the thicket composed of cases of infectious disease was cleared away, many other menaces to the health of school children began to stand out more clearly. These were, for the most part, medical problems —for example, defects of vision, hearing, and teeth, and malnutrition— which called for more refined techniques than simple observation. School health services, in most places where they were set up, were considered to be the sole responsibility of physicians, nurses, and dentists, and great reliance was placed upon the periodic school medical examination as a means of finding children in need of professional attention.

However, the results of concentrating on the purely medical aspects of the school health service were disappointing. Generally speaking for the country as a whole, in most schools routine health examinations became little more than cursory and superficial inspections of the students to meet the demands of legislation or to assure the public of the school's interest in the health of the children. Certainly there was little educational value either for the students or their parents in such hurried inspections. Moreover, it sometimes happened that children in serious need of attention were not discovered, and the records of a substantial proportion of children known to have severe uncorrected defects were lost somewhere in the shuffle of inefficient filing systems.

The importance of putting the teacher back into the observation post from which she had been withdrawn in the advancing front of the routine medical examination was first publicly recognized in 1924 by Dr. James Frederick Rogers, then consultant in hygiene of the U.S. Office of Education. In his pamphlet "What Every Teacher Should Know about the Physical Condition of Her Pupils," [1] Dr. Rogers paid tribute to the "unique, first-line position" of the teacher in the health observation of school children and pointed her out as "the 'keystone' of the health examination service." The practical information given in this historic pamphlet for use as a guide in the continual health appraisal of children by their teachers has since been amplified and presented in many different forms in other publications.[2]

The Astoria Study

In the early 1930s, an increasing number of educational and health authorities felt that something was wrong somewhere along the straight pathway which ideally should have led from the detection of remediable defects in school children to their correction. This uncomfortable feeling was crystallized in the report of a study[3] made in 1932–1933 in the New York City schools. The situation pictured in this report was recognized as reasonably representative of the situation in the country as a whole—at least in the large urban centers. The recommendations made in this and earlier studies were given successful field testing in the Astoria Health District demonstration study[4] sponsored by the Department of Health and the Board of Education of New York City.

In the four-year Astoria study, interest was focused on the role of the teacher in the school-health-service program. New York City teachers were already expected to observe children for departures from good health and to refer those in obvious need of attention to the nurse or the physician serving the school. Building on this foundation, methods were worked out for making the teachers' continuing observations a vital part of the school program for maintaining and improving the children's health. As a result, the health observation of school children became

[1] Pamphlet 68 (revised 1945), Federal Security Agency, U.S. Office of Education.

[2] One of the most recent is the pamphlet entitled "Health Appraisal of School Children" (3d ed., 1961), a Report of the Joint Committee on Health Problems in Education of the National Education Association and the American Medical Association.

[3] "Physical Defects—the Pathway to Correction," American Child Health Association, New York, 1934. (A study of physical defects among school children in New York City, conducted by the research division of the American Child Health Association in cooperation with the Department of Health and the Department of Education, supervised by a special advisory committee, and financed by the Metropolitan Life Insurance Company.)

[4] Dorothy B. Nyswander, "Solving School Health Problems," Commonwealth Fund, New York, 1942.

teacher-centered rather than physician-centered or nurse-centered. Instead of the routine periodic medical examination of all children, the "Astoria plan" of school medical service calls for the examination of each child when he enters school, either by the school physician or his family physician, and thereafter only when the observations of teacher or nurse, or both, indicate that he is in need of further medical attention. It was found during the study that examinations by physicians of children referred by teachers as needing medical attention showed that eight out of ten such children actually had health problems. This was a striking demonstration of the efficiency of alert, informed teachers in recognizing "something wrong" when they see it.

The Astoria plan as used in the New York City elementary schools influenced school health programs in many parts of the United States and Canada. The fundamental role of the teacher in the school health program is currently emphasized on the value-defining, policy-making level by national organizations interested in school health.[5] It would be difficult now to find a manual on school health services or school health examinations issued by state health or educational authorities, or both, which does not emphasize the value of the teacher's observations in detecting signs and symptoms that indicate the need for medical, dental, or other specialized care.

THE ART OF OBSERVING CHILDREN

In general, observation means the act of noticing or paying attention to things perceived through the senses. We observe the shape and colors of a tree (things seen), the rustle of leaves (things heard), the odor of a rose (things smelled), the savor of salt (things tasted), the texture of cloth (things felt). Everything we know about the outside world and the people in it, all the experiences that teach us and guide us, come to us through observation.

Practically all of us observe the appearance and behavior of others and form opinions based on our observations. "He looks tired," "She looks happy," "He acts scared," "She's too fat," "He's too thin"—these are only a few of the things we think or say which show that we are constantly appraising someone's state of health or state of mind.

But what are such observations worth? Do they serve any useful purpose? That depends upon what makes an observation worth while. Is it vague or specific? Is its significance understood and appreciated? Is it an idle observation or one that can be put to work for the benefit of the person observed?

A woman sitting opposite a child on a bus might think to herself, "That

[5] See "Suggested School Health Policies" (3d ed., 1958), Joint Committee on Health Problems in Education of the National Education Association and the American Medical Association.

child looks pale and thin." But this observation has no value in getting something done for the child, because the child means nothing to the observer.

A visitor in the home of identical twins might say to their mother, "My, those children look so much alike that I don't see how even you can tell them apart." And the mother might find it difficult to explain why it is that she can easily tell Johnny from Jimmy. "If they were your children," she might say, "you would notice many ways in which they are different." In effect she would be saying that her powers of observation have been sharpened by her love and interest. It is interest in a particular child, then, that largely determines whether the things we notice about that child are specific enough to convey a real meaning for us. But even interest is helpless if the knowledge and understanding necessary for intelligent observation are lacking.

Standards of Comparison

A little girl on first hearing the story of the creation exclaimed, "My, Adam must have been happy that first morning when he saw the sun come up." She had grasped the idea that Adam, observing the first sunset, had no way of knowing there would be a sunrise. And we cannot appreciate the significance of what we observe in children without something to go on—some standard of comparison based on knowledge and experience. Of course, we have a general idea of the look of health—rosy cheeks, bright eyes, glossy hair, firm flesh, rounded contours, sturdy legs, good posture. We speak of "radiant health," or of a person being "aglow with health," and think we know what we mean when we say it. But if we come right down to cases, how can we be fairly sure that the plump, rosy-cheeked child is healthy and the thin, pale child undernourished? What do we have to go on? Suppose we look at Tommy Brown through the eyes of his mother, his teacher, and his doctor.

The Mother's Yardstick. To his mother, Tommy is unique. She does not compare him objectively with other children, because to her there is no comparison. However, she has learned how Tommy looks and behaves when he is healthy and happy, or, as she might say, when he is "like himself," and that knowledge furnishes her with a yardstick for checking up on what she observes. Either Tommy is like himself—as he is when she knows that he is well and happy—or unlike himself—as he is when he is ailing and fretful.

The Teacher's Yardstick. Tommy's teacher, like his mother, has an opportunity to become familiar with his appearance and behavior from day to day. Through constant association the child makes a distinct impression on her. She forms an opinion of his learning ability, his attitude toward his work and his playmates, his behavior in the classroom and on the playground. She is in a position to note changes for the worse in her picture of the child at his best. But she also has a more objective yardstick than that of his parents. Tommy shares her interest and attention with thirty children or more. She is sensitive not only to changes that make Tommy look or act unlike himself, but also to individual differences that may or may not throw him too far out of line with what she has learned through training and experience to expect of children of approximately his age in the way of behavior and learning ability.

The Physician's Yardstick. The physician's interest in a child who is brought to his attention for a routine medical examination or because of a particular illness or physical defect is based largely on his obligation to deliver the professional verdict and recommendations for which he is consulted. Is Tommy physically sound and well nourished? Or is there something wrong? And, if so, what? In making his examination the physician constantly compares his findings with what he knows to be normal for healthy children of approximately that age. There are, for example, normal chest sounds, normal body temperature, normal vision, and so on. And there are typical sets of signs and symptoms to guide him in making a diagnosis if he finds any marked departures from normal.

Of the value of the physician's observations there can be no doubt. Just as an astronomer with a telescope can make many more observations about the heavens and learn far more about a particular star than the casual stargazer can, so the physician with his trained eyes and ears and fingertips and precision instruments and tests can make many more observations about the body and learn far more about the physical condition of a particular child than a layman can. And not only that—what he observes means far more to him than it would to the untrained observer. Anyone can listen to heart sounds through a stethoscope, but only a physician can interpret the meaning of those sounds. Anyone can observe visible signs of trouble in the body, but only a physician can identify a particular disease or defect and tell it apart from any number of others that may resemble it.

The Value of Teacher-parent Observations

In the last analysis, the only way in which we can be sure of getting the correct answer to our question, "Is this child healthy?" or, if he seems ill, "What is the matter with him?" is to ask the doctor.

What then are the observations of parents and teachers worth? Are they to be considered unemployable or can they be put to work?

Getting Medical Attention for Children Who Need It. First of all, how is a child to get to the doctor when he needs medical attention? Under ordinary circumstances the family physician depends almost entirely on parental observation as a means of reaching his child patients when they need him. For that reason alone, parents should know what to watch for in the way of specific signs and symptoms as a means of sharpening the natural keenness of observation occasioned by their love and interest. And when the child goes to school, still another "seeing eye" is focused on him.

The chief value of the teacher's observations, as far as getting a child to the doctor for needed medical attention is concerned, lies in the fact that a teacher is likely to be more objective than the parents. A mother may actually be too close to a child to notice a slowly developing defect. Progressive loss of hearing is commonly referred to as a "thief in the night," creeping up on one unawares. The same may be said of the insidious development of nearsightedness or of malnutrition or of certain diseases, such as rheumatic fever, tuberculosis, and diabetes. Also, children like everyone else have little personality quirks, and these are often so familiar to parents that they may quite effectively disguise a developing defect. "But he has always been like that—he never pays attention," a mother might say in reply to the suggestion that lack of attentiveness may indicate loss of hearing. Even obvious signs of trouble, such as decayed teeth (especially "baby teeth"), poor posture, chronic "sniffles," excessive overweight, and behavior difficulties of various kinds, may be disregarded at home either because "familiarity breeds contempt" or because such conditions do not seem to have any appreciable direct effect on the child's general health.

At school, on the other hand, an objective measure of accomplishment is set up in the welter of emotions that surrounds practically all children. A teacher is bound to be puzzled if a particular child does not seem to be making the progress he himself has led her to expect of him, or if he seems very different compared with others in his group. And she has the welfare of the whole class to think of as well as the welfare of each child in it. Is the behavior of one or two children upsetting the morale of the group? Is Tommy's running nose or the sore at the corner of Jane's mouth "something catching"?

In a school with a well-organized health service, the teacher has an opportunity to discuss all such problems with the school nurse or school physician. In schools without such facilities, she may carry her concern directly to the parents. In either case she is able to perform a real and lasting service for the child by calling attention to departures from good health which might otherwise have been neglected.

Helping the Doctor to Understand the Child. The second important contribution of the observations of parents and teachers to a child's welfare is the light they throw on the doctor's search for the best way to help the child.

The human body has often been compared to a machine, which can be checked by a doctor as a piece of machinery can be checked by a skilled mechanic to make sure that there is "no sand in the gearbox," no loose or missing or damaged parts. But the comparison breaks down when we think of the body as made of living stuff subject to the innumerable delicate adjustments occasioned by the interplay of body, mind, and spirit. This interplay is what makes us individuals—each one of us a person unlike all other persons—whose health status cannot be determined simply by objective procedures like urinalyses and blood tests and measurements of heart capacity and reactions to the knee-jerk test, and so on.

The difference between the human body in general and the human body in particular is what makes the difference between the study of medicine as a science and the practice of medicine as an art. And that is why unlikeness to self—to the way in which a person usually looks and acts—is an important finding from a medical practitioner's point of view. No patient likes to be treated as if he had been newly created in the waiting room to satisfy a doctor's curiosity. And no physician can do his best for a patient who is a closed book in everything that cannot be determined by rule of thumb. But the modern physician often does not have the opportunities open to the old-time family doctor to know his patients inside out. He has to depend more than his predecessors did on secondhand observation to get the information that will enable him to do his best for us and our children; he has to ask questions, and we have to know the answers.

Any mother who has been present at a medical examination of her child knows the sort of questions the doctor asks: "When did you begin to notice that she was losing weight?" "How is his appetite?" "Has his face always twitched like that?" "Is he naturally pale?" "Does his head ache in the morning or at night?" "How long has he been troubled with constipation?" And so on. The doctor is trying to get a picture of the child as he usually looks and behaves so that he can appraise the importance of what he observes. And for that he must depend upon those who are constantly with the child.

The teacher can perform for the school nurse and school physician the same services that the mother performs for the private physician, not only in selecting children who need medical checkups, but also in giving information that she is in a good strategic position to obtain. Also, she may be of great service in getting needed information to the private physician by sharing her observations with the parents. Upon the information given by those who know the child well, coupled with what he finds out for himself, the doctor bases his diagnosis and decides on the treatment. And just as the mother at home cooperates best with the doctor when she knows what he hopes to accomplish, so the teacher is best able to give the child the supervision and guidance he needs in school when she has learned from doctor and nurse what the child's health problems are and how they can be solved.

Learning to Be a Good Observer

In order to decide whether a child who is not obviously ill needs medical attention, training in observation is necessary. This means cultivation of the knack of observing what a person not medically trained can observe.

Practicing Observation. An easy first step in acquiring this knack is to look for just one thing in the children encountered during a day. For example, if you look only for freckles, you will be surprised to find how quickly you become aware of freckles and the pattern of their distribution on the face. You may watch for the color of eyes until you find yourself automatically noticing eye color in children. Other easy exercises in observation, which may be compared to the simple finger exercises one learns when playing the piano, include noting the number of children in a class who wear glasses or the number who write lefthanded.

The next step is comparable to playing one's first "piece" on a musical instrument. It consists of the unobtrusive observation of individual children for five minutes or so, with the object of describing afterward from memory each child's face and body build and gait. This method has proved useful in the formal training of teachers in the art of observation. Opportunities are made for a group of teachers and a school physician to watch children for a certain length of time. Then each teacher writes down her impressions of each child. Later in a group conference the physician reviews the teachers' descriptions and points out any significant observations which have been missed.

The final and most important step is practice in observation for the specific purpose of detecting departures from good health. Since this implies familiarity with normal appearance and behavior, it is necessary to define what is meant by "normal."

What Is "Normal"? In a great many different situations, our conception of normality is based upon what is conspicuously familiar. It is a conspicuously familiar fact, for example, that the mean body temperature of the great majority of healthy persons is 98.6°F (see Reactions to Internal Temperature Changes, in Chap. 7). So the "normal" mark is set at 98.6° on our clinical Fahrenheit thermometers.

In a large group of persons of a certain age, the height of the majority will be within a few inches above or below the mean, or average, height of the group. The ordinary range in height at various ages is so familiar that we can tell at a glance whether a person is unusually tall or unusually short. The same is true of weight and body shape. Going on what may be called our feeling for normality, we can readily tell whether a person is unusually thin or unusually fat, unusually well shaped or unusually misshapen. Our conception of what is right and proper in the way of behavior is also based upon our experience with the sort of behavior that is conspicuously familiar at various ages. It is all right—"normal"—for a child to be childish, for example, but not for an adult.

Day-by-day Observation of Particular Children. In observing a child, we use both our familiarity with normality and its standard variations, won by lifelong experience in observing the people around us, and our familiarity with that particular child's usual appearance and behavior.

The teacher in her day-by-day association with her children learns how each one looks and behaves when he is well. It may take some time to gain this knowledge, but once acquired it makes a great difference in the ease with which significant changes in appearance and behavior are recognized. To illustrate what is meant by the sort of knowledge that underlies the common expression, "He is not the same child," observe the pictures of Jane in Plates 1 and 2.

In Plate 1 you see Jane as her teacher sees her when she is healthy and happy. Her face glows with life. The color of her skin and lips is good. She looks rested but alert, ready to join eagerly in the day's activities.

By treasuring her impressions of Jane as a picture of health, the teacher has a basis for comparison in her careful and unobtrusive observation of Jane's appearance and behavior from day to day. She knows that as clouds change the look of a sunny landscape, so illness changes the look of a healthy child.

In Plate 2 you see the changes from her usual appearance which her teacher noticed when Jane returned to school after an illness. Her face now looks drawn and tired. Her pink cheeks have become sallow and her clear eyes dull with circles beneath. Her usually glossy hair now lacks luster, and her happy rested expression has been lost. Just by looking at her and observing her behavior, her teacher can tell that she is not yet ready to take full active part in the school program.

Time and Place of Observation

The system of daily health inspection in schools grew out of the methods adopted in the latter part of the nineteenth century to deal with the appalling prevalence of communicable disease among school children, especially in the larger cities. The control of communicable diseases was then such an imperative problem that practically everything else was ignored. When trachoma, diphtheria, and a host of other dangerous infections were rampant, no one had time to look for or to bother with deviations from good health that were not catching or seriously crippling. It is as if a gardener should come upon a garden choked with weeds, which had to be cleared away before any attention could be paid to less obvious, but no less important, menaces to the health of the flowers.

Those days fortunately are far behind us, thanks to the extraordinarily rapid progress in preventive medicine and to the work of all those who have made it possible for children to benefit by immunization procedures and other measures for controlling the spread of communicable disease. As a result, there is time today to explore possibilities that would not occur to teachers confronted with cases of gross medical neglect. Tony, who is not making good progress in school, may have no obvious physical condition like trachoma or scabies to explain his backwardness. Yet his teacher, in her concern for Tony's well-being, is on the alert for signs that may indicate that something connected with his health is affecting his learning ability.

Formal Inspection. Although the state of emergency that occasioned the deputizing of teachers as inspectors of school children for signs of communicable disease no longer exists, except possibly in epidemics, the habit of devoting a period at the beginning of each day for the formal inspection of the children by the teacher still persists in many school systems. The inspection is made in a good light and usually while the pupils are seated. Points of observation include the skin of the forearms, hands, face, and neck (for cleanliness, signs of skin infection, rash, signs of scratch marks, etc.); hair and fingernails (for "nits," neatness, and cleanliness); teeth and gums (for cleanliness, bleeding or inflamed gums); ears (for cleanliness, discharge from ear canal); nose (for nasal discharge); and clothing (for cleanliness and neatness, possession of handkerchief or paper tissues).

A daily formal inspection of this kind has its advantages and also its disadvantages. Among its advantages is the guarantee that the children will be observed attentively for at least five minutes or so at the start of the day, just as a formal period of health instruction is a guarantee that provision for guiding children in the ways of health will be included in the curriculum. Probably its chief disadvantage is the chance that it may be embarrassing to individual children. Another is the psychological effect on both teacher and children. Upon its completion it is apt to be dismissed from the mind as something over and done with for the day. The child has "passed" so to speak; the teacher has done her duty—so on to the reading, writing, and arithmetic.

Informal Inspection. In informal morning inspections, the teacher observes each child as she says "Good morning." She stands with her back to the light and looks at the child unobtrusively, but with a purpose. Just as she notes whether his hair is combed and his face washed, so she makes a quick estimate of his facial expression. Is it happy and smiling? Or is it unusually pale or sad? Does he look tired or rested? Is his nose running? Are his eyes clear and bright? Or droopy-lidded? Or inflamed?

Children who seem to need a closer inspection as evidenced by this quick once-over may then be looked at carefully in as good a light as possible. If the teacher notices signs and symptoms which in her opinion require the immediate attention of a doctor or nurse, she will then follow the procedures for referral that are in operation in the school. For example, it may be routine to send the child directly to the nurse or physician serving the school, or to refer him to the principal, who will seek the advice of the physician or nurse, or to send the child home with an explanatory note.

Keeping health inspection informal—not making an issue of it—increases the chances that it will become a continuous process throughout the school day, because there is nothing about it to suggest a dead end— a job done. There are many ready-made opportunities throughout the day to make worth-while observations without involving extra time and effort on the teacher's part. For example, what posture does the child assume as he sits in his seat? Does he slump down or slouch over? How far from his eyes does he hold his book when he reads? Is his position cramped when writing? What does he choose to eat from the menu in the school lunchroom? If he brings his lunch, what are the contents of his lunch box? Does he spend an adequate time in eating? Or does he "swallow his lunch whole" so as to have more time for play? Does he play happily with others? Or is he unduly quarrelsome? Or does he hang back from entering group games?

Parental Observation. When the child is in school he is removed for part of his day from the solicitous observations of his parents. However, the times and opportunities for observation open to parents cover many important factors connected with the child's health or health habits. Parents, for example, should "look at" their children carefully, but informally and unobtrusively, while they are eating breakfast. Are their appetites as good as usual? Do they appear rested, alert, ready for the day's activities? Are there any signs of the sniffles which might indicate that they should stay at home? Before they leave for school one question that usually arises is whether they are dressed suitably for weather conditions. After school parents should be on the lookout for signs of unusual fatigue, unhappiness or discouragement, poor appetite at supper, and so on, which might indicate poor adjustment to school or some physical condition that needs medical attention. It is better to learn by indirection how a child feels than by nagging him with direct questions.

THE CHILD AS A WHOLE

At first sight a child is only what he appears to be on the surface. Just as the passengers on a ship, observing an iceberg, see only the unsubmerged tenth, so the teacher meeting a child for the first time observes only the unsubmerged part of his personality—his body build and posture; his facial features and expression; the coloring of his skin, hair, and eyes; his tone of voice and diction. She gets what is called "a first impression," which may be good or bad according to the child's appearance and manner and their impact on her own personality.

First impressions are important if they indicate that a child differs radically from most other children in the group in appearance or behavior (see Identifying Children with Emotional and Social Problems, in Chap. 9). Ordinarily, however, it is as unwise for one human being to trust a first impression of another human being as it would be for a ship's captain to trust the impression that there is no more to an iceberg than what he sees floating on the ocean. Of course, no iceberg can begin to compete with a human being in complexity and uniqueness. To appraise the whole child correctly on better acquaintance—the nine-tenths below the surface as well as the one-tenth above—the teacher must have a working knowledge of human beings in general and what makes them tick, as well as of that particular child.

The Child and Heredity

By "personality" we mean the person as a whole—body, mind, and spirit working together as a unit. Each person at any one time is the unique product of the personality he inherited from his parents as modified by the dynamic exchanges between himself and his environment.

Chromosomes and Genes. With few exceptions, every cell in the body of every person contains a complete blueprint of that person. This blueprint consists of perhaps 50,000 pairs of genes grouped within the cell nucleus in chains called *chromosomes.* The genes are tiny particles of matter that determine hereditary characteristics and regulate the chemical processes of life. The chromosomes are threadlike bodies whose form and structure are distinct only during the period when the nucleus of a cell is dividing to make two new cells (mitosis). They have a strong affinity for certain dyes, hence their name chromosomes, which in Greek means "colored bodies." The body cells of the higher animals contain two complete sets of chromosomes, one set inherited from the father and one from the mother. Up to the year 1956 the majority of geneticists concluded that there were forty-eight chromosomes in every cell of the human body. In that year, investigators using new techniques established the number of human chromosomes as forty-six, that is, two complete sets of twenty-three each, one set coming from the father and one set from the mother. How the genes located on the chromosomes transmit their coded hereditary information to the cells is a very complex story which is now unfolding but is still far from complete.

Every child ordinarily receives a pair of genes related to the same factor, one from his father and one from his mother. Each pair may consist of two similar genes or of two different genes. If the pair consists of two different genes, one dominates the other. The "dominant" gene, as it is called, expresses itself by determining which one of two contrasting parental traits appears. The other gene, called "recessive," remains hidden or latent. The eye color of a child, for example, is determined by the pairing of the eye-color gene inherited from his father with the eye-color gene inherited from his mother. If both genes in the pair are brown-eyed genes, the eyes will be brown; if both are blue-eyed genes, the eyes will be blue. But if one gene in the pair is a brown-eyed gene and the other a blue-eyed gene, the eyes will be brown because the brown-eyed gene is dominant and the blue-eyed gene is recessive. The recessive gene, however, will not be changed in any way by the presence of the dominant gene. Ordinarily genes do not change. In the next generation a recessive gene may be paired with another recessive gene related to the same factor and so have a chance to express itself.

Individual Uniqueness. What we know about genetics at the present time suggests that so diverse are the kinds of genes present in human beings that no two individuals, with the exception of identical twins, can be exactly alike in their hereditary makeup. Since a child receives his hereditary endowment from his parents, it is only natural that we often see obvious similarities between parents and children. It is not only the kinds of genes that a child inherits, however, but also the combinations in which they occur that determine the child's characteristics. Since a redeployment, or reshuffling, of genes takes place in each generation, it is also natural that we often see wide divergences between parents and children.

Dominant genes tend to express themselves no matter what the combination in which they occur. As most so-called "superior" traits seem to be expressions of dominant genes, parents with a superior genetic endowment will tend to transmit this to their children. But the process of redeployment also permits the birth of a defective or inferior child to superior parents as well as the appearance of a superior child from a dubious family background.

Hereditary Defects and Diseases. Recessive genes, as we have seen, can express themselves only when a child receives a double dose of a particular recessive gene which has been carried in hidden form by his parents. Certain severe physical and mental defects that can be inherited continue to appear only because in each generation normal carriers of the recessive defective genes by chance marry each other. This sets the biological stage for the birth of a defective child. Such a child will not be born, however, unless he happens to receive the defective genes responsible from both his parents. The more moderate degrees of hereditary mental defects appear to be due to the action of multiple genes, both dominant and recessive.

It is good to know that great progress is now being made in the recognition and successful treatment by diet, hormones, drugs, or surgery of certain defects or illnesses that have a hereditary basis. Later on in this book the reader will learn of several such medical achievements.

Mutations. The fact that genes ordinarily are passed on unchanged from generation to generation does not mean that they cannot be altered. When a changed gene occurs, a transformation, or "mutation," of the characteristic which it determines takes place. The changed, or mutated, gene continues to reproduce itself and appears in the descendants of the person with the first mutated gene for as long as the hereditary line is continued or until another mutation occurs. Some mutations can have desirable effects. Other mutations, however, can be most undesirable, especially those that produce abnormal genes responsible for hereditary defects and diseases. Mutated genes appear to be produced spontaneously by environmental influences, and thus environment may be said to have the power of striking at the very roots of life.

In 1927 H. J. Muller discovered that mutations of the fruit fly can be produced experimentally by bombarding the flies with X rays. Since then there has been a growing concern over the possible genetic consequences of our exposure to increasing amounts of radiation. We receive a certain amount of radiation from the natural radioactivity of the atmosphere, the earth, and the body itself. From man-made sources, the average individual receives a slightly larger dosage. At present the bulk of this radiation comes from medical and dental use of X rays. Another fraction has resulted from the radioactive fallout produced by nuclear weapons testing in the atmosphere. The partial test-ban treaty offers hope that this source of radiation will be controlled.

With respect to medical and dental exposure, it is difficult to conceive of the practice of modern medicine and dentistry without recourse to X rays. Improved X-ray techniques, adequate safeguards, and more careful selection of persons for X-ray examination and treatment are now reducing these man-made radiation hazards to a minimum.

The Child and Environment

A child's equipment and potentialities at birth are continually being modified by the forces and things, the people and events, to which he is exposed. Strictly speaking, environment is everything to which a living organism is able to respond. In the case of a human being, it includes all the animate and inanimate sources of stimuli that arouse in him the sensations of seeing (unless he was born blind), hearing (unless he was born deaf), tasting, touching, smelling, pain, heat and cold; the air he breathes, the food he eats, the water he drinks; the customs (things he should do), the taboos (things he should not do), the demands, criticisms, rewards, punishments, promises, and ideals of the people with whom he comes in contact.

If we were not safe in saying that personality is unique on the basis of heredity alone, we should not go far astray in claiming that a child's environment after birth would serve to make him different from all other children. Even children brought up in the same family cannot be said to have the same home environment because home conditions are constantly changing. The first child, for example, has a different environment from that of the second, if only through the difference in the size of the family. Birth and death, marriage and divorce, fluctuations in family income with their effect on living standards, moving from one street or community to another, visits of relatives and friends—these are only a few of the events that may profoundly influence one child and have little or no effect on another, because of difference in age or experience or temperament or some other factor at the time they occurred.

Heredity versus Environment. Whatever may have the greatest effect —unchangeable heredity or changeable environment—in influencing human destiny, it is certain that the individual is a product of the two and that the environment from the moment of conception is the factor most readily controllable. The eugenists—people who specialize in the science of being well born—hold out hopes for an improved mankind in the selection, through the regulation of mating, of the genes we pass on. A program of this kind is not so simple as it sounds.

It must be remembered that recessive defect-producing genes are very widely scattered in the population at large. Probably no one is completely superior. Most of a superior individual's genes may be good, but he may have a few recessive ones that would result in the outcropping of undesirable traits in his descendants. A child may have perfectly good genes and be unable to develop his genetic potential because of a poor environment, although children generously endowed with intelligence or special talents may break away from bad influences and succeed in spite of them. This is amply illustrated by the careers of many famous men and women. On the other hand, a child with a relatively poor inheritance may make a success of his life if he is brought up in a good environment. Who can say that one person's success is due to "good" genes and another person's failure to "bad" genes until all persons have been brought up in environments that enable them to make the best of what they have?

The Child Himself

In spite of the emphasis laid here on heredity and environment as determiners of personality, it would be a mistake to assume that its form and pattern are merely the passive result of the child's physical and mental inheritance and the imprints made upon him by everything coming into his body or acting on it from without. It must be remembered that his body is equipped at every point with sensitive nerve endings that supply him with information about the external world, and with a skeleto-muscular system that enables him to bring himself into active contact with a wide variety of objects and events. Even as a tiny baby he is capable of the purposeful activity required to modify the impressions made upon him by his environment. By his cries in protest against discomforts caused by unpleasant sensations, for example, he gets needed attention—his diaper changed, his hunger satisfied, a pricking pin removed, or an extra blanket supplied.

As time goes on, the internal changes incident to his own growth and development and the accumulation of new experiences enable him to bring even greater pressure to bear on the unending series of external forces with which he is continually bombarded. As a result, the child, already roughhewn by heredity, gradually acquires attitudes, tastes, and behavior patterns that are peculiarly his own. He himself then will have the last word about how he shall be modified. Within the limits set by his inborn constitution and by the raw materials in his environment, he will become the architect of his own body, of his own character. If this were not so, there would be no point in trying to give children the incentives and the knowledge that will help them to take advantage of their opportunities for the best possible growth and development.

Physiological Sameness

Although the personality of every human being is unique, the bodies of all healthy human beings are built and work pretty much alike within normal variations. It is of great importance to keep this fact in mind in observing children. Upon it are based everything we know and teach about the human body and its care and everything that tells us whether a child is healthy or needs medical attention.

What would be the sense of telling children what they need in the way of food and what foods supply these needs if each body differed from every other body in its food requirements? And how could any doctor examining a child find "something wrong" if there were no universal right—if it were natural for each child to possess a stomach or a heart or any other organ that was constructed and worked differently from every other child's?

The many different signs and symptoms that may indicate that something is wrong physically all have a background of physiological sameness. Even when the trouble is primarily due to some form of emotional or social maladjustment, characteristic physiological signs may appear.

FOR REVIEW AND DISCUSSION

Under this heading at the end of each chapter readers will find tests and questions which will give them opportunities to review what they have learned and to express their own ideas in class discussion.

1. Suppose you are on the affirmative side in a debate on the following question: Resolved that the teacher occupies a strategic position as an observer of the health status of school children. Make an outline of the talking points you would use.

2. Unobtrusively observe a strange child in a public conveyance or waiting room and afterward write a description of his appearance and behavior. Later observe and describe in writing a child you know well— a member of your family or a child in a class you are teaching. Compare the two descriptions. Which one is fuller and better? Why?

3. Have different members of the class play the roles of parent, teacher, and physician in a panel discussion of these questions:

   a. In what ways do the observations of a child by his parents, by his teacher, and by his doctor differ from one another? What makes these differences?

   b. Of what value to the physician are the observations of a child patient's parents and teacher?

4. Tell the difference between the words or terms in each of the following pairs:

   a. Chromosomes and genes
   b. Recessive genes and mutated genes
   c. Eugenists and geneticists
   d. Heredity and environment

5. Suppose you are on the negative side in a debate on the following question: Resolved that heredity is the sole determining factor in personality development. Outline the arguments you would use.

SELECTED REFERENCES

The Human Body and Healthful Living

Best, Charles Herbert, and Normal Burke Taylor: *The Human Body; Its Anatomy and Physiology,* 4th ed., Holt, Rinehart and Winston, Inc., New York, 1963. (A text for laymen which supplies a firm grounding in physiology without being too technical about it. Specific sections will be listed as references in the chapters of this book to which they apply.)

Davis, Arthur S., and Warren H. Southworth: *Meredith's Hygiene,* McGraw-Hill Book Company, New York, 1954. (A textbook for college students.)

Glemser, Bernard: *All about the Human Body,* Random House, Inc., New York, 1958. (An interesting book with clear, simple drawings.)

Langley, Leroy L., and Emanuel Cheraskin: *The Physiology of Man,* 2d ed., McGraw-Hill Book Company, New York, 1958.

Miller, Benjamin F., and Ruth Goode: *Man and His Body,* Simon and Schuster, Inc., New York, 1960. (Describes the wonders of the human mechanism.)

Scheinfeld, Amram: *The Human Heredity Handbook,* J. B. Lippincott

Company, Philadelphia, 1956. (Explains the "how" and "why" of inherited characteristics.)

Scheinfeld, Amram: *The New You and Heredity*, J. B. Lippincott Company, Philadelphia, 1961. (An easy-to-read, well-illustrated book on human heredity.)

Schifferes, Justus Julius: *Essentials of Healthier Living*, John Wiley & Sons, Inc., New York, 1960. (A stimulating college textbook covering all important topics in personal, family, and community health.)

Turner, Clair E.: *Personal and Community Health*, 12th ed., The C. V. Mosby Company, St. Louis, 1963.

Medicine and Public Health

Fishbein, Morris: *The Handy Home Medical Adviser and Concise Medical Encyclopedia*, Doubleday & Company, Inc., Garden City, 1963.

Hilleboe, Herman E., and G. W. Larimore (eds.): *Preventive Medicine*, W. B. Saunders Company, Philadelphia, 1959.

Maxcy, Kenneth F.: *Rosenau Preventive Medicine and Public Health*, Appleton-Century-Crofts, New York, 1956. (A classic text in public health.)

Mustard, Harry S., and E. L. Stebbins: *An Introduction to Public Health*, 4th ed., The Macmillan Company, New York, 1959.

Smillie, William G., and E. G. Kilborne: *Preventive Medicine and Public Health*, 3d ed., The Macmillan Company, New York, 1963.

Periodicals

Teachers who wish to keep abreast of developments in fields related to personal and community health and safety will find the following publications helpful:

Accident Facts. A valuable classified compilation of accident statistics, issued annually by the National Safety Council.

Canada's Health and Welfare. Issued monthly in English and French by Information Services Division, Canadian Department of National Health and Welfare.

Child Study. Child Study Association of America.

Children. Issued bimonthly by the U.S. Department of Health, Education, and Welfare, Children's Bureau.

Journal of the American Association for Health, Physical Education, and Recreation. Issued monthly by the Association.

Journal of School Health. Issued monthly by the American School Health Association.

National Parent-Teacher. Issued monthly by Parent-Teacher, Inc.

Public Health Reports. Issued monthly by the U.S. Department of Health, Education, and Welfare, Public Health Service.

Recreation. Issued monthly, except July and August, by the National Recreation Association.

Safety Education. National Safety Council.

School Life. U.S. Department of Health, Education, and Welfare, Office of Education.

Science News Letter. "The Weekly Summary of Current Science," Science Service.

Statistical Bulletin. Issued monthly by the Metropolitan Life Insurance Company.

Today's Health. Issued monthly by the American Medical Association.

Understanding the Child. Issued four times a year by the National Association for Mental Health.

Government and National Voluntary Agencies

The agencies listed here have available educational material on a variety of subjects related to health and safety. Organizations with special areas of interest are listed at the end of the chapters concerned with that area. For information regarding available materials, write to the organization. The addresses of these organizations, and of others mentioned in this book, are given at the end of the book.

American Council on Education
American Medical Association
American Public Health Association
Equitable Life Assurance Society
John Hancock Mutual Life Insurance Company
Metropolitan Life Insurance Company
National Health Council
National Public Relations Council of Health and Welfare Services, Inc.
National Safety Council
Public Affairs Committee
Science Research Associates
Science Service
U.S. Department of Health, Education, and Welfare: Children's Bureau; Office of Education; Public Health Service

Many state and city health and education departments also offer free or inexpensive material in the field of health and safety.

Chapter 2   THE TEACHER AND THE

SCHOOL HEALTH PROGRAM

School Health Education
Healthful School Living
School Health Services
The Major Health Problems of Children and Youth

The function of the school is education, and health, by definition, is a state of being. What has *health* to do with reaching educational objectives? Actually, the two are so intimately interwoven that one cannot flourish without the other. Those who are primarily interested in education have gone on record as giving health a prominent place in the galaxy of educational objectives.[1] Those who are primarily interested in health have long realized that education is essential to the development of good attitudes toward health and good personal health behavior as well as to the understanding, appreciation, and support of public health work.

After health had been established as one of the objectives of education it became clear that three main ways of approaching this goal were open to the school. These three approaches are known as school health education, healthful school living, and school health services. The teacher has responsibilities related to each one.

SCHOOL HEALTH EDUCATION

The need for health education is based upon the fact that no one who has reached the age of reason can be kept healthy and safe solely by what is planned and done for him. His continued well-being depends in large part upon what he himself knows and feels and thinks and does. School health education is the process by which children are given opportunities to acquire the knowledge, attitudes, skills, and habits upon which their present and future well-being will in large part depend.

Health Knowledge

There is an impressive body of knowledge that has to do with conserving, promoting, and protecting health in all its many aspects—physical,

[1] In 1918 a committee of the Commission on the Reorganization of Secondary Education appointed by the NEA issued a report entitled "Cardinal Principles of Secondary Education." In that report, health was first named a "primary objective of modern education." The report was published by the Bureau of Education of the U.S. Department of the Interior.

mental, emotional, social, and spiritual. This knowledge is drawn from practically every area of learning, but more especially from the sciences that deal with human beings—physiology, psychology, sociology, and medicine.

A rich and variegated stock of usable health knowledge helps to enlarge young people's understanding of themselves and others and of health itself in terms of total fitness for living. Many health practices would seem unreasonable, arbitrary, or foolish without scientific knowledge to give them validity. From our own experience we know that facts have power to act as deterrents or incentives in matters that affect health. What thirsty person on a country hike, for example, would refrain from drinking the clear, cool water from a pond unless he had learned why he shouldn't? Or who would give thought to his daily diet beyond getting enough to satisfy his hunger unless he had learned what he needs to get from food in order to keep healthy?

Knowledge that has to do with the promotion of health and the prevention of disease has no power to make its possessors use it, but there is no question of the power it gives to those who *do* use it to improve and protect their own health and that of their fellow citizens. We need only to look backward for a hundred years or so to see what a tremendous difference scientific knowledge and its use have made in the prevention of disease and the prolongation of life. Let us not forget that generations of human beings have perished for lack of the information with which every schoolboy and schoolgirl can now be equipped.

The subject matter of health education is made up of everything in this area of knowledge that the majority of students can learn and utilize in their progress from the first grade through the twelfth. Here is a brief summary of what they should have learned before leaving high school:

1. Enough about the functions and makeup of the body to understand how factors such as food, sleep, exercise, stress, choice of work, and recreation affect physical and mental fitness

2. Enough about the drives that influence human behavior to understand what is needed for emotional and social fitness

3. Enough about communicable disease, alcoholism, and drug addiction to help in fighting them

4. Enough about accidents to help in their prevention

5. Enough about first-aid procedures to know "what to do till the doctor comes"

6. Enough about disabling or handicapping conditions to know how to prevent them or to adjust to them

7. Enough about the relationships between personal, family, school, community, and world health to understand individual responsibilities for protecting the health of others

Making Health Education Work

According to Alfred North Whitehead's definition, "Education is the acquisition of the art of the utilization of knowledge." If we accept this definition, it is easy to see that motivation is one of the teacher's biggest problems. It is always possible to pump enough knowledge into the minds of a class to enable most of its members to pass on into the next grade and eventually to graduate. But what is the point of doing this unless the students at the same time acquire the art of applying what they learn?

Specifically, so far as health education is concerned, there is a very intimate relationship between knowledge and its use. In studying health the student is studying something that affects himself—his own life, his own body and mind, his personal relationships with his environment. Yet it is no easy task to get him to apply what he learns to himself.

Individuals now living in our country are on the whole healthier and can expect to live longer than their predecessors in former times, but for that they have to thank the research scientists, physicians, and public health workers who do for them what they cannot do for themselves. There are, however, a great many ills that could be avoided and a great deal of positive, radiant health that could be enjoyed if individuals would take the responsibility for doing for themselves what only they can do. To awaken this sense of responsibility in our young people, it is necessary to relate health to the things that they want to do and to be. In effective health teaching the accent is placed not on health as an end in itself but rather on health as a means of helping each individual to reach his attainable goals.

It is for the teacher to inspire and motivate her students to live in accord with the scientific principles upon which desirable health attitudes and practices are based. She does this partly by her own example—by exemplifying in her own personality and behavior the values she wishes her students to absorb. She does it too by finding important applications for health knowledge in the daily lives of individual students and by relating its uses to the needs, interests, and aspirations of each one.

Health Education in Elementary Schools

Most elementary schools now make definite provision in the curriculum for education in health and safety. The classroom teacher is responsible for the teaching of health as she is for the teaching of all other subjects. It is recommended in *Suggested School Health Policies* that the amount of time allotted to health education be at least equal to that devoted to other major areas.[2]

[2] *Suggested School Health Policies,* 3d ed., Joint Committee on Health Problems in Education of the National Education Association and the American Medical Association, 1958.

Health teaching in the elementary school is directed largely toward the development of health habits and wholesome attitudes toward safe and healthful living. The interested, resourceful teacher helps the children to gain experience through using what they learn in a great many school activities, for example, playground activities; eating lunch in school; the use of drinking water, handwashing and toilet facilities; and preparation for special procedures, such as weighing and measuring, periodic health examinations, and vision and hearing tests.

Opportunities to learn the scientific facts upon which healthful living and disease prevention are based are introduced at the appropriate grade levels in the elementary school. Ideally, they are geared to the interests and intellectual appetites of the majority of children who have reached that level. Visual and auditory aids, graded health textbooks or health readers, models, and other instructional material may be used to good advantage. Also, there is scarcely a subject or unit activity that cannot contribute facts or concepts to vitalize health teaching. There must be careful planning, however, preferably with the advice and assistance of a school health educator or school health coordinator, to develop a unified program of instruction for the elementary grades.

Health Education in Junior and Senior High Schools

Health may be taught in secondary schools as a required, independent subject; or an allied subject, notably biology, may be elected instead of health; or health may be correlated with other areas of learning, such as physical education and home economics, with which it obviously has many ties. The procedure of choice, however, is the provision of a specific health course for all students. The main reason is related to the need for giving the study of health in all its aspects a coherence and relevance which for most students it would otherwise lack. The health course gives students opportunities to acquire from many different sources, and to apply here and now, knowledge, concepts, and understandings that are essential to the protection and improvement of health and the enrichment of life.

Another reason for an independent health course in the secondary school is related to the fact that certain aspects of health and safety education are matters of national concern. Whenever anything harmful to health or dangerous to life is identified, there has been a tendency to pass a law requiring the schools to do something about it. Statutes on the books of nearly every state require the teaching of the evil effects of alcohol and narcotics. A movement is now on foot to pass laws to alert young people to the dangers of cigarette smoking. Driver education, fire prevention, sanitation, communicable disease control, and some other specific areas of health or safety education have been made required school subjects in various states. Physical education laws have also been passed as a result of the recognition in recent years of the great need for increasing the physical fitness of the nation's youth.

Current health- and safety-instruction laws mean that room must be found for many diverse subjects in the already crowded curriculum of most secondary schools. If they are not to be given haphazard or catch-as-catch-can treatment, there must be some sort of unifying force. Increasingly this is being found in an independent course in which students are enrolled for the specific purpose of studying health in all its aspects. In junior high school the minimum time allotment for the study of health recommended in *Suggested School Health Policies*[3] is a daily period of two semesters during the seventh, eighth, or ninth grade and, in the senior high school, two semesters preferably in the eleventh or twelfth grade.

Correlation. The provision of an independent health course does not mean that the teachers of other subjects cannot take a valuable part in health education. The fact that the subject matter of health is drawn from practically every area of learning means that the teachers of other subjects can often contribute relevant knowledge or furnish suitable learning situations. Experience has shown that the most effective correlation takes place when the health teacher or a health coordinator has an opportunity to review with other teachers the possibilities of correlating health with their subjects and to work out a give-and-take which is satisfactory to all. A well-conceived plan guards against wasteful duplication of subject matter.

The Health Teacher. It is considered highly desirable that the health teacher should be a specialist in health education just as the teachers of other subjects in high school are specialists in their fields. But what is considered desirable is not always possible. The biology teacher, the general science teacher, the physical education teacher, the athletic coach, perhaps any teacher whose work load is not already too great, may be charged with the teaching of health. It is not essential for a health teacher to be a specialist in the field, but it is important at the start to have a working knowledge of the subject matter. Health is the product of right ways of thinking and living, and these right ways are for the most part applications of the sciences that deal with human beings.

The attitude toward health which the teacher expresses in her looks, manner, and character often carries more weight than what she teaches. Here are the most frequently mentioned qualities of the successful health teacher:

Good physical and mental health
Emotional stability
Integrity of character

[3] *Ibid.*

A warm, friendly, outgoing manner
An attractive appearance, confident bearing, and pleasing voice
Ability to get along well with others
A sense of humor, resourcefulness, and enthusiasm

In cataloguing these virtues there is no intent to imply that in order to be a good health teacher it is necessary to be a sort of superman who never gets sick or has off days like ordinary mortals. It is done only to suggest that health teaching is more likely to be effective when the teacher can demonstrate in her own person that health is associated with what everyone likes most about other people.

HEALTHFUL SCHOOL LIVING

The term "healthful school living" covers just about everything that makes it possible for students, teachers, and all other school personnel to live healthfully and safely during the school day. This applies both to the school plant and its operation and upkeep and to the emotional and social climate of the school.

The Physical Environment

Factors in the physical environment conducive to health, safety, and learning include all the facilities, equipment, and services required to ensure favorable living and working conditions. The following environmental conditions are those most frequently emphasized:

Lighting in line with present-day standards for classrooms, study halls, and other locations in the school building

Maintenance of appropriate *ventilation,* whatever the means used (window-gravity ventilation or mechanical ventilating systems)

A safe and abundant *drinking water supply* with sanitary dispensing equipment (bubble fountain or paper cups)

Adequate *hand-washing facilities* (hot and cold running water, soap, and paper or individual towels) and *sanitary toilets*

Adjustment of seats, desks, and tables to *postural needs* of their users

Special *provisions for safety* in the design, upkeep, repair, and use of the gymnasium, playground apparatus, science laboratories, and school shops

Reliable *fire protection* and frequent fire drills

An attractive *school lunchroom* or cafeteria with the necessary equipment for the proper care of food supplies, for preparing and serving wholesome, well-balanced lunches, and for sanitary dishwashing

Well-planned and properly equipped *health service units* with separate rest and isolation rooms for boys and girls

School buses kept in excellent condition and operated by well-qualified, careful drivers

Emotional and Social Environment

The provision of a wholesome emotional and social environment depends primarily upon the policies and personalities of the administrative and teaching staffs. Kindly, just, understanding teachers interested in students as individuals can create the atmosphere necessary for good emotional and social development.

The following environmental factors are most frequently mentioned as playing an important part in conditioning the emotional and social climate of the school:

Organization of the school day so as to avoid undue fatigue and stress and to provide time for outdoor games and other physical activities

Classroom procedures that encourage desirable teacher-pupil and pupil-pupil relationships and that discourage excessive competition, too rigid discipline, and overemphasis on marks and attendance records

Adaptation of programs to students' abilities and the use of methods of promotion that stimulate each student to do his best

Constructive interpersonal relationships of both the teaching and the nonteaching personnel

Teachers who show unflagging interest in the well-being of every student and whose conduct of the class is kind, firm, understanding, consistent, and friendly

Perhaps the most important health factor in the school environment is the teacher. Teachers naturally are concerned with the living and working conditions of their own students. They know how a cheerful, healthful, livable school environment affects physical and mental well-being. It is the teacher's awareness of the living conditions in the classroom—of stuffiness or draftiness, of glare on the chalkboard or dimness in far corners, of Tom's foot in the aisle or of Mary's pencil on the floor—that leads to the righting of many environmental wrongs. It is knowing students well enough as individuals to apprehend what's bothering them—that Jim is brooding because he is only five-foot-three, for example, or that Alice needs practice in learning the right way to get the attention she craves—that enables the teacher to extend a friendly helping hand.

A Cooperative Enterprise

Provision for healthful school living is an important responsibility of the board of education and the school administrator. But teachers, custodians, other school personnel, and the students themselves have a great deal to do with maintaining and, when necessary, improving the environment of their school. In communities where school buildings are antiquated or poorly planned or equipped, experience has shown that alert, interested teachers, parents, and pupils, with the help of ingenious, cooperative custodians, can find ways to make the most of the facilities available and provide others that are lacking. It is hardly necessary to add that the maintenance of favorable environmental conditions in any school plant, no matter how well designed and adequately equipped, requires the cooperative effort of all those who live and work in it. Teachers share with custodians the responsibility of making sure that students use properly the facilities provided for safe and healthful school living. From kindergarten through high school there are innumerable opportunities for boys and girls to take part in activities that give them experience in doing what must be done to keep their surroundings clean, orderly, and attractive.

Educational Value of a Good Environment

All teachers want well-lighted, well-ventilated, clean, attractive, un-crowded classrooms because in such surroundings they and their students can work most comfortably and efficiently. But a good school environment is also a special part of a larger and more comprehensive picture. It furnishes the teacher with opportunities to emphasize the relationships to health, safety, and comfort of environmental factors such as lighting, ventilation, sanitation, and good housekeeping. Convincing boys and girls that good environmental conditions are worth working for is one of the most important objectives of school health education.

An attractive healthy environment gives all students opportunities to appreciate and enjoy pleasant surroundings. It shows that the school is meeting the environmental standards recommended in the study of health. The students find no disillusioning contrast between what they learn and the example set by the school. Most important of all, it provides students with the means of practicing what is recommended, always washing hands before eating and after toilet, for example, or always having a proper light to read by, or always eating a good lunch, or always wearing safety glasses when exposed to eye hazards in the school shop or laboratory.

SCHOOL HEALTH SERVICES

The need for school health services is based on the fact that no one can get rid of an already existing infection or chronic illness merely by knowing and practicing the rules of healthful living. The child who learns in school that milk is an excellent source of the calcium necessary for building good teeth can drink milk till the cows come home without having a single decayed tooth restored to health. No amount of hand washing and sneezing into a handkerchief is going to cure Johnny's cold. No waiting for the green light will set Mary's broken leg, nor will wearing rubber boots on rainy days repair the damage already done to Frank's heart by rheumatic fever.

Existing departures from good health are hard problems that health education alone cannot solve. Yet they interfere with the process of education itself. In varying degrees they endanger the child's present—and, possibly, future—well-being. If contagious, they are a menace to the whole group. In any school, at any time, there are bound to be children who, for some reason, are not up to par; or who are suffering from a specific disability, such as poor eyesight or loss of hearing; or who appear to be "coming down with something," which may or may not be catching; or who have skinned their knees or cut their fingers or injured some other part of their bodies.

School-health-service Activities

The major objectives of a school health service are the health maintenance and the health improvement of school children. School-health-service activities include complete medical examinations or health appraisals; dental examinations and cleaning of teeth; screening tests for vision and hearing; conscientious follow-up after medical and dental examinations, to assure the correction of any adverse conditions discovered; communicable disease control; first aid in case of emergencies; and health counseling and guidance. To provide all the students in a school with everything they need in the way of health care and supervision requires the services of many different professionally trained persons—physicians, public health nurses, dentists, dental hygienists, psychologists, and other specialists. What is provided in actual practice depends upon the resources available in the school and community. The kind and amount of specialized services found in different schools range all the way from complete coverage in large urban school systems to no specialized services in remote, one-room schools.

The chief concern of the physicians, dentists, nurses, and other professionally trained personnel who are serving the school is rightly the actual carrying on of health-service activities. But they are finding out that they achieve much better results when they take time to get acquainted with the boys and girls and their parents, to explain what they are doing clearly and simply as they do it, to volunteer praise where it is due, to give reasons for their recommendations to parents, teachers, and others responsible for acting on them, and to develop and maintain effective working relationships with private physicians and other individuals or groups in the community concerned with meeting health and welfare needs.

Administration. Responsibility for carrying on the health services in a school varies by states or by different communities within one state. In some places the health department is responsible; in others, the department or board of education; in still others, the health and education departments jointly. Whatever may be the administrative status of the school health service, its operation is closely related to the school program as a whole. The core of our thinking regarding the goals, organization, and functioning of a good school-health-service program is the conviction that health service in a school must be a cooperative undertaking in which members of the teaching staff and members of the health-service staff work together as one team instead of considering themselves as members of two different teams. Also, the school team must work with the parents and with organized groups and individuals in the community who are interested in giving school children opportunities to stay healthy or to obtain needed medical, dental, nursing, or other specialized care.

Health Examinations. The recognition of the strategic position occupied by the teacher in her day-by-day association with her students is making possible the gradual evolution of a more efficient plan for health appraisals than the old one based on the idea that "every child should be given an annual routine health examination." The trend now is to have children examined and given booster immunizations, preferably by the family physician, before they enter school and then to provide three or four additional examinations at important stages in the child's progress through school. For example, these examinations might take place (1) upon entering the intermediate grades (grade 4); (2) upon entering junior high school (grade 7); (3) upon entering senior high school (grade 10); and (4) possibly in the year before graduation from high school. Dental supervision, of course, must be given more frequently.

In between these routine examinations any student whose appearance or behavior suggests to the teacher or nurse, or both, that medical attention is needed is referred for immediate interim examination.

Reducing the number of routine examinations given in schools for apparently normal and healthy young people makes it possible for the school physician to give more time to students in need of special attention. Also more time is available for making the periodic health examination an on-the-spot educational experience for children and parents in a highly teachable situation. In many elementary schools the parents are notified that their child is to be examined and are invited to attend the examination. The nurse confers with the teacher and the mother beforehand to obtain information that may furnish the physician with valuable leads as he makes his examination. During or after the examination the mother and the teacher have an opportunity to talk over the findings with the physician and nurse and to discuss plans for follow-up procedures.

This close working together of all those most intimately concerned with the child's well-being will enable teachers and parents to appreciate the significance of their observations and to gain confidence in their powers of observation. And it will supply the physician and nurse with clues to guide them in doing their part in safeguarding the health of the child.

For high school students it is now considered best to make the health examination a highly individualized affair. It often takes great skill to break down the reluctance of adolescents to talk about troubling health problems and worries. Physicians who serve secondary schools usually have gained this skill. Alone with the physician and with plenty of time, adolescent youngsters may be encouraged to air their worries and reach a better understanding of themselves and of their parents and of other people, too.

Cumulative Health Records. Teachers share with the school physician and other health specialists serving the school in the preparation of the student's cumulative health record, which in many school systems is begun in kindergarten or first grade and continued from grade to grade. This record, which is, in effect, the youngster's school health history, contains all significant information bearing on his health. It has been called "the focal point on which all communications between teacher, family, physician, dentists, and nurses are centered."

Communications from the teacher include observation of the young person's appearance or behavior which in her opinion—often bolstered by that of the nurse—indicates that "something is not right." In many schools it is up to the teacher to make and to record the results of periodic height-weight measurements and screening tests for vision, hearing, and speech and also to note the causes of absences as they are reported. She or the nurse or both may also record what they have learned in interviews with parents about the home situation as it affects the child's well-being. The information entered in a student's health record is of special value to a physician whose acquaintance with the youngster is limited to occasional contacts in school.

Communications from the physician which go into the cumulative health record include a report of what he finds each time he examines the youngster and a statement of what he thinks should be done to improve the child's health. The findings and recommendations of the physician, when properly interpreted to the teacher, throw light on aspects of a young person's appearance or behavior or rate of growth which puzzled the teacher enough to report them.

Working with Parents. It is a well-recognized function of the school health service to help parents and students to understand individual health needs as revealed in school health records. The physician serving the school may readily identify a source of trouble or he may find that further medical study is necessary in order to get the information required for a definite diagnosis. It is not part of his duty to give or prescribe treatment or to carry on extensive investigations. Parents are responsible for their children's health. The school may provide services which the parents are unable or unwilling to provide, such as periodic medical examinations, dental prophylaxis, and adequate lunches. But when it comes down to getting the treatment that is needed, the parents and students, with the advice of their physician, must make the decisions. This does not mean that the school feels justified in washing its hands of the matter when its personnel has done the spadework of finding and reporting to parents things that need attention.

Parents whose children have always been looked after by the family physician may very well be puzzled or hurt or angered by the implication that they are neglecting their child's health needs. These parents, in specially arranged interviews with the teachers and health specialists, may be agreeably surprised to learn how much school people can contribute to an understanding of their children. And they may be impressed, too, with the fact that exchanges of information between the school and the family physician depend largely upon them.

Except in critical emergencies, the school communicates with a child's physician only through his parents. The physician makes his recommendations to the parents, who are primarily responsible for the child's health. Yet the school may be of great help in getting the physician's recommendations followed. Perhaps there is need of adjustment in the young person's school program and his out-of-school activities. Perhaps eating habits should be improved. He may need more or less exercise or more sleep. Some physical, mental, or emotional handicap may have to be considered in planning his work and recreation. A private physician can count on the school to help parents in carrying out his recommendations if the teachers and health specialists know what they are.

Children whose families do not have physicians and dentists of their own may go without needed medical and dental care for a variety of reasons. Unless a youngster is unmistakably ill, it may be difficult to convince his parents that he is not "doing all right." In some cases, parents do not know how to go about getting a reliable doctor or what services are provided by the health department clinics and voluntary agencies.

Within almost any community there are resources which can be tapped to meet most health problems. The cooperative teamwork of all concerned —school people, local medical and dental societies, official and voluntary community agencies—is the heart and soul of efforts to interpret urgent health needs to parents, encourage them to take action, and help them find ways and means of securing treatment or other needed attention for their children.

Educational Value of School Health Services

As a specialist in education the teacher is primarily concerned with ways in which the students' experiences with health-service activities can be used in the classroom to make health education meaningful and functional. In preparation both for medical examinations and for screening tests of various kinds, there are innumerable opportunities, depending upon the age of the students, for the teacher to correlate previews of the procedures to be followed with the subject matter of history and the biological and physical sciences. After all the returns on examining and testing procedures are in and duly entered on the students' health records, the recommendation of the examiners furnish a rich store of educational leads to the teacher, who, alone or in cooperation with the nurse or health counselor, is responsible for the health guidance of individual students.

The small emergencies, like minor injuries, and the big emergencies, like epidemics, which call the forces of the school health service into action also are "good grist at hand" to keep the mill of health education going. The school nurse sees children when they are sent to the health service unit by the teachers for an accidental injury or suspicion of illness. If she is alert to the educational opportunities in such situations, the child not only gets the necessary attention but also suggestions as to how the mishap might have been avoided or why cuts and scratches are cared for with aseptic precautions or why coming to school with a cold is not a good idea. In the control of communicable disease the school health staff works closely with the community health department. The practical details of this cooperation may be made the subject of special reports or class discussions on what a health department does to safeguard the health of all citizens. Also the policies and procedures of the school for dealing with emergencies arising out of accidental injury and of ways in which the school is cooperating with the civil defense authorities of the community may be reported in connection with safety education and training in first aid.

THE MAJOR HEALTH PROBLEMS OF CHILDREN AND YOUTH

Child health problems today are in several respects radically different from those which confronted parents and teachers earlier in the twentieth century. The most important change has been the great reduction in the death rate for school-age boys and girls (Fig. 2-1).

The savings in life represented by this reduction are in large part the fruits of the amazingly brilliant and productive work done during the early 1900s in controlling the infectious diseases. Although diseases in this category are still important causes of illness among school-age children, there has been a very marked decline in deaths from those that took the heaviest toll of young lives earlier in the twentieth century. This decline has been so great that, in the current list of the five leading causes of death in the school ages, accidents now hold first place in every age group and malignancies (especially leukemia) hold second place (see Table 2-1).

Five Leading Causes of Death

1. *Accidents.* The fact that accidents are now by far the greatest threat to life and limb in childhood and youth, and an important cause

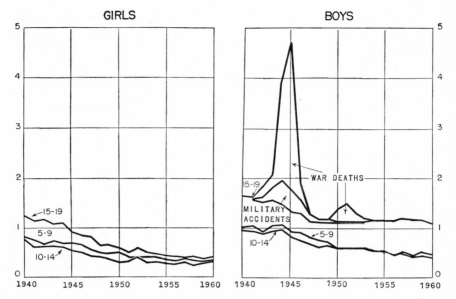

FIG. 2-1. Death rates per 1,000 in school-age girls and boys, by age group, 1940 to 1960. (*Metropolitan Life Insurance Company, industrial policyholders.*)

of death at all ages, clearly indicates the need for intensifying safety education in the home, in the school, and in the community. The rising rate of motor vehicle accidents involving teen-age drivers is of particular interest, especially since there is increasing evidence that teen-age drinking is a factor. (See Teen-age Drinking as a Social Problem in Chap. 9.)

Each year accidents take the lives of more than 13,000 children between the ages of five and nineteen, as the figures in Table 2-2 show.

Motor vehicle fatalities account for almost half the number of accidental deaths of school-age children. At ages five to nine years, three of every five motor vehicle deaths are the result of children being run over or hit as they play on or cross streets, highways, and driveways. At ages ten to fourteen years, only one-fourth of the motor vehicle fatalities are among pedestrians. At these ages, deaths of bicyclists in collision with motor vehicles are at their peak.

In the high school and college age group, when young people begin to drive, motor vehicle accidents take an even higher toll. The driver-education courses now given in public schools are one attempt to help solve this problem, and, according to the National Safety Council,[4] these courses are beginning to pay off. The Department of Motor Vehicles of New York, for example, found that a group of drivers with driver education had one-third fewer traffic violations and one-fifth fewer accidents than a comparable group of drivers without driver education.

[4] *Accident Facts*, 1963 edition, National Safety Council.

In Michigan, where driver education is required for everyone under eighteen who applies for a driving license, driver-education graduates of Lansing public schools were found to have accidents only half as fre-

Table 2-1

THE FIVE LEADING CAUSES OF DEATH IN THE
SCHOOL AGES, IN THE UNITED STATES, 1962

Cause of death	Death rate per 100,000
Ages 5–9	
Accidents	18.1
Malignant neoplasms	7.7
Congenital malformations	3.5
Influenza and pneumonia	2.5
Diseases of heart	0.9
Ages 10–14	
Accidents	18.0
Malignant neoplasms	6.1
Congenital malformations	2.8
Influenza and pneumonia	2.0
Disease of heart	1.2
Ages 15–19	
Accidents	48.9
Malignant neoplasms	7.7
Suicide	3.8
Homocide	3.7
Congenital malformations	2.8

Source: National Center for Health Statistics.

quently as the national average for drivers in the same age group. Also, these young drivers had 20 per cent fewer accidents than older Lansing drivers—in contrast to the usual experience in other parts of the country,

Table 2-2

SCHOOL-AGE ACCIDENTAL DEATHS, 1961

Age group	Number of deaths	Rate per 100,000
5–9	3,468	18.1
10–14	3,249	18.8
15–19	6,648	49.1

Source: *Accident Facts*, 1963 edition, National Safety Council.

where younger drivers often have about twice as many accidents as older drivers.

Drowning is an important cause of accidental deaths among children five to fourteen years old. Boys are the most frequent victims, with the death rate from drowning for boys four times that for girls. In this age group drownings increase in relative importance among both sexes with age. Not only do the older children participate more often in swimming, boating, and other sports, but also they are increasingly permitted to do so on their own.

Fires and explosives account for one-tenth of the total number of accidental deaths among children at ages five to fourteen years. Among girls at ages five to nine years this cause ranks second only to motor vehicle accidents. A considerable number of casualties are due to firearm accidents, particularly among the older school-age boys. Thus, at ages ten to fourteen years, 12 per cent of the accidental fatalities among boys result from the careless use of firearms.

Although falls are an important cause of nonfatal injury among children, they account for only 3 per cent of the fatal injuries.

Of particular interest to school personnel are fatal injuries in competitive sports. Although precise figures are not available, injuries are quite common and the annual toll includes many severe injuries as well as a number of deaths.

Football accounted for 108 deaths in the United States during the five-year period 1955–1959, according to data issued by the American Football Coaches Association. As Table 2-3 shows, of this total eighty-one sustained their injuries in activities directly associated with the game, such as tackling and blocking; tackling was responsible for more than one-fourth of the fatalities directly connected with the game. The twenty-seven deaths indirectly attributable to football were caused by heat stroke, heart failure, and other conditions.

Table 2-3

NUMBER OF ACCIDENTAL DEATHS FROM FOOTBALL
UNITED STATES, 1955–1959

Type	Direct	Indirect
Total	81	27
College	7	4
High school	51	18
Professional and semiprofessional	5	1
Sandlot	18	4

Source: Dr. Floyd R. Eastwood, Chairman, Committee on Injuries and Fatalities, American Football Coaches Association.

Fifty-one of the eighty-one deaths directly associated with football were among high school players. The annual rate of fatal injury averaged about 1.7 per 100,000 for the students playing high school football, who number about 600,000. Among the 66,000 players who participated in college football, the rate was slightly higher.

The hazard of fatal injury in baseball is relatively small. In the past five years, relatively few fatalities have occurred in amateur baseball, although more than two million boys participate in the sport annually as members of scholastic teams, the Little League, American Legion Junior, and similar organizations. The infrequent instances of fatal injury resulted from various mishaps. A few players were hit on the head with a ball while they were batting or running bases; one player was killed when his head hit the base as he was sliding "home"; and another was killed when, playing as infielder, he was struck on the head with a batted ball during practice.

Occasional fatalities also occur in other competitive sports, such as basketball, skiing, and ice hockey, but there are no overall figures either on injuries or deaths for these sports.

The incidence and severity of injuries sustained in competitive sports can be decreased by players having proper equipment and facilities and good instruction and supervision; by adequate health examinations of athletes; and by prompt medical attention for injuries. Sports authorities have instituted a number of safety precautions but, although these measures have borne fruit, competitive sports can be made even safer than they are now.

The team approach is the newest development in attempts to prevent accidents—now the nation's No. 1 public health problem. The leader of the team on a national level is the National Safety Council. Cooperating with it on the local, state, and national level are the professions of medicine and public health, the schools, police and fire departments, industrial and business concerns, governmental agencies, and many voluntary organizations interested in health and welfare.

2. *Malignancies.* All forms of cancer are included under the general heading "malignancies." Cancer today is second only to diseases of the heart and arteries as a cause of death in the population as a whole. The rise in the death rate for cancer in recent years is explained partly by the fact that many more people than formerly are now reaching the ages when cancer is most likely to develop. But cancer also is the leading cause of death by disease among school children. Part of the explanation lies in better diagnosis and in the fact that the number of deaths from communicable diseases in the school ages has become very much lower. There is, however, an actual increase in the number of cancer deaths in childhood and youth resulting from the long-term upward trend in the mortality rate and the rapid growth of the child population. Currently, about 4,000 cancer deaths occur annually at the ages under fifteen, or nearly 50 per cent more than a decade ago.

Leukemia is the most common form of cancer in childhood, being responsible for nearly half the total death toll from malignancy under age fifteen. The leukemia death rate is at a peak in the age group one to four and decreases during the school ages (see The Leukemias in Chap. 10). Cancers of the nervous system, chiefly of the brain, are the second most frequent form of cancer in childhood. Other fairly frequent sites of malignancy are the kidneys and bones.

Children afflicted with cancer generally live only a short time, often less than a year. Consequently, the frequency of new cases, and the total of existing cases, parallel the number of deaths from the disease. Such differences as do exist between incidence and mortality for the various types of malignancy reflect variations in the ages at onset and the rapidity with which the disease runs its fatal course.

Cancers in children are treated by means of X rays or radioactive substances, surgery, hormones, and various chemicals. Chemotherapy appears to offer great promise in the management of common childhood cancers. Some of the chemicals developed to date have been helpful in alleviating symptoms and prolonging the lives of children with leukemia. A large and intensive research program has been organized to discover or develop chemicals which will destroy cancer cells without harming normal cells. At the same time, fundamental research goes on at an accelerated pace to find the cause of cancer. The outlook for progress in the control of cancer in children is increasingly hopeful, but the battle is far from won.

3. *Congenital Malformations.* Congenital malformations are abnormalities in the structure of the body which are present at birth. In a sample study of 5,500 infants born alive, about 7 per cent were found to have some type of congenital malformation. The most serious types are deformities of the heart or great blood vessels which interfere with the heart's action or impose an added work load on the heart.

More than seventy out of a hundred babies born with congenital malformations die in their first year of life; about eight more die at ages one to four. In the school ages the number of deaths decreases but even so congenital malformations hold third place as a cause of death at ages five to fourteen years, with congenital heart defects as an important contributing cause of diseases of the heart at ages five to nineteen. (Congenital heart and blood-vessel defects in children and the great advances being made in their surgical correction are discussed in Chap. 10. Congenital crippling, or orthopedic, defects are discussed in Chap. 18.)

4. *Influenza and Pneumonia.* With the exception of rheumatic fever, pneumonia, with influenza as its most common precursor, is the only infection that has continued to be a leading cause of death among children from the year 1900 until now. Currently it ranks fourth as a cause of death at ages five to fourteen.

Great progress has been made in the treatment of pneumococcal and other bacterial pneumonias since the introduction of chemotherapy. Less success has been obtained in the treatment of the virus pneumonias.

Influenza can be a cause of death in its own right; it is most feared, however, because it so often paves the way for pneumonia, especially in older persons and in persons with ailments of the heart and other chronic conditions. (More information on influenza and pneumonia is given in Chap. 11.)

5. *Diseases of the Heart.* Congenital heart defects and rheumatic fever are responsible for the great majority of deaths from heart disease in the school ages. The cause of rheumatic fever has not yet been demonstrated but we know that attacks are triggered in susceptible children by a streptococcal infection, usually "strep" sore throat. The chief characteristic of rheumatic fever is its tendency to recur, with the danger of heart damage increasing with each recurrence. Rheumatic heart disease has become much less frequent since the sulfa drugs and penicillin have made it possible to avert recurrent attacks of rheumatic fever. (More information on rheumatic fever and rheumatic heart disease is given in Chap. 10.)

Stories of High Achievement

There are two reasons for reviewing some of the twentieth century's outstanding public health achievements. First, these "success stories" demonstrate what cooperation and intensive efforts can do. Second, they remind us that the price of continued control of these threats to life and health is unflagging vigilance and constant effort.

1. *Tuberculosis.* "The Captain of all these men of death that came against him to take him away, was the Consumption, for it was that that brought him down to the grave." So wrote John Bunyan in his *Life and Death of Mr. Badman.* "The consumption," or tuberculosis as we call this disease today, still held the unenviable distinction of being "captain of the men of death" in the early 1900s. Its demotion to a place far down in the ranks of the causes of death by disease has been called one of the "most spectacular medical and social achievements in history."

As short a time ago as 1930 tuberculosis was one of the leading causes of death in school-age children. It led all other causes of death among girls from ten to nineteen years of age. Among boys it rated third as a cause of death at ages ten to fourteen and second at ages fifteen to nineteen. Today tuberculosis does not appear on any list of leading causes of death in the United States at any age. This remarkable achievement is due largely to:

Intensive campaigns of education, especially in schools, about the cause and manner of spread of tuberculosis
Extensive case-finding programs
Great advances in methods of treatment, especially with the use of drugs
The general improvement in living and working conditions which has helped both to reduce the opportunities for the spread of tubercle bacilli and to build up better resistance against them

Although all the devoted individuals and agencies who have worked so hard to wipe out TB have cause for rejoicing in the progress made so far, there is certainly no cause for complacency. The National Tuberculosis Association estimates that about thirty-five million Americans are infected with tubercle bacilli and that by the end of the 1960s about 250,000 persons will develop active tuberculosis. Even in this country, which has the lowest death rate from tuberculosis, U.S. Public Health Service officials say that it will take another generation before TB can be eradicated.

The problem is largely one of finding new cases and checking up on old ones to be sure that arrested cases are not reactivated. Every untreated active case is a source of infection from which the seeds of the disease (tubercle bacilli) can be scattered in ever-widening circles. A school-bus driver in New York state, for example, was found to have active TB. Tuberculin testing of all children in the school revealed that sixty children who had not even been exposed to the active case reacted positively and of those exposed, eighty-five children were infected. In an Illinois town a twelve-year-old boy was diagnosed as having advanced tuberculosis in both lungs. Tuberculin testing of all school children revealed that more than 20 per cent reacted positively. Stories like these show the need for the periodic tuberculin testing of all children and young adults with an annual chest X-ray examination for those whose test is positive. (For further information on the tuberculin test, see Tuberculosis in Chap. 11.)

2. *Communicable Diseases of Childhood.* Diphtheria, measles, scarlet fever, and whooping cough (the big four among the communicable diseases of childhood) took a heavy toll of child life in the early twentieth century. In 1930 these four diseases together ranked second as a cause of death among children five to nine years of age and sixth at ages ten to fourteen. Today they have almost reached the vanishing point so far as being a cause of death is concerned.

Diphtheria once returned year after year in devastating epidemics, closing schools and inspiring terror in every parent or teacher who heard a child complain of a sore throat. With diphtheria toxoid available for making susceptible children immune from diphtheria, any community, if it wishes, can now ensure the disappearance of this disease. Many large cities where immunization of children has been universally and continuously practiced have proved this point.

Whooping cough and measles, although less dangerous than diphtheria, often have damaging consequences, especially in young children. An effective vaccine against whooping cough has long been available, and a more recently developed vaccine against measles promises control and early eradication of an often complicating illness that strikes almost all American youngsters.

Scarlet fever is a member of a group of infections caused by bacteria known as hemolytic streptococci (see Scarlet Fever and Streptococcal Sore Throat in Chap. 11). There are no immunization measures available for protection against streptococcal infections, but penicillin is effective in treatment and in the prevention of serious complications—notably rheumatic fever and acute inflammation of the kidneys.

3. *Poliomyelitis*. This disease has never reached the status of an important cause of death, but its ability to cripple the young and healthy has made it one of the most feared of all the childhood diseases. Fortunately we now have the power to bring polio to an end "as it were a tale that is told." With the introduction of Salk killed-virus vaccine in 1954 and of Sabin live-virus vaccine in 1962, there is good reason to believe that polio is definitely on the way out. (More information about poliomyelitis is given in Chap. 8.)

4. *Gastrointestinal Infections*. Typhoid fever, diarrhea and enteritis, and other milk- and water-borne infections were once high-ranking causes of death in infancy, childhood, and youth. Now they are disappearing, largely as a result of the work of public health sanitarians who have succeeded in safeguarding water and milk supplies over large areas.

In these stories of high achievement we can discern both a footnote of encouragement and a footnote of warning.

A Note of Encouragement. It is encouraging to learn what has been accomplished in controlling once common causes of death and disability in childhood and youth by the discovery and application of medical knowledge. Although there are still several diseases—leukemia, for example—which can make us sick at heart, there is no longer the generally hopeless attitude that prevailed before medical research began to show tangible results. Medical old-timers, in their reminiscences, have told us of the gloom pervading the medical wards in contrast to the cheerfulness of the surgical wards in the period when medicine was stymied and surgery was forging ahead. Now, the gloom is lifting. There is every reason to believe that the day will come when both medicine and surgery will have the means at hand to deal with most, if not all, of the chief causes of early death.

A Warning Note. The warning note is struck by the realization that memories are short and that it is easy to forget what an ebbing menace —diphtheria, smallpox, tuberculosis, for example—was like when it was at the flood. Yet forgetfulness would be disastrous if it should lead to neglect of the safeguards and precautions now available for controlling preventable disease. Even though some diseases—smallpox, typhoid fever, and diphtheria, for example—have almost been wiped out as causes of death, there can be no letup in efforts to hold what has been won. There are still so-called "islands" of children who have not been immunized from diphtheria, tetanus, whooping cough, and polio; yet only thoroughgoing immunization of each succeeding generation of children will permit the eventual eradication of these diseases. To let the strong walls of immunization crumble, to dismiss the public health watchmen responsible for preventing disease, prolonging life, and promoting health through organized community effort; to let nature take its course in conditions for which physicians have lifesaving drugs and surgical procedures, would put us back to where our ancestors were a hundred years ago.

Tales of Woe

The fact that the death rate is declining among school children does not mean that there has been a comparable reduction in illness, physical defects, and accidental injuries. The Paradise of Children would indeed return to earth if there were some way of getting completely rid of colds and sore throats, chicken pox and mumps, upset stomachs and broken bones, decayed teeth and impetigo, head lice and poison ivy, allergies and obesity, and all the other minor and major afflictions of the young. Although many of these afflictions are not ordinarily serious, some of them may interfere with a child's education or lead to worse trouble later on. Others may be blessings in disguise by immunizing children from infections that might have serious consequences later in life.

Still other problems are giving growing concern to physicians, educators, and indeed to all those who are interested in the welfare of young people. Among them are cigarette smoking and the problems that are considered to be symptoms of serious moral and social ills. They include the increasing incidence of venereal disease in adolescence, the growing number of teen-age pregnancies out of wedlock, and the rising rate of juvenile delinquency, narcotics addiction, and drinking in the school ages (see Chap. 9).

Healthier Children for Healthier Adults

In efforts to improve physical and mental fitness in the later years of life, physicians are now seeking in the records of the earlier years clues to the infirmities of middle and old age. Who can estimate the effects on body or mind, or both, of the insults and injuries that may have been sustained in bouts with illness, or in unhappy experiences at home or in school, or in substandard nutrition, or in efforts to compensate for some undiscovered physical defect? Children's bodies and minds, by and large, are pretty tough if their heritage is good, but sometimes unfavorable environmental influences are tougher.

It would be impossible to protect all children from environmental impacts that may or may not leave scars on their developing personalities. What the school *can* do through health education and health services, in cooperation with home and community agencies, is to reduce the chances

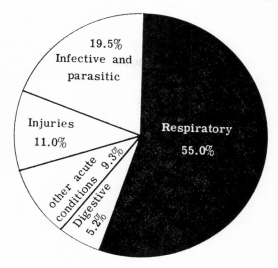

Fɪɢ. 2-2. Causes of school absence among children under fifteen for year ending June 30, 1961. (*Illness among Children, U.S. Department of Health, Education, and Welfare, 1963.*)

of infection, injury, malnourishment, and the development of neurotic trends; to encourage immunization and other protective measures; to recognize and work for the correction of remediable defects and conditions; and to help those children who are irretrievably handicapped to make as good an adjustment as possible to life as they must live it.

Leading Causes of Acute Illness among School Children

Since 1957 the National Survey Division of the Public Health Service has been collecting data on illness in the United States general population. Reports based on these data furnish statistical evidence regarding the leading causes of illness among school children.[5] Of particular interest to teachers and school nurses is the effect of illness on school attendance (Fig. 2-2). In the year ending June, 1961, the days lost from school because of acute illness among children in the six to sixteen age group totaled 156,914,000; this represented an average loss of four days per child. The number of days lost from acute illnesses will naturally fluctuate from year to year as epidemics come and go.

Respiratory Infections. Respiratory infections are universally recognized as the chief illnesses responsible for school absences. They include the common cold, tonsillitis, influenza, pneumonia, and pulmonary tuberculosis. Of these, the common cold is by far the worst offender. The picture here has not changed a great deal over the years. The respiratory virus infections (notably colds and influenza) probably cause as many absences today as in the school days of the fathers and grandfathers of the current crop of children. But the bacterial invasions of the lungs which are so

---

[5] *Illness among Children,* Children's Bureau Publication No. 405, U.S. Department of Health, Education, and Welfare, 1963, p. 7.

often invited by these infections are not nearly so potentially dangerous to life as they once were. Although pneumonia is still rated among the leading causes of death at ages five to fourteen, far fewer children are getting it and dying of it, thanks largely to the use of the sulfonamides and antibiotics in its prevention and treatment. (See Chap. 11 for more information on respiratory diseases.)

Common Childhood Diseases. Teachers may expect that the so-called "common childhood diseases" will continue to be a steady cause of school absences. In the early 1960s these diseases were measles, German measles, mumps, chicken pox, and streptococcal infections (scarlet fever and "strep" sore throat). These diseases are respiratory diseases in the sense that they are for the most part air-borne. Direct passage through the air from person to person is the easiest and quickest way for germs to travel from the sick to the well. The respiratory passages are the portals both of entry and of exit for the droplets in which they are chiefly spread. Contact with infected persons also affords opportunities for reasonably rapid but indirect transportation by way of hands or objects freshly soiled with infectious discharges.

With the development of measles vaccine (1962) and its widespread use, it is believed that measles as a cause of absence can eventually become negligible. There is no sure way to prevent outbreaks of streptococcal infections but prompt medical attention can work wonders in protecting youngsters from their serious consequences, notably rheumatic fever and acute nephritis. That is why it is so important to refer children who complain of sore throat to the school doctor or nurse.

No way yet is available for preventing German measles, mumps, and chicken pox but reduction in the sickness rate of these diseases is not a matter of great public health concern and is even considered unwise by some physicians. There is something to be said for the old belief that it is better to let children of school age have ordinarily mild contagious diseases and get them over with rather than to make a great effort to protect them from illnesses that are usually far more serious when contracted later in life. This is particularly true of German measles and mumps. German measles occurring in an expectant mother within the first three months of pregnancy may result in serious congenital defects in the child. Mumps occurring after puberty may be complicated by inflammation of the sex glands (see Mumps, in Chap. 14).

Accidental Injuries. Loss of life is not the only measure of the extent of the accident problem. Accidental injuries also are a leading cause of disability. Indeed they are the third most common cause of school absences. They include fractures, dislocations, sprains, wounds, lacerations, contusions, and many superficial injuries.

Data from the United States National Survey[6] for the two-year period

_____
⁶ *Ibid.,* p. 10.

July, 1959, through June, 1961, revealed that children aged six to sixteen had an average annual loss of 3.9 days from school as a result of accidental injuries. Girls tended to stay out of school because of injuries more than boys; the average was 4.5 days lost from school for girls compared with 3.7 days lost by boys. However, for the age group fifteen to sixteen, boys remained out of school because of injuries an average of 8.5 days per year, compared with only 3.7 days for girls.

Digestive Disorders. Digestive disturbances as a group constitute the fourth most important cause of illnesses among school children. Stomachache, nausea and vomiting, diarrhea, and constipation, to name the most common, are really symptoms. They may indicate a temporary gastrointestinal upset or some more serious condition for which the digestive system may or may not be directly to blame.

Acute gastrointestinal upsets are very common in childhood, largely because many children have not learned discretion in eating or drinking or have formed poor eating or bowel habits or have especially sensitive stomachs or bowels. "Green-apple stomachache" is symbolic of children's experiments with excessive amounts of indigestible foods. And any adult who has had much to do with children is familiar with the spells of vomiting, or colic, or diarrhea that so often occur after periods of fatigue or overeating, especially of sweets.

The principal diseases in the gastrointestinal group for which bacteria or viruses are responsible include bacillary dysentery, infectious hepatitis (acute catarrhal jaundice), and food infections and food poisonings. Appendicitis also is still a common disease among children of school age, but it is not nearly so deadly as it used to be. Education of the public in "what to do till the doctor comes" when symptoms of appendicitis develop, and the use of antibiotics in combatting peritonitis, account largely for the drop in the death rate from this dangerous infection. (See Chap. 13 for more information on gastrointestinal disorders.)

Other Acute Conditions. A fairly large group of acute disorders is composed of several different ailments and conditions, each of which is comparatively rare as a cause of absence. High-ranking disorders in the miscellaneous group are acute skin conditions, such as impetigo and ringworm.

Chronic Conditions among School Children

Data from the U.S. National Health Survey for the period July, 1959, through June, 1961, indicate that restricted activity due to certain specified chronic conditions accounted for nearly thirty-three million days lost annually from school among children in the age group six to sixteen[7] (see Fig. 2-3). This figure represents three days lost for each child with at least one chronic condition. The conditions reported include hay

[7] *Ibid.*, pp. 12–22 and Table 21, p. 80.

fever, asthma, and other allergies; chronic sinusitis, chronic bronchitis, and other chronic diseases of the respiratory system (excluding tuberculosis); heart disease and other circulatory diseases; defective speech, hearing, and vision; and orthopedic impairments, especially those involving the legs and hips. The data so far collected indicate that far and away the chief chronic conditions responsible for school absences are the respiratory allergies, notably asthma, and the chronic respiratory diseases. The two groups account for more than half of the days lost from school because of chronic conditions.

In addition to children who are absent from school for varying lengths of time because of some chronic illness or defect are the large number of children with decayed teeth, mild nutritional deficiencies, and other conditions that do not usually restrict activity. Also there are many children who show marked deviations from normal behavior which later may lead to serious mental ill health.

We have taken a quick and somewhat casual look at the health problems that are most common in childhood. It is not by any means a complete review of all the ills of the flesh and the spirit to which teachers should be alerted. It is well to remember also that the eyes and ears of true observers are not blind and deaf to all but the majorities and the averages. It is no comfort to the person with a rare disease or condition to know that it is rare. Knowing from training and experience what can be expected of healthy children in a certain age group in the way of appearance and behavior, the teacher will be guided by what she personally sees and hears, no matter how ordinary or how extraordinary a deviation from the average or normal may be.

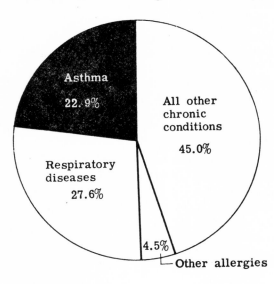

Fig. 2-3. Days lost from school because of chronic conditions among children between six and sixteen for the year ending June 30, 1961. (*Illness among Children, U.S. Department of Health, Education, and Welfare,* 1963.)

FOR REVIEW AND DISCUSSION

1. What would you think or say, if you were present at a discussion in which any of the following statements were made?

    a. The home should be exclusively responsible for a child's health.
    b. Teachers already have too much to do to have responsibilities connected with the preparation of cumulative health records.
    c. The teaching of health in secondary schools can best be accomplished through correlating with other subjects rather than through an independent health course.
    d. In the teaching of health it is not necessary to have a working knowledge of the subject matter so long as the students are provided with an approved health textbook or health reader.

2. Select the correct ending for each of the following incomplete sentences:

    a. The part of the school health program in which motivation is most important is (1) school health services, (2) health education, (3) healthful school living.
    b. The leading cause of death among children of school age is (1) accidents, (2) leukemia, (3) congenital malformations.
    c. One of the diseases that can be eradicated by immunizing each succeeding generation of children is (1) tuberculosis, (2) scarlet fever, (3) diphtheria.
    d. The leading causes of acute illness in school children are: (1) respiratory infections, (2) digestive upsets, (3) malnutrition.
    e. It is safer to have the following infectious diseases in childhood than in adult life: (1) typhoid fever and smallpox, (2) rheumatic fever and scarlet fever, (3) German measles and mumps.

3. Write, or discuss in class, your answers to the following questions:

    a. How is recognition of the teacher's ability to detect in her students significant departures from health helping to evolve more efficient plans for school health examinations?
    b. How has the discovery that infectious diseases are carried by microorganisms made possible the control of such diseases?
    c. What once common infectious diseases are now comparatively rare? What measures are currently being used to combat each disease mentioned?

SELECTED REFERENCES

The School Health Program

American Medical Association, Department of Health Education: *Physicians and Schools; Report of the Eighth National Conference on Physicians and Schools*, the Association, Chicago, 1961.

Cromwell, Gertrude E.: *The Nurse in the School Health Program*, W. B. Saunders Company, Philadelphia, 1963.

Florentine, Helen G.: *The Preparation and the Role of Nurses in the School Health Program*, The National League for Nursing, New York, 1962. (A report prepared for the use of administrators, educators, and students; presents guidelines prepared by an interdisciplinary committee.)

Grout, Ruth E.: *Health Teaching in Schools*, 4th ed., W. B. Saunders Company, Philadelphia, 1963.

Johns, Edward B., and others: *Health for Effective Living*, 3d ed., McGraw-Hill Book Company, New York, 1962. (A basic health education text for college students.)

Means, Richard K.: *A History of Health Education*, Lea & Febiger, Philadelphia, 1962.

National Education Association–American Medical Association Joint Committee on Health Problems in Education, Washington, D.C.: *Health Appraisal of School Children*, 1957.

Health Education, 5th ed., 1961.

Healthful School Living, 1957.

School Health Services, 1953.

Suggested School Health Policies; A Charter for School Health, 4th ed., 1962.

Nemir, Alma: *The School Health Program*, W. B. Saunders Company, Philadelphia, 1959. (Emphasizes the role of teachers in fostering and promoting a good school health program in relationship to the total curriculum.)

Oberteuffer, Delbert: *School Health Education*, 3d ed., Harper & Brothers, New York, 1960.

Smith, Helen Norman, and Mary E. Wolverton: *Health Education in the Elementary School*, The Ronald Press Company, New York, 1959.

Strang, Ruth M., and Dean F. Smiley: *The Role of the Teacher in Health Education*, The Macmillan Company, New York, 1951. (One of the earliest and best books in this field.)

Turner, Clair E.: *School Health and Health Education*, 4th ed., The C. V. Mosby Company, St. Louis, 1961. (A standard text by one of the pioneers of the health education movement.)

Health Problems of Children and Youth

Accident Prevention Can Be Learned, Metropolitan Life Insurance Company, New York, 1962.

Illness among Children, U.S. Department of Health, Education, and Welfare, Children's Bureau Publication No. 405, 1963.

White House Conference on Children and Youth, Golden Anniversary, 1960:

> *Focus on Children and Youth,* a report of the Council of National Organizations on Children and Youth.
>
> *Children in a Changing World,* a book of charts.

Three reports on *The Nation's Children,* edited by Eli Ginsberg, Columbia University Press, New York, 1960, covering:

1. *The Family and Social Change*
2. *Development and Education*
3. *Problems and Prospects*

Wright, Beatrice A.: *Physical Disability—A Psychological Approach,* Harper & Brothers, New York, 1960.

Organizations

National Education Association
National League for Nursing
National Safety Council

Chapter 3　GROWING UP PHYSICALLY

The Pattern of Growth
Skeletal Growth and Development
Muscular and Fatty Tissue
Stages and Rates of Growth
Measuring Physical Growth and Development

There is no subject more complex than that of human growth and development. It can be discussed in this chapter only to the extent of giving teachers some idea of what should be kept in mind in observing the physical progress of school children toward maturity.

By strict definition, physical growth is limited to increase in size, and development to increase in complexity. Growth is an affair of time and space—children grow chronologically and dimensionally. Development also proceeds with age, but its relationship to increase in size varies greatly according to the process involved. A tremendous increase in complexity can take place with very little increase in size. There is, for example, a very close correlation between the head size (breadth and height from the ears up) of a three-month-old baby and a seventeen-year-old boy or girl, but there is a vast difference in the complexity of the brain at these two ages. On the other hand there can be considerable increase in size with very little or no increase in complexity. For example, the leg (from the knee to the floor) is nearly four times as long in a seventeen-year-old boy or girl as in a three-month-old baby, but practically no increase in the complexity of leg structure takes place between these two ages.

THE PATTERN OF GROWTH

Growth is an expression of the tremendous power generated by the union of sperm and egg. As scientists have not yet been able to create living cells from inorganic chemicals, growth which is a power belonging to life can be studied only by observing how some of its results are achieved. Just so, without being able to duplicate the effects created by an artist, we can watch him at work and form some idea of his technique.

The process of physical growth has a beginning and an end. Beginning with the first mitosis, or division of the fertilized egg into two cells, growth stops when full maturity has been achieved. The stoppage of increase in size is fully as important as its start. If we find it hard to think of ourselves as having once been microscopically small, our imaginations bog down completely at the idea of ever being infinitely large. Our only example of runaway growth—cancer—is a solemn reminder of the biologic necessity for keeping a tight rein on increase in size and for bringing it to a halt when maturity is reached.

If growth and development are defined in terms of progressive maturity, then it is evident that different parts of the body become adult —that is, mature—at different times. At birth or shortly after, an individual needs the services of almost all his body organs. Therefore we find that with a few exceptions—the sex glands, for example—an individual's organs are functionally mature even in early life. An organ must reach a certain size in order to function. After that it may keep on growing but usually does not grow a great deal. The internal ear is adult in size at birth. The olfactory apparatus in the nose reaches almost adult dimensions at the age of six months. The cranial cavity, which holds the brain, is nearly as large as it will ever be when a child is six years old. The eye, on the other hand, is usually not fully developed until age nine or ten.

The body framework, as a whole, is not fully mature until the third decade of life, but its various components have their own pattern of growth. In general these components, which together make up stature, consist of the head and neck, the trunk, and the lower limbs. The head and neck and the trunk are most fully developed at birth, because they contain all the organs upon which life depends; hence they need to grow less than the legs. At birth the legs make up only about 33 per cent of stature; at one year, 35 per cent; at six years, 45 per cent; and at seventeen years, 48 per cent. Of the three segments, the head grows at the slowest rate, because it is closest to adult proportions at birth and at two years of age is nine-tenths as big as it will ever be. Vertical growth in the arms and legs is comparatively greatest during grade school age, and in the trunk during high school age when the sex organs are reaching maturity.

So we see that, in growing, the body does not expand symmetrically as a bubble expands with an increase in the volume of its contents. It has a definite growth pattern, with different parts having their own time schedules for coming to maturity.

SKELETAL GROWTH AND DEVELOPMENT

Growth is motivated by forces contributed partly by heredity and partly by environment. In the germ cell, to which both parents contribute, is laid away each individual's growth pattern. But no matter what potentialities in the way of body build and physical stamina a child may have inherited, his actual size and shape and physical condition at any one time will show the marks left by any defects in structure that may have been present at birth (a congenital heart or blood-vessel defect, for example), the important illnesses and accidents he has suffered recently, the kinds and amounts of food he has eaten, the physical activities he has engaged in, and many other environmental factors.

How Bones Grow

Hereditary influence is chiefly responsible for the so-called body types —the tall slender type at one extreme, the short and stocky type at the other, with an intermediate or "average" type in between. These variations in body build are largely determined by the size, shape, and density of the skeleton.

A newborn baby's skeleton is partly bone and partly cartilage. The shafts of the bones of the arms and legs, of the bones of the feet, and of the fingers and toes, for example, are well developed, but the ends are masses of cartilage which present in a general way the shape of the future bone. As the child grows older, ossification centers, called *epiphyses*, appear in the masses of cartilage as points of spongy bone. These juvenile pieces of bone, or epiphyses, gradually spread until at last they unite with the large, or parent, bone. With the fusion of the epiphyses, growth stops.

By taking X-ray pictures of the bones of large numbers of children at various ages, it has been possible to demonstrate with considerable accuracy not only the average time at which the various ossification centers make their appearance but also the average age when these centers (epiphyses) unite with the parent bone. The skeletal age of the child as

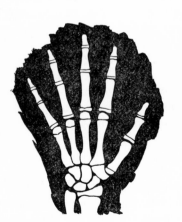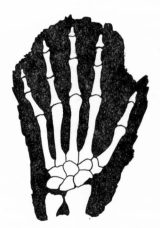

Fig. 3-1. Drawings made from hand-wrist X rays (back view) of two boys, each of whose chronological age was close to fifteen years. Yet the hand at the left shows a skeletal age of thirteen and a half years as compared with a skeletal age of nearly seventeen years shown in the hand at the right. Notice especially the differences in the wrist bones.

revealed by the X ray is considered to be a more accurate indicator of progress toward bodily maturity than is chronological age. A fifteen-year-old boy, as Fig. 3-1 shows, may have a skeletal, or developmental, age ranging all the way from thirteen to seventeen years.

Hormonal Influences

Every child is born with his pattern of growth, but hormones produced by several different endocrine glands are chiefly responsible for executing this design (see The Endocrine System in Action, in Chap. 6). These hormones activate and control skeletal growth and, through their influence on sex maturation, bring it to a stop after adolescence. Variability in the functioning of the endocrine glands concerned results in variable amounts of the hormones they produce and consequently in the wide differences in body build and the many variants in body type and rate of skeletal growth that are readily observed in any large group of children.

The known hormones that control the growth of the skeleton are secreted by the anterior pituitary, the thyroid, the gonads, and the cortex, or outer portion, of the adrenals.

During infancy and early childhood the spread of ossification centers in the bones is activated directly by the growth-promoting hormone of the front (anterior) portion of the pituitary. As the time of puberty approaches, another anterior-pituitary hormone works indirectly against the first by stirring up the gonads. The gonadal secretion speeds up bone growth, with the result that the epiphyses unite in a relatively short time and growth stops. The thyroid enters the picture through the influence of its hormone, thyroxine, upon energy metabolism, that is, all the chemical processes by which food and oxygen are transformed into heat and energy.

Some of the possible variations in body build and appearance which may be produced by the overactivity or underactivity of the endocrines that influence growth will be discussed in Chap. 6.

Influence of Diet

In forming bone, the bone cells are dependent upon the bone-building materials supplied in food. These materials are the salts of calcium and phosphorus, which are combined to form calcium phosphate. Vitamin D is required for the utilization of calcium and phosphorus by the bone cells, and ascorbic acid (vitamin C) is necessary for the composition of intercellular cement, which affects the structure and the strength of bones as well as those of other tissues.

If babies and children fail to obtain adequate and balanced supplies of calcium, phosphorus, and vitamin D, the bones do not calcify normally and rickets is the result. The typical rickety child—bowlegged, knock-kneed, or pigeon-breasted—once served as a dramatic reminder of the important part played by diet in skeletal growth. Rickets has become a rare disease in our country largely because the diet of so many babies and children is supplemented with some good source of vitamin D (see Rickets in Chap. 18).

Influence of Posture

Continual faulty posture during the growth years affects skeletal growth by changing the normal stresses to which the weight-bearing bones are subjected. Such changes may contribute to the development of certain orthopedic defects such as lateral spinal curvature (see Posture and Its Appraisal in Chap. 18).

Influence of Physical Defects and Illnesses

Congenital defects, chronic illness, bone injuries, and even acute attacks of common childhood diseases, such as severe diarrhea, measles, whooping cough, and mumps, sometimes delay the formation of various ossification centers beyond the time at which they usually appear. In most cases such delays are only temporary. In any event children in whom ossification centers fail to appear in the proper time sequence are not to be considered abnormal but merely delayed in their progress toward skeletal maturity.

MUSCULAR AND FATTY TISSUE

The body and the pace of physical growth are set by the forces that bring the skeleton to maturity. But the bulk and modeling of the tissues that cover the bony framework also influence body dimensions and estimates of nutritional status. Height—from the top of the head to the soles of the feet—is practically skeletal height, but the width and girth of various parts of the body reflect the bulk of the muscles and the relative fullness or emptiness of the fat deposits just beneath the skin (subcutaneous fat). Normally muscle tissue constitutes approximately 40 per cent of body weight, and fatty tissue constitutes from 10 to 15 per cent.

Influence of Skeletal Build

The type of skeletal build with which a child is endowed appears to be related in some measure to the amount of tissue with which his bones are padded and operated. The two healthy six-year-old girls shown in Plate 3 illustrate this point. Jean is a tall child with big bones, and Frances is a delicate-looking child with small bones. Jean's large bony framework requires large muscles for its operation, while Frances's lighter framework requires smaller muscles. Also Jean is well equipped, skeletally speaking, to carry a relatively large amount of subcutaneous fat, whereas Frances is built for light loads.

Factors Influencing Muscular Development

Aside from constitutional factors, food and activity are the most important factors in muscular growth and development. Food supplies the raw materials, and activity leads to the building of extra material into the system. Hence the kinds and amounts of food a child eats and the extent to which he uses his skeletal muscles in work and play will have a great deal to do with the comparative heaviness or lightness and the comparative strength or weakness of his musculature.

Factors Influencing Fat Deposits

The amount of subcutaneous fat is the most variable factor affecting the proportions and weight of the body. Fat is found in every cell, tissue, and organ, but in certain regions great numbers of specific fat-containing cells are normally packed closely together to form adipose tissue. These groups of fat cells are the storehouses of fat, or fat depots, of the body (see How the Body Uses Food, in Chap. 12).

A certain amount of fat is found in all children who are reasonably well nourished. Excessive thinness or excessive fatness, no matter what may be its origin or nature, is not normal. The body in its wisdom would never on its own initiative reduce its store of fat below the danger point or hamper its movements and run the risk of shortening its life because of an excess of fat.

Some thin children who look as if they needed to be fattened up rapidly gain very slowly, while some roly-polys who look as if they needed to reduce may continue to gain rapidly. A history of leanness or obesity in the family seems in many cases to accompany a tendency to remain thin or to put on weight at every twist and turn in life's journey. Constitutional type and makeup and the degree of activity of different children seem to go hand in hand. The high-strung, strenuous child tends to be wiry and thin. He seems to burn up (metabolize) his food at a faster pace than does the more placid, easygoing type of child.

Usually there is nothing to worry about in these constitutional variations. This is especially true when they are brought about by differences in individual timetables of development. The little fat boy with well-padded hips may have an unawakened or sluggish endocrine system, which later on will become functionally mature, with the result that at seventeen or eighteen he has become as streamlined as his peers. The thin wiry child may begin to fill out during the puberal cycle. Whether medical intervention is necessary in cases of this kind or whether a policy of watchful waiting is indicated is, of course, for the physician to decide. Increased knowledge of the individual differences in growth and development has helped pediatricians to be a little more casual, a little less concerned, about some of the constitutional variations in degrees of fatness and rates of development.

On the other hand, more than a moderate degree of overweight in children and young people interferes with exercise and play, limits participation in the normal activities of the group, and may result in personality difficulties. And more than a moderate degree of under-weight may be responsible for chronic fatigue, poor physical endurance, and lower resistance to infection.

Sudden loss of weight or marked change in an established rate of growth may be a sign of some physical disturbance, for example, diabetes, rheumatic fever, or tuberculosis. Sudden gain in weight, in a very few cases, may accompany a glandular disorder. By and large, however, eating too much or too little is the direct cause of excessive fatness or excessive leanness. (See Overweight and Underweight, in Chap. 12.)

STAGES AND RATES OF GROWTH

Very roughly the stages of growth are divided into four periods: prenatal, preadolescent, adolescent, and postadolescent. By far the most rapid growth takes place in the prenatal period. During these nine months, the biologic forces that motivate growth and development work at tremendous speed, adding inches to stature and pounds to weight and bringing about rapid increases in complexity of structure, for example, forming the four-chambered heart of the infant from the simple pulsat-ing tube of the embryo. At birth the individual has grown from an imponderable zygote, or fertilized egg, into a ponderable infant weigh-ing seven or eight pounds, more or less, and measuring about twenty inches from top to toe. And from a single dependent cell he has devel-oped into an exceedingly complex multicelled organism with all his equipment for living an independent existence either actually or po-tentially present.

Following birth the biologic workmen slow down. Their remaining task is to put on the finishing touches—to bring their masterpiece to the perfection of maturity. But there is no hurry about this. For a number of years the rate of growth gradually slows down before speeding up again in preparation for puberty. Yet the biologic workmen do not lie down on the job altogether. Indeed, according to the yardstick and the scale, they seem to be putting on a very creditable performance.

Rates of Gain in Height and Weight

In Fig. 3-2 are shown the yearly gains in weight and height of the average boy and girl for each year from birth to seventeen years of age.

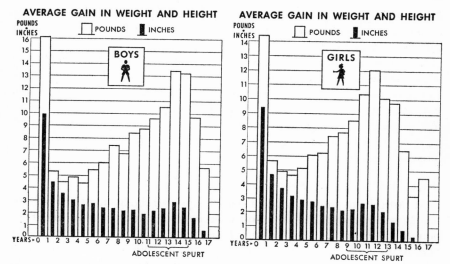

Fig. 3-2. Yearly gains in pounds and inches of the average boy and girl from birth to seventeen years.

They indicate that gain in height progresses at a rapidly decelerating rate from birth to age two, and at a slowly decelerating rate from two to nine in girls and from two to eleven in boys. The rate of gain in weight during these childhood years, before the start of the puberal cycle, decelerates rapidly to age two years, decelerates very slowly from age two to age three, and thereafter picks up speed. From nine years to twelve years in girls, and from eleven to fourteen in boys, gain in both height and weight progresses at an accelerating rate and then begins to decelerate until terminal size is reached. This happens at age sixteen in the average girl and age seventeen in the average boy, but there are many individual variations.

The Puberal Cycle

The anterior pituitary ushers in the onset of puberty by stimulating the production of the internal secretion of the gonads, or sex glands. The gonadal hormones are responsible for the emergence during puberty of the characteristic differences in body structure (secondary sex characteristics) which distinguish members of the male sex from those of the female. At the beginning of the puberal cycle there is a spurt in growth because the gonadal secretion speeds up skeletal growth, particularly in the long bones. On the average the puberal cycle begins in girls at nine years and in boys at eleven years. For the average girl the peak in puberal growth comes in the twelfth year, and for the average boy in the fourteenth year. The rapid spurt of growth at adolescence is followed by a fairly sudden stoppage of the spurt, because the activity of the gonadal secretion causes the epiphyses of the bones to unite in a relatively short time.

The influence of the internal secretion of the gonads is extremely important in physical growth and should be kept in mind in interpreting the growth curve during the puberal cycle of individual boys and girls. Excessive gonadal secretion, for example, may accentuate the rapidity of the spurt but balance it by an earlier fusion of the long bones. Under-secretion usually results in a late puberty with slower growth over a longer period of time.

Height and Weight Differences in Boys and Girls

At birth the average boy has a slight edge over the average girl in both height and weight. The superiority of boys amounts to only about ¼ pound and ¼ inch. This tendency for boys to be a little taller than girls persists through the tenth year, but in the eleventh year the girls over-take the boys, and their stature continues to exceed that of boys up to age fourteen. The boys then pass the girls and in the end top them by more than 4½ inches (see Fig. 3-3).

Sex differences in weight are negligible or nonexistent from birth up through ten years, although the boys tend to be slightly heavier than the girls. At eleven years the average girl overtakes the average boy and continues to put on weight more rapidly until the end of the fourteenth year, when she begins to drop behind. On the average the boys at ma-turity are about 19 pounds heavier than the girls.

Since the average girl starts her adolescent spurt two years earlier than the average boy, it is natural to find many girls in junior high school who are taller than boys of their age. In some cases this may constitute a social or emotional problem, which can usually be solved by giving boys and girls an understanding of the principles of growth. It will be com-forting to the boys to learn that their slight inferiority in height is

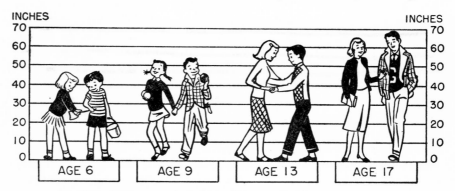

FIG. 3-3. Differences in height of boys and girls at various ages.

almost certain to be temporary. And the girls will be glad to know that there is great likelihood that the "boy-taller-than-girl" ideal will eventually be realized.

Overlapping of Age and Size

In computing an average, or mean, for body dimensions at various ages, we find that the majority of children at each age are within a few inches or pounds above or below the average. However, the range of height and weight for the whole group will be wide. For example, the average height for a large group of healthy fourteen-year-old boys may be 65 inches, with most of them ranging from 3½ inches above to 3½ inches below. But the actual range in height for the whole group may be from 56 to 73 inches. In the same way, the average weight for a group of 100 healthy thirteen-year-old girls may be 100 pounds, with fifty of them weighing between 90 and 110, but the range of weight for the whole group will be much wider than this.

Physical growth takes place at such widely different rates in different individuals that two healthy young persons, separated in chronological age by several years, may measure the same in any one or more body dimensions. For example, it is not unusual to find a boy of ten and a boy of fifteen weighing the same, or a girl of eleven and a girl of sixteen being equally tall. Every teacher is familiar with these overlappings of age and size. She has only to look around her classroom to note that the variations in stature of the majority of the children of approximately the same age are not great, but that a few children will be noticeably shorter or taller than the average.

When "Outsize" Is a Problem

The physical measurements of boys and girls have little or no relationship with their mental measurements. As a child passes from infancy to maturity, mental ability increases progressively with age but not with size. It has been found that the correlations between IQ and stature and IQ and weight are far too low to have much if any significance. Since this is so, in one grade there may be a few little chaps, several big huskies, and a great many in-betweens, all falling close to one another in chronological age and mental age. It sometimes happens that the exceptionally big husky boy at one extreme or the little runt at the other seems to himself and others to be "out of his class." This is only one of the many psychological problems that may arise as a result of being "outsize" as regards physical size or shape.

The physician may find that the hereditary pattern of growth or some other unchangeable constitutional factor appears to explain exceptionally small or large size for age or exceptionally slow or rapid progress in growth. In this case the most useful observation the teacher can make is to note whether being outsize—small or large—is having an unfavorable influence on the child's total development. If the physician's findings indicate that marked deviations from the average are likely to be permanent, the child's problem may be solved by helping him to organize his life on the basis of a frank acceptance of his physical characteristics.

In most cases, however, outsize, especially during adolescence, is temporary. Few adolescents know that wide variations from the average are compatible with normality. Most of them have the fixed idea that deviations from the average are abnormal. Consequently an adolescent may become anxious and unhappy when his companions are maturing more rapidly than he is. For this reason the fact that many different states and modes of growth and development are all normal must be made clear to him. A teacher or school nurse may be able to improve a worried adolescent's emotional attitude toward himself by a patient, clear explanation of the facts of growth and of individual variations in growth and sexual maturation. But a young person may need more reassurance than this if his doubts regarding his normality are producing a great deal of anxiety. A doctor in whom he has confidence is best fitted to remove such doubts by repeated explanations and discussions of the facts of growth and development.

MEASURING PHYSICAL GROWTH AND DEVELOPMENT

Extensive studies during recent years have added greatly to our knowledge of how children grow and how the individual members of any group may be expected to deviate from the average, or mean, at various ages in body size, build, relative amounts of different tissues, nutritional state, and rates of growth. Body measurements are useful in appraising the physical status of a child at the time they are taken and in evaluating the progress made in the intervals between successive measurements. Much attention has been given to the selection of a system of body measurement for use in spotting children in need of medical investigation because of considerable deviation from normal growth patterns.

Height and Weight

The two measurements which are easiest to make and which have been made most consistently in checking up on a child's nutritional status and rate of growth are height and weight. Height is a measure of length —up-and-down size—and weight is a measure of mass. Since growth means an increase in size and bulk, and all healthy children grow, we expect a healthy child to become progressively taller and heavier as the years pass.

Height-weight-age Tables. The most common use to which measurements of height and weight in school have been put is to determine the appropriateness of mass (weight) to length (height) at successive ages. When school weighing and measuring first became popular a generation ago, it was considered desirable to have some standard of comparison for the individual child. For that reason, tables were devised showing average weight for height and age. In constructing such tables the average, or mean, weight for height at various ages of very large numbers of children were computed, and the average weight for a particular height, age, and sex were then set up as the standard of comparison for any boy or girl of that height and age.

It would be rare indeed for the weight of an individual child to be exactly the same as that arrived at by averaging the weights of thousands of children. All that can be expected is that his weight will fall within the weight range of a substantial fraction of the total number of children of his age and height measured. Hence, in using height-weight-age tables a child is considered to be overweight or underweight only if his weight is from 10 to 15 per cent above or below the mean weight reported for each height at different ages.

The use of tables of this kind has several disadvantages. One is the tendency to accept the average as the ideal or normal. After the anatomical dimensions of large groups of children have been tabulated and averaged, we have simply a collection of mathematical averages of weights for height at various ages. Because a child is within the weight range of the majority of those who were measured to arrive at the average does not mean that he is "normal" or that his weight is optimum. He is only average. He represents what is, not necessarily what ought to be. Yet a child who is much smaller or larger than the average is apt to be disturbed about it, fearing that something is wrong with him.

Another disadvantage in the use of average weight for height and age tables is the impossibility of determining which of the groups of tissues are involved in marked deviation from the average. Is it the relative lightness or stockiness of the skeleton? the relative bulkiness or thinness of the muscles? or the relative leanness or fatness of subcutaneous tissue? It is easy to see that mistakes may be made in appraising a child's health status if these factors are not taken into consideration in deciding whether or not a child is excessively thin or excessively fat. If the weights of the two six-year-old girls shown in Plate 3, for example, were compared with the average weight for their height, big-boned Jean might be classified as overweight and small-boned Frances as underweight. Yet both girls have been given a clean bill of health by the physician who examined them, because his physical examination was supplemented by a knowledge of their inherited body build and health history.

Height–weight–age–body-build Tables. In an attempt to allow for body build in comparing a child's weight with average weight for height and age, tables of weight in relation to age, height, and body type have also been worked out. Classifications of body build fall into three main groups: "tall, slender type," "average (medium) type," and "short, stocky type." It must be remembered, however, that there are many gradations in body build, or physique. The classification into which a child falls will depend upon the characteristics that are predominant. Without other measurements besides height and weight, it is often difficult to guess to which group a child belongs.

The trunk, with its powerful bone structure and tightly packed organs, contributes more to weight than do the head and limbs. Hence, a child with a long and roomy trunk, with broad shoulders and wide pelvis, would be classified as having a heavy frame irrespective of total height. And a child with a medium or short trunk would be classified as medium or slight in build, depending upon the ruggedness or delicacy of his skeleton.

Height-age and Weight-age Curves. By calculating the average, or mean, height and weight at various ages of very large numbers of children, and plotting average height and average weight separately against age, it is possible to construct charts showing average, or mean, height-age and weight-age curves for boys and girls together with normal variations from these averages. Examples of such charts prepared by Howard V. Meredith from data collected at the Iowa Child Welfare Research Station, State University of Iowa,[1] are shown in Figs. 3-4 to 3-7. You will note that each of the graphs shows five "normative zones" for height: tall, moderately tall, average, moderately short, and short; and five "normative zones" for weight: heavy, moderately heavy, average, moderately light, and light. The normative zones in these charts furnish a pattern that may be used in checking up on the individual child's growth pattern. This is done by noticing the zone of location of the child's height and weight points as they are plotted on his individual chart. If a child's height and weight points do not fall in corresponding zones (as tall and heavy, or short and light), or if a child's height or weight jumps abruptly from one zone to another in the course of successive measurings, the child should be referred for medical investigation.

Wetzel's Grid. Another method of revealing trends in growth through the use of height and weight measurements is the grid developed by Norman C. Wetzel, known as Wetzel's grid [2] (Fig. 3-8).

In the graph forming the first panel of this grid, the vertical scale is

[1] Reproductions of these charts are available in booklet form. Each booklet is designed for recording the growth in height and weight of a single child. The booklets may be obtained from the American Medical Association or the National Education Association. For addresses of these organizations, and of others mentioned in this book, see the list at the end of the book.

[2] *Grid for Evaluating Physical Fitness in Terms of Physique (Body Build) Development Level and Basal Metabolism,* published by NEA Service, Inc.

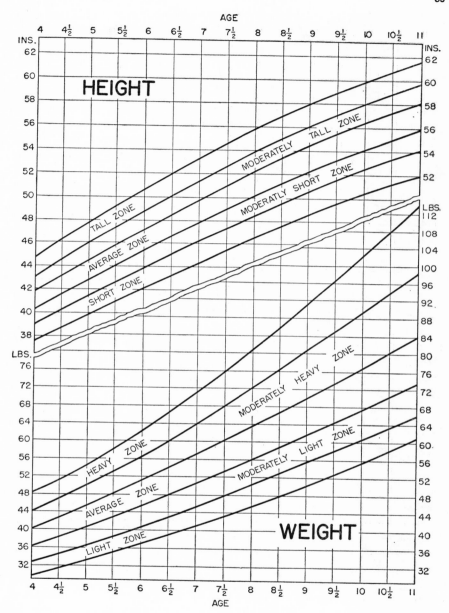

FIG. 3-4. Physical growth record for boys, ages four to eleven. (*Howard V. Meredith, reproduced by courtesy of American Medical Association.*)

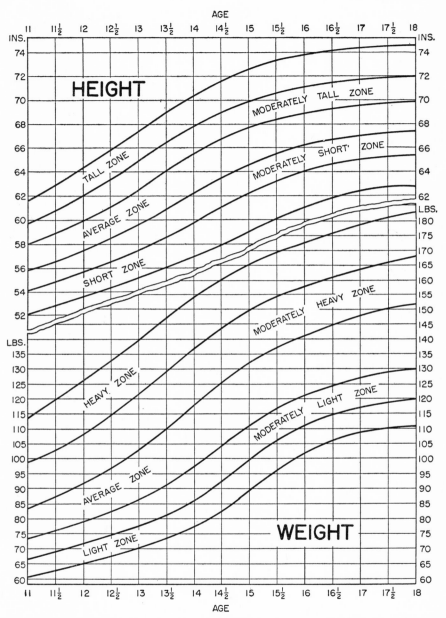

FIG. 3-5. Physical growth record for boys, ages eleven to eighteen. (*Howard F. Meredith, reproduced by courtesy of American Medical Association.*)

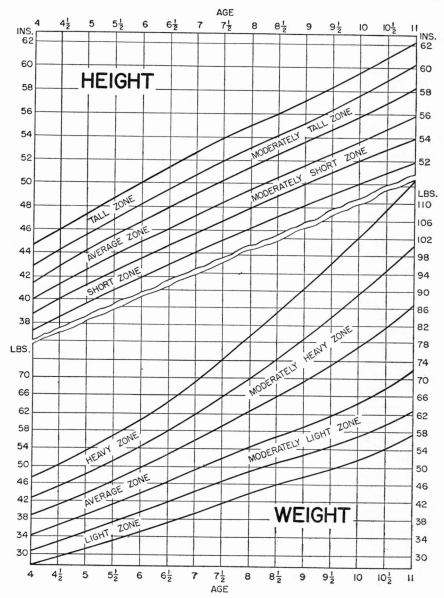

FIG. 3-6. Physical growth record for girls, ages four to eleven. (*Howard V. Meredith, reproduced by courtesy of American Medical Association.*)

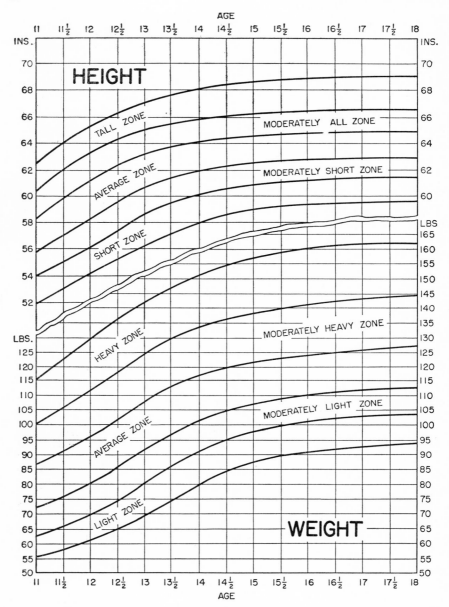

Fig. 3-7. Physical growth record for girls, ages eleven to eighteen. (*Howard V. Meredith, reproduced by courtesy of American Medical Association.*)

assigned to weight (pounds) and the horizontal scale to height (inches). When the child's weight is plotted against his height on this panel, a point is located which falls into one of several "physique channels" (see Fig. 3-9) that traverse the graph obliquely from top to bottom. These channels are designated at the top by symbols. The more obese and stocky types are at the left of the channel system (A_4, A_3, A_2), the medium (A_1, M, B_1) in the center, and the thinner lighter types (B_2, B_3, B_4) at the right. The curve plotted from successive measurements represents the child's channel course. This curve tends to follow the particular physique channel that corresponds to the child's body build. The tendency to follow a particular channel is due to the tendency in health to preserve the same physique, or shape, at successive ages. Hence, if a child moves out of his established channel, a change in his nutritional or health status is indicated.

The graph forming the first panel also contains numbered developmental-level lines which cross the channel lines at regular intervals. Each level represents a different size, that is, a different value of body surface. The numbered level at which a height-weight point is located measures the child's size (body surface area). The direction of the course taken by the child through the channel system is the result of change in size with respect to change in shape.

In summary, the channel system serves three purposes:

1. It identifies the child's physique, or body build, by the channel in which the various weight-height points fall.

2. It measures the child's size by means of the developmental levels at which these points are located.

3. It acts as a direction finder for ascertaining the trend or direction of the child's own development.

In the second panel a field is provided for determining speed of development. On this graph, size (developmental level) is plotted from the vertical scale, and age from the horizontal scale. The curve plotted for the individual child from successive points in this panel is called his "auxodrome," or age schedule of development. A set of standard auxodromes (blue curves for boys, red curves for girls) shows how many children at any given age (expressed as a fraction of the total number at that age in the general population) may be expected to have reached a given developmental level. Thus it is possible to recognize whether a child's developmental level is high or low in relation to the normal distribution of size for age and also to detect deviations from its expected course.

In a third panel the developmental-level lines are correlated with an energy scale which indicates the basal heat production in calories per day at each level. Daily fuel requirements of the child are approxi-

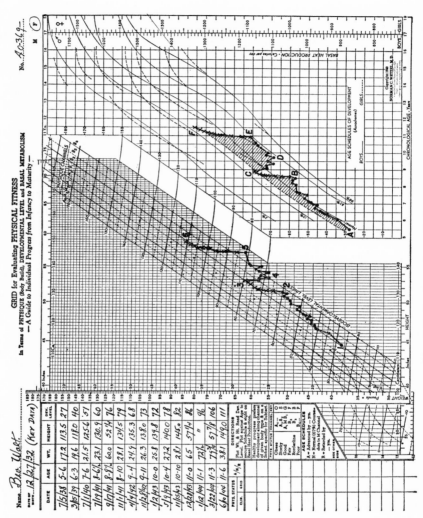

FIG. 3-8. See legend on facing page.

mately twice his basal heat production. These developmental-level–calorie relationships form the basis for planning additional dietary allowances in the medical treatment of malnutrition.

The principles upon which Wetzel's grid has been constructed lie in the realm of advanced mathematics, but the teacher or nurse making height-weight measurements can easily learn to plot them in the channel system, read the developmental level, and then plot developmental level against age in the second (right-hand) panel. The physician inspecting the grids of a number of children can readily select those which indicate deviations from the expected patterns of growth.

Skeletal Stockiness, Muscular Bulk, and Subcutaneous Fat

The three tissues that have the greatest influence on body build, stature, and weight are the skeleton, the musculature, and the subcutaneous fat. Hence, in addition to measurements of length and mass (height and weight), measurements of the stockiness of the skeleton, the bulkiness of the musculature, and the quantity of subcutaneous tissue have been found helpful in the appraisal of a child's physical status.

Various measurements for determining the magnitude of these three attributes have been proposed by investigators who have carried on extensive studies relating to the appraisal of the physical status of

---

FIG. 3-8. Wetzel's-grid record showing two episodes of simple growth failure (malnutritional type), plotted from the data tabulated in centimeters (height) and kilograms (weight). (*Reproduced by courtesy of Normal C. Wetzel.*)

Channel course: This child's normal body type, first observed at point 1, falls between physique channels B_1 and B_2. Segments 1–2 and 3–4–5 of her actual channel course represent moderate and severe departures from true channelwise direction (indicated at 1, 3, and 6) with corresponding losses of physique from her own B_1, B_2 body type. Segments 2–3 and 5–6 indicate recovery responses following treatment started at 2 and 5. Physique was completely restored at 3 and 6.

Auxodromic progress: The child's "own," or "expected," auxodrome (age schedule of development) is represented by the broken line *ACF*. The line *ABCDEF* is the child's actual auxodrome.

The slowing down, or lag, in speed of development, corresponding with the losses of physique shown in her channel course, is measured by the vertical difference between the expected auxodrome (*ACF*) and the actual auxodrome (*ABCDEF*). At *B*, for example, the level actually reached is 57, whereas according to the child's expected auxodrome it should be 74. Therefore, her lag in speed of development at *B* amounts to 17 levels. At *E* it amounts to 22 levels. Segments *B-C* and *E-F* of the actual auxodrome show speed-up during the first and second recovery phases, with complete return to her own schedule at *C* and *F*. Failure in both episodes continued to increase until definite action had been taken at 2 (in channel course), *B* (in auxodrome) and 5, *E* to investigate causes and to remedy them.

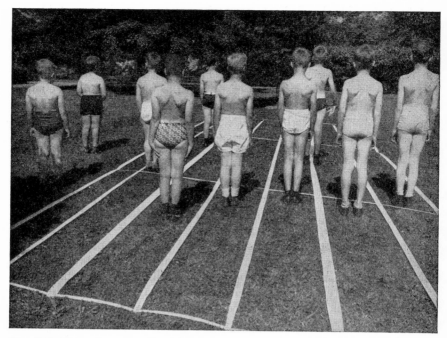

FIG. 3-9. These boys are lined up in their respective physique channels (ranging from A_4 at the left to B_3 at the right) to illustrate the value of Wetzel's grid in determining body type. Observe the striking physical differences in the boys at approximately the same developmental level (level 95). (*Reproduced by courtesy of Normal C. Wetzel and Science Illustrated.*)

children. One set of measurements is that of Harold C. Stuart and Howard V. Meredith.[3]

In addition to body weight and standing height, the measurements selected by these authorities are chest circumference and hip width (pelvic breadth at the crests of the ilia, that is, the upper edges of the hipbones) to indicate the degree of skeletal stockiness, and leg girth (the greatest circumference of the calf) to indicate the bulkiness of the musculature. The method suggested for estimating subjectively the thickness of the skin and subcutaneous tissue is to draw together and elevate between the thumb and index finger a double layer of skin and subcutaneous tissue (*a*) in the region slightly below and a little to the side of the left shoulder blade, and (*b*) in the region immediately above the top of the left hipbone. Ratings of the thickness of subcutaneous tissue are made according to a scale extending from 1 plus (+) at the

[3] Harold C. Stuart and Howard V. Meredith, "Use of Body Measurements in the School Health Program," *American Journal of Public Health*, vol. 36, no. 12 (December) 1946.

lower end to 5 plus ($+++++$) at the upper end. To make these ratings, Stuart and Meredith point out, familiarity with the range of individual differences in given sex-age groups is required, as well as considerable experience in making judgments of subcutaneous tissue in the regions specified.

On the basis of measurements of large numbers of healthy American boys and girls in the school ages, Stuart and Meredith have constructed a table giving selected percentiles[4] (10, 20, 50, 75, and 90) at each half-year interval from five to nineteen for each of their recommended body measurements. The percentiles for weight and height are given in Table 3-1.

What the Teacher Can Observe

The various systems of body measurements of school children have been described both because teachers should be aware of the developments in this field and because many of them may be called upon to assist in the taking and recording of such measurements for the use of the physician in making school health examinations. Measuring height and weight at stated intervals is often a duty of the teacher, and her subjective estimate of nutritional state is an observation that can be of great help in getting medical attention for children who need it. It is considered best to leave to the physician the interpretation of individual deviations from the body measurements given in tables or charts that show average or normal growth patterns. Such discrepancies must be viewed in the light of the child's medical and social history and a thoroughgoing evaluation of his physical status and growth progress.

Classroom Weighing and Measuring. The primary interest of the teacher in height-weight measurements lies in the light they throw upon the child's progress along his or her own pathway of development. All healthy children grow. The easiest way to keep track of their progress in growing is to keep a record of height and weight for each child and note from successive measurements the child's gain or lack of gain. The record may be kept in the form of height-age and weight-age curves, which the child himself may help to plot, as in the physical growth records shown earlier in the chapter (Figs. 3-4–3-7); or on Wetzel's grid, if that system of recording height-weight measurements has been adopted by the school

[4] By "percentile" is meant the expression of values in terms of per cent. The percentile rank of a child in a group of children arranged in order of magnitude in respect to a certain attribute indicates that child's superiority over children in the group with a lower percentile rank and inferiority to children with a higher percentile rank. For example, a child with a percentile rank of 75 in respect to height is taller than 75 per cent of his group and shorter than 25 per cent. If his percentile rank is 50, he occupies the middle position; hence, his height is medium or average (the mean). If his percentile rank is 25, he is taller than 25 per cent of his group and shorter than 75 per cent.

Table 3-1

GAINS IN WEIGHT (lb) AND HEIGHT (in.): AGES 6 TO 18 YEARS

Age	Girls					Boys				
	Light and short (Percentile 10)	Moderately light and short (Percentile 25)	Average (Percentile 50)	Moderately tall and heavy (Percentile 75)	Tall and heavy (Percentile 90)	Light and short (Percentile 10)	Moderately light and short (Percentile 25)	Average (Percentile 50)	Moderately tall and heavy (Percentile 75)	Tall and heavy (Percentile 90)
6 years										
Weight	39.9	42.9	46.5	50.2	54.2	40.9	44.4	48.3	52.1	56.4
Height	43.5	44.5	45.6	47.0	48.0	43.8	44.9	46.0	47.5	48.6
6½ years										
Weight	42.2	45.5	49.4	53.3	57.7	43.4	47.1	51.2	55.4	60.4
Height	44.7	45.7	46.9	48.2	50.0	44.9	46.0	47.5	49.0	50.0
7 years										
Weight	44.5	48.1	52.2	56.3	61.2	45.8	49.7	54.1	58.7	64.4
Height	46.0	46.9	48.0	49.5	50.7	46.0	47.3	48.9	50.0	51.0
7½ years										
Weight	46.6	50.6	55.2	59.8	65.6	48.5	52.6	57.1	62.1	68.7
Height	47.0	48.0	49.3	50.7	51.9	47.2	48.6	50.1	51.5	52.7
8 years										
Weight	48.6	53.1	58.1	63.3	69.9	51.2	55.5	60.1	65.5	73.0
Height	48.0	49.1	50.4	51.8	53.0	48.4	49.8	51.1	53.0	54.0
8½ years										
Weigh	50.6	55.5	61.0	66.9	74.5	53.8	58.3	63.1	68.9	77.0
Height	49.0	50.0	51.4	52.9	54.1	49.5	50.8	52.3	54.0	55.1
9 years										
Weight	52.6	57.9	63.8	70.5	79.1	56.3	61.1	66.0	72.3	81.0
Height	50.0	51.0	52.3	54.0	55.2	50.5	51.8	53.3	55.0	56.0

9½ years										
Weight	54.9	60.4	67.1	74.8	84.4	58.7	63.7	69.0	76.0	85.5
Height	51.0	52.0	53.4	55.0	56.3	51.4	52.7	54.3	56.0	57.1
10 years										
Weight	57.1	62.8	70.3	79.1	89.7	61.1	66.3	71.9	79.6	89.9
Height	51.8	53.0	54.5	56.1	57.5	52.2	53.6	55.2	56.8	58.0
10½ years										
Weight	59.9	66.4	74.6	84.1	95.1	63.7	69.0	74.8	83.4	94.6
Height	52.9	54.1	55.8	57.4	59.0	53.1	54.5	56.0	57.8	59.0
11 years										
Weight	62.6	69.9	78.8	89.1	100.4	66.3	71.6	77.6	87.2	99.3
Height	54.0	55.2	57.0	58.7	60.3	54.0	55.3	56.7	58.7	59.7
11½ years										
Weight	66.1	74.0	83.2	94.0	106.0	69.2	74.6	81.0	91.6	104.5
Height	55.0	56.3	58.3	60.0	61.8	55.0	56.3	57.8	59.6	60.9
12 years										
Weight	69.5	78.0	87.6	98.8	111.5	72.0	77.5	84.4	96.0	109.6
Height	56.0	57.4	59.6	61.6	63.2	56.0	57.1	58.9	60.0	62.1
12½ years										
Weight	74.7	83.7	93.4	104.9	118.0	74.6	80.6	88.7	102.0	116.4
Height	57.4	58.7	60.7	62.6	64.0	56.9	58.0	60.0	61.8	63.6
13 years										
Weight	79.9	89.4	99.1	111.0	124.5	77.1	83.7	93.0	107.9	123.2
Height	58.7	60.0	61.8	63.5	64.8	57.7	59.0	61.0	63.3	65.0
13½ years										
Weight	85.5	94.6	103.7	115.4	128.9	82.2	89.6	100.3	115.5	130.0
Height	59.5	60.8	62.3	64.0	65.3	58.8	60.2	62.5	64.8	66.5
14 years										
Weight	91.0	99.8	108.4	119.7	133.3	87.2	95.5	107.6	123.1	136.9
Height	60.2	61.4	62.8	64.4	65.7	60.0	61.6	64.0	66.3	67.8
14½ years										
Weight	94.2	102.5	111.0	121.8	135.7	93.3	101.9	113.9	129.1	142.4
Height	60.7	61.8	63.0	64.3	66.0	61.0	62.7	65.0	67.2	68.7

Table 3-1 (Continued)

GAINS IN WEIGHT (lb) AND HEIGHT (in.): AGES 6 TO 18 YEARS

Age	Girls					Boys				
	Light and short (Percentile 10)	Moderately light and short (Percentile 25)	Average (Percentile 50)	Moderately tall and heavy (Percentile 75)	Tall and heavy (Percentile 90)	Light and short (Percentile 10)	Moderately light and short (Percentile 25)	Average (Percentile 50)	Moderately tall and heavy (Percentile 75)	Tall and heavy (Percentile 90)
15 years										
Weight	97.4	105.1	113.5	123.9	138.1	99.4	108.2	120.1	135.0	147.8
Height	61.1	62.1	63.4	65.0	66.1	62.1	63.9	66.0	68.1	69.5
15½ years										
Weight	99.2	106.8	115.3	125.6	139.6	105.2	113.5	124.9	139.7	152.6
Height	61.3	62.3	63.6	65.2	66.4	63.0	64.8	66.8	68.8	70.1
16 years										
Weight	100.9	108.4	117.0	127.2	141.1	111.0	118.7	129.7	144.4	157.3
Height	61.5	62.1	63.8	65.3	66.5	64.0	65.8	67.5	69.5	70.7
16½ years										
Weight	101.9	109.4	118.1	128.4	142.2	114.3	121.6	133.0	147.9	161.0
Height	61.5	62.3	63.9	65.3	66.6	64.6	66.3	68.0	70.0	71.1
17 years										
Weight	102.8	110.4	119.1	129.6	143.3	117.5	124.5	136.2	151.4	164.6
Height	61.5	62.4	64.0	65.4	66.7	65.2	66.8	68.4	70.1	71.5
17½ years										
Weight	103.2	110.8	119.5	130.2	143.9	118.8	125.8	137.6	153.6	166.8
Height	61.5	62.4	64.0	65.4	66.7	65.3	66.9	68.5	70.3	71.6
18 years										
Weight	103.5	111.2	119.9	130.8	144.5	120.0	127.1	139.0	155.7	169.0
Height	61.5	62.4	64.0	65.4	66.7	65.5	67.1	68.7	70.4	71.8

Source: Harold C. Stuart and Howard V. Meredith, "Use of Body Measurements in the School Health Program," American Journal of Public Health, Vol. 36, No. 12 (December) 1946.

medical service; or on a simple record form which provides spaces for noting height and weight (and other body measurements if they are made) at successive intervals.

Although frequency of measurement varies in different schools, it is recommended that children be weighed every month and measured for height three times a year—preferably in September, January, and May. Weight should be taken with the child wearing as little clothing as is practicable and without shoes. Height should be measured with the shoes removed.

Failure to gain weight over a period of one or two months rarely has significance in elementary school children because most preadolescent youngsters naturally fail to gain in this period. Approximately 10 per cent of elementary school children, however, fail to gain for three successive months between September and May. Failure to make any gain in a three-month period is nearly always a sign that something is wrong, either because of poor health habits or because of a disease or some other condition that needs medical attention. Children who fail to gain for three successive months, and children who suddenly or persistently make excessive gains, should be called to the attention of the nurse or physician. At the time of making this referral a report should be given of the child's progress in school, the standard of living to which he is accustomed, and any other information that the physician may find significant in making a medical judgment about the child.

Continuous records of height and weight without reference to a standard table have specific value in several ways:

1. They make it possible for school personnel to screen out youngsters for medical examination because of discrepancies between height and weight status or because marked changes have occurred in their individual growth patterns between successive measurement periods.

2. They can be used to point out to the child the relation between growth and health. Thus, while they are not diagnostic in a clinical sense, they are a good educational device.

3. They can be used as an incentive to encourage the child to keep in good condition or to build up his health. His growth record is something the child can see and understand. In most cases it is a mirror revealing the relationship between growth on the one hand and nutrition, sleep, rest, and exercise on the other. By keeping track of his progress the child can see that his physical growth is closely bound up with his health habits. This provides one way of appealing to the child to take some of the responsibility for his health.

4. The records are of interest to parents, who naturally like to have evidence of their child's progress. They may be helpful to the parents in arousing the child's pride in his health and in winning his cooperation in matters that affect his health. Hence they provide a valuable medium

of health education through which the teacher, the parent, and the child can collaborate regularly in a matter that is of importance to each one of them—the child's present and future well-being.

FOR REVIEW AND DISCUSSION

1. Match each word or term in Group A with the word or term in Group B which you associate with it.

Group A	Group B
1 Epiphyses	4 Growth-promoting hormone
2 Rickets	8 Energy metabolism
3 Anterior pituitary	7 Overactivity
4 Puberty	5 Fat depots of body
5 Adipose tissue	2 Vitamin D deficiency
6 Auxodrome	3 Activation of gonads
7 Hyperfunction	1 Ossification centers
8 Thyroxine	6 Wetzel's grid

2. Select the correct ending for each of the following incomplete sentences:

   a. To determine a child's developmental age it is necessary to know his (1) birth date, (2) his skeletal age, (3) his height and weight.
   b. The average height of a large group of fourteen-year-old boys was found to be 64 inches; this means that (1) all normal fourteen-year-old boys are 64 inches tall; (2) most of the boys in the group are 64 inches tall; (3) the heights of all the boys were added and divided by the number of boys measured in order to determine the average.
   c. Periodic weighing and measuring gives valuable information about the growth and development of school children because it shows what progress each child is making according to (1) his own growth record, (2) the gains made by other children in the class, (3) the measurements given in a height-weight-age table.

3. How would you help a youngster who

   a. Is painfully conscious of being much smaller or larger than others in the class?
   b. Thinks that something must be wrong with him because he is maturing less rapidly than his friends are?
   c. Is embarrassed because the girl he likes best in junior high is taller than he?
   d. Has failed to gain in weight over a period of three months?

SELECTED REFERENCES

Breckenridge, Marian E., and E. L. Vincent: *Child Development; Physical and Psychological Growth through Adolescence,* 4th ed., W. B. Saunders Company, Philadelphia, 1960.

Gesell, Arnold L., and Frances L. Ilg: *The Child from Five to Ten,* Harper & Brothers, New York, 1946.

Gesell, Arnold L., and others: *Youth; the Years from Ten to Sixteen,* Harper & Brothers, New York, 1956.

Hurlock, Elizabeth B.: *Adolescent Development,* 2d ed., McGraw-Hill Book Company, New York, 1955. (Covers all aspects of development—physical, mental, social, and emotional.)

Lane, Howard, and Mary Beauchamp: *Understanding Human Development,* Prentice-Hall, Inc., New York, 1959. (A good text on physical growth, as well as mental, emotional, and social aspects of development.)

Rand, Winifred: *Growth Development of the Young Child,* 6th ed., W. B. Saunders Company, Philadelphia, 1958.

Stuart, Harold C., and Dane G. Prugh: *The Healthy Child,* Harvard University Press, Cambridge, Mass., 1960. (Covers physical, psychological, and social development.)

Wilkes, Edward T.: *Family Guide to Teenage Health,* The Ronald Press Company, New York, 1958. Part I, *Growth and Development.*

Organizations

Association for Childhood Education

Child Study Association

Children's Bureau, U.S. Department of Health, Education and Welfare

Chapter 4 GROWING UP EMOTIONALLY AND SOCIALLY

Psychological Makeup
Phases and Aspects of Emotional and Social Development
Characteristics and Needs of Children by Age Groups
Emotional Needs of All Children

When children are old enough to enter school, they are already complex personalities. Each one is the unique product of his biologic, intellectual, and emotional constitution modified by an infinite variety of influences springing from his environment.

Constitution is what is born into the tissues and remains with the individual throughout his life. We know that inborn factors determine individual differences in the ability to resist disease, privation, and the effects of the passing years. We know, too, that inborn differences in intellectual ability exist and can be measured. But who can say what factors are inherent in newborn babies which account for variations in the amount of trouble, happiness, and anxiety they will have in dealing with their environments?

The inheritance of tendencies to emotional or mental instability has been intensively studied, but so far there is little scientific evidence to indicate whether such tendencies exist and, if so, what they are. We do know, however, that individuals vary greatly in their capacity to stand up emotionally under the discipline and stress of living. We know, too, that these variations arise under a surprisingly wide latitude of environmental conditions. Poverty, hardship, and neglect on the one hand; wealth, ease, and loving care on the other, have produced their quotas of failures and successes. We can safely surmise that there seems to be a wide margin of safety in the emotional growth of children.

PSYCHOLOGICAL MAKEUP

In discussing mental, emotional, and social development, we are concerned primarily with that part of the personality known as the *psyche*, or mind. Psychologists in studying the mind have found it helpful to conceive of it as occupying three levels—the unconscious, or subconscious, mind on the lower level, the conscious mind on the middle level, and the conscience on the upper level.

The Conscious Mind

All the mental activities that a person knows about and can control go on in his conscious mind. They are based upon the impressions left by past experiences in the association, or memory, centers of his brain. When a person is confronted with a new problem or a new situation, for example, the memory of what he has already learned comes to his aid. Every experience in life has added to his stock of knowledge to draw on in thinking and acting. That knowledge is right there in the conscious part of his mind where he can readily get at it.

The Unconscious Mind

Other things go on in the mind, however, of which the individual is not conscious and which he cannot control. This type of mental activity is based upon the impressions left by all those past experiences which he does not consciously remember. The storage place of all such impressions is the unconscious mind. Largely they serve as emotional ties linking us with our forgotten past. We may like or dislike a person at first sight, for example, because he reminds us of someone we liked or disliked long ago. Or some of our present fears and anxieties may be echoes of our responses to unfortunate early experiences with whatever it is that is making us afraid and anxious.

The Development of Conscience

Within the unconscious mind at birth are powerful instinctual drives or forces which seek for expression. Not only do these inner forces war among themselves, but also they come eventually into conflict with forces in the outside world. These outer forces seek to mold the child into an acceptable member of the family and the society into which he was born. The child's ego, the part of his personality that he knows as "I, myself," emerges during this process. An essential part of ego formation is identification with the wishes and ideas of the parents. The parents are always giving, the child always taking and putting together in his own mind, the various pieces of the picture of what is expected of him as a responsible member of society. Naturally the ego is weaker than it will be later when the child is able to think and function independently and when his own ideal of what he wants to be becomes firmly established.

As the child grows older the parents cannot always be with him to remind him that some things are wrong and must not be done, and some things are right and must be done. To overcome the feeling of insecurity that arises from not being able to remember what is right and what is wrong, the child erects a mechanism that operates automatically to keep him on the right track. This mechanism is called the conscience. At first, the child's conscience is the reflection of his parents' consciences.

But as the child gains more knowledge of the moral concepts and behavior ideals of the society in which he lives, his conscience takes on substance and becomes an integral part of his personality.

The conscience is a very important part of personality. It acts as a traffic policeman to push back down into the unconscious mind all the powerful impulses, drives, and desires of which it does not approve. As the struggle takes place below the level of consciousness, the individual is not aware of what is going on, but he does consciously experience the emotions associated with it.

The Drama of Personality Development

With the arrival on the scene of the conscience, the stage is set for the lifelong drama of personality development. The central figure in the struggle—the hero—is the ego. The instinctual impulses of aggression and sexuality arising from the unconscious mind threaten individuality by urging the ego to be too independent and grasping—too self-centered and selfish. The cultivated impulses arising from the conscience threaten individuality by urging the ego to be too dependent upon social dictates, too self-effacing and submissive. The happy denouement of this struggle is the development of a well-balanced and mature personality—an individual with a profound sense of personal worth combined with a lively sense of responsibility toward others.

PHASES AND ASPECTS OF EMOTIONAL AND SOCIAL DEVELOPMENT

We now know a great deal about the phases of emotional and social development through which the child passes before physical maturity is reached. As a baby he is helpless. He has no capacity to give; he can only receive. He is wholly dependent upon others to meet his needs. If he is loved and properly cared for he does not have to wait long for the relief of tension caused by discomforts such as hunger, cold, and pain.

A little later, however, he does have to learn to wait. Little by little he finds that the pleasure of relieving the inner tensions set up by his instinctual needs and urges must be postponed for the attainment of some greater or more distant good. The acquirement of toilet habits, which usually begins toward the end of the first year, is emblematic of the child's introduction to the training that grooms the human being for social acceptance. Giving up the satisfaction of wetting and having a bowel movement when and where he pleases wins for the child his parents' approval, which eventually gives him more satisfaction than the immediate relief of tension.

Learning to Meet the Requirements of Social Living

Every child at each stage of his development has pleasures, desires, and purposes upon which he wants to act "right here and now." Taking action, however, may conflict with what is considered right and proper by his own developing ego or by outside authorities. In postponing action, or in directing his energies into more acceptable channels, or in repressing unworthy impulses for the sake of the more solid lasting satisfaction represented by his own or outside approval, he gains practice in dealing realistically with the forces that influence him. In this process, however, he is bound to experience the pangs of frustration.

The easier and pleasanter dealing with reality is made, the quicker the child will learn, and the fewer will be his feelings of frustration and resentment against authority. Each success in learning new skills in living strengthens his ego and makes him better able to take the next step forward in his development.

Many of the things required of the child are in line with his own needs and desires. He overcomes his feelings of frustration fairly quickly because of his pleasure in finding that the new patterns of behavior are preferable to the old. For example, the child must learn eventually to feed, wash, and dress himself. At first he may feel disappointed or hurt when his mother does not give him all her attention. But he finds that being able to do things for himself gives him a pleasant feeling of independence. Even though it may take him two or three times longer than it would take his mother to button his coat or to tie his shoelaces, he insists upon doing it. Walking all by himself frees him from the restraining hand that often keeps him from going where he wants to go. And so the tremendous effort required in learning to walk alone is worth it—it is made gladly.

However, there are many requirements that seem to interfere with the child's freedom or threaten his ego. The time comes when he must begin to give up the satisfaction of having his playthings all to himself. He learns that certain things and certain persons are inviolable. There are, for example, things which he may not take without permission or without paying for them, things which he may not touch or even go near. He learns that the penalty for kicking, biting, hitting, or otherwise assaulting grown-ups and younger children is much greater than for similar encounters with children of approximately his own age.

As the child grows older and his environment widens, he comes up against many other requirements that force him to give up his freedom to do as he pleases. To be socially acceptable he finds, for example, that in playing and working with others he must take turns, obey the rules of the game, refrain from crying even when hurt, go to school regularly although sometimes he'd much rather be somewhere else, be on time when he feels like loitering, walk in the school corridors when he'd rather run, keep still in the classroom when he wants to talk, and so on.

The child learns to meet many such requirements because he has been convinced that failure to do so will delay or block the coming of some greater good, or will seriously handicap his personal well-being. However, he seldom meets them with equanimity. We have all seen the prototype of Shakespeare's boy "creeping like snail unwillingly to school" because he has learned that the fruits of truancy are less appetizing than the fruits of attendance.

Also, the child often experiences overwhelming emotions such as anger or fear when he is frustrated or confronted with the unknown. Experience gradually teaches him that it is safer or nicer or wiser to keep such feelings bottled up. So he learns to control overwhelming emotions—to be angry or afraid inside and not show it, to be frustrated and not sulk or weep. During the learning process, however, his feelings often spill over. This is natural, because it takes time to learn to repress strong feelings successfully or to divert them into channels of constructive activity (see Frustration, in Chap. 9).

As the child grows up he is expected to put away such childish things as temper tantrums, or fits of sulkiness, or crying. On the surface, at any rate, he is expected to have worked out the adjustments that make possible what we label adult behavior, but the impulses that aroused childish behavior cannot be thrown away or given away. Like the dolls and the tin soldiers in the attic, they remain unclaimed in the lost-and-found department of his mind as reminders of the child he once was. More often than he realizes, they influence his conscious thoughts and actions.

Importance of the Teacher's Role

When a child enters school most of his ways of responding to social requirements have already been determined. The teacher becomes an unusually important person in his life. During school hours at least she is the embodiment of the authority which hitherto has resided only in the parents or other adults in position of authority in the home. If the emotional atmosphere and standards of conduct of the home have made possible the successes which foster a strong sense of personal worth, the teacher can concentrate on serving the child's intellectual needs and on helping him to make the adjustments necessary to live and work happily with others of his own age. Unfortunately, however, the teacher often has the more difficult task of counteracting trends developed by an unwholesome emotional environment. Some children are unwanted, and most of those who are, know it. The relation with the teacher may be the child's first experience of being wanted. The teacher's acceptance of him as an important and valuable person can do much to heal the wounds of rejection. Through her own emotional stability, warm friendliness, fairness, and sense of humor she may do much to counteract the emotional instability and the antagonism toward authority mirrored in the behavior of children who have been dealt with inconsistently or without affection and understanding.

CHARACTERISTICS AND NEEDS OF CHILDREN BY AGE GROUPS

Although each child is unique, he has many things in common with others who are in his same stage of physical, mental, emotional, and social growth. The more things the teacher knows about the age group to which her children belong, the surer will be her judgment in dealing with them as individuals. It is important to keep in mind, however, that children of about the same chronological age may differ greatly in levels of maturity.

Primary Children

Children from six to eight years of age have a great need for close personal attachments and for encouragement in their attempts to reach adult standards of behavior. This is the age of "bringing things to teacher," of waiting eagerly for the word of thanks or the word or nod of approval, of enjoying the feeling of being liked and understood. The friendly, sensitive, and perceptive teacher will create in the classroom the genial social climate which will help primary children to develop to the best of their potentialities.

Mental Development. Perhaps the most outstanding mental characteristics of six-year-olds are their curiosity and their eagerness to learn. However, their attention span is limited. Six-year-olds are usually enthusiastic in beginning something but may need to be encouraged and helped to finish it. Many activities of short duration, which can be changed quickly, are needed to keep these children interested and busy.

Indecisiveness is another typical characteristic of the six-year-old. Confronted with two equally desirable courses of action, he has great difficulty in making up his mind. For this reason, it is considered unwise to place him in too many situations in which he must make choices or decisions. Routine—doing the same things at about the same time during the day—removes the necessity for making some decisions and helps to give the child a feeling of security.

At age seven, thinking about things begins to assume importance in mental development. The seven-year-old takes time out to mull things over in his mind. His private inner life is beginning to take shape within the framework of the gregarious, active life he leads at home and in school. For that reason the seven-year-old is prone on occasion to dream, to brood, to talk to himself, to sulk, to be heedless and inattentive. Seven-year-olds also are developing capacity for self-criticism. They are eager to do well and have almost a perfectionist attitude toward their work. In writing and drawing they are apt to use their erasers as much as their pencils in their striving to improve what they have done.

The impulse to reach out toward new experiences and new achievements is perhaps the most important factor in the intellectual growth of eight-year-olds. In obeying it the child is forced to think, to experiment, to select, to discard, and to evaluate himself in comparison with others. The horizons of his thinking are expanding to take in a past when he wasn't around and to envision a future peopled with others who will come after him.

Curiosity about people and places outside of his own immediate environment illustrates the eight-year-old's expanding sense of time and space. He enjoys tales of "far away and long ago." He begs his parents and grandparents to tell him stories about the things they did when they were boys and girls. He is interested in the way of life of children living in other parts of his own country and in other parts of the world. This is a good time to cultivate friendly feelings toward other lands and peoples by emphasizing likenesses as well as differences.

Emotional Expression. Six-year-olds are nearing the close of the period of emotional development characterized by strong motor responses to anger, fear, and frustration, such as fighting, excessive restlessness, and rudeness. During the year they become happier and more enthusiastic about doing things they enjoy. Outright emotional explosions, such as temper tantrums, or fits of crying, begin to decrease. Sometimes it may be possible to distract a child when emotional storm warnings appear. At other times it seems that nature must run its course.

At age seven, children have their emotions under better control than at age six. They are more likely to withdraw into themselves when hurt or angry than to show their feelings by aggressive behavior. The "sulks" seem to have taken the place of temper tantrums as a typical reaction to frustration. This does not mean, however, that seven-year-olds will not stand up for what they consider to be their rights. They may get into fights with other children on the playground, but more often they will walk off and refuse to play.

Seven-year-olds are prone to worry largely because of their anxiety to make a good showing in their work and to hold their own with other children. Some of them may need considerable reassurance about their school progress during the year and also some help in dealing with play situations that they are not yet able to handle satisfactorily.

Eight-year-olds are more outgoing in the expression of their feelings than are seven-year-olds and tend to react to frustration with aggressive behavior or an "I don't care" attitude. In spite of their seeming nonchalance, however, tears may be very close to the surface or even overflow when they are corrected or rebuked or teased by adults. They criticize one another freely, however, without evoking hard feelings. They are eager for praise and sometimes deliberately court it by asking leading questions, such as, "That's not so good, is it?" or "I didn't do so well, did I?"

Eight-year-olds are losing many of the fears they had earlier and are not inclined to worry so much. But some of them may still worry if they feel that they are not making good progress in their schoolwork or are not holding their own with the other children or are not coming up to adult standards of behavior. Sometimes they worry in the midst of an activity for fear that it "won't come out right." Some sensitive children of this age go through agonies of mind if the memory of a terrifying experience is kept bottled up.

Social Development. When children enter the first grade, they are in or approaching the period of social development characterized by keen competition and an impulse to experiment, to investigate, and to show off. Normally, these children are strongly motivated by the desire to be leaders, to be first, to feel important, and to be considered important. Some six-year-olds, however, already may show a tendency to what is called withdrawing behavior. Instead of being self-assertive, boastful, and noisy, they are likely to be submissive, shy, timid, solitary, and dreamy. They seldom get into trouble with parents or teachers. Yet the habit of withdrawal has more dangerous implications for the future mental and emotional health of the child than the habit of defiance (see Chap. 9).

Most six-year-olds like to think that they are helping mother and teacher. They can take on easy routine chores at home and help with various classroom tasks such as passing out papers, erasing the chalkboard, taking out and putting away books and work materials, and caring for plants and pets in the classroom. Their manifest enjoyment of responsibility, however, should not lead grownups to expect too much of them or to exert too much pressure.

Children at age six cannot be expected to assume full responsibility for getting to places or doing things on time. They are learning to tell time, but their sense of time is immature. They will need to be reminded frequently that it is time for bed, for example, or for getting up or for starting for school or for washing their hands before meals.

The seven-year-old has gained a good idea of what is considered right and proper by his parents and teacher, and he is sensitive to their approval and disapproval. Talebearing is common at this age because it provides a way of winning adult approval of one's own goodness. At the same time the seven-year-old wants to be approved and accepted by the children in his group. Sometimes this makes for conflicts, since the group may applaud, or at least condone, aggressive behavior that adults find annoying or even downright naughty. The shy withdrawn child may find that the other children do not want him around because he is uncertain as to what they want him to do or because he does not know how to do it.

Seven-year-olds feel closer to the adult world than do six-year-olds, and it is hard for them to take adult criticism or teasing with good grace. On the other hand they are amenable to friendly suggestions for improvement in their behavior because they are seeking approved standards of behavior, and knowing what is expected of them helps to give them a sense of security.

Seven-year-olds, like six-year-olds, cannot be depended upon for consistent help at home or in school. Except for easy short-term chores, they may make a good start but seldom have the staying power to reach the finish line under their own power. Their sense of time is still immature and they are inclined to dawdle. But they know that there are certain things like getting to school and going to bed that should be done on time.

Eight-year-olds are seriously striving to meet adult standards of behavior. They are more willing to take the blame for naughty acts and give fewer alibis and excuses than at earlier ages. Their sense of right and wrong and their ability to distinguish fact from fancy are becoming more clearly defined. They may still tell "tall stories," but with a discernible twinkle in the eye. Their brand of humor is often expressed in fooling adults or in trying to catch them in mistakes.

Eight-year-olds can assume responsibility if it is not made too exacting and burdensome. But they have not yet reached the stage of wanting to see a job through from start to finish; they are apt to get bored with one activity and want to shift to another. They still need reminders about getting to places and doing things on time. When asked to do something, "Wait a minute" might almost be called the watchword of eight-year-olds.

Play Relationships. Sex differences in play begin to assert themselves at about age six. Some six-year-old boys may already be thinking of the little girls and their games as silly, and some of the little girls may look upon boys and their activities as too rough. However, boys and girls need the experience of working and playing together, and in the first grade it is seldom that differences in strength or interest will call for separate activities.

Group games are beginning to become popular, but many six-year-olds may still be unable to get along well in playing with their classmates. Some may be too rough or too bossy in their play. Others who are less aggressive or more timid may need protection until they learn how to take care of themselves in rough-and-tumble games. Many six-year-olds have a carry-over from the possessiveness and individualism which characterized their play at younger ages. These children still need some opportunity to play alone, in twosomes, or in small groups. Group activities, such as playing tag or hide-and-seek, in which a child may leave the group without disturbing the play, provide experiences in playing together without demanding too much in the way of good social behavior.

As a rule seven-year-olds play well together, but the spirit of competition is greater than at age six. Sex differences in play are becoming established, although most boys and girls enjoy playing together in group games. There may be some cases of boy-girl friendships, but usually children of this age choose friends of the same sex.

At age eight, boys and girls are definitely drawing apart in their play activities. This is the period when boys, especially, begin to form gangs or clubs. Passwords, a secret language, a secret meeting place, and membership rules drawn up by themselves have great fascination. At this age, however, clubs of this kind are usually mushroom growths of short duration. Girls also may form secret societies, but more often they get their greatest satisfaction from chums or "best friends."

Games of all kinds—both outdoor games and table games—in which there is a strong element of competition, are entered into with zest by third-graders. The desire to win is intense, and a certain amount of bickering over whose turn it is and what is and what is not fair is to be expected.

Preadolescence

Beginning about the ninth or tenth year, physiological age becomes much more significant than chronological age in respect to mental, emotional, and social development. This is because children are due for one of the great changes which periodically take place during life. This change is the passage from childhood into adolescence.

Adolescence, which lasts roughly for about ten years, begins with puberty. The whole period extending from birth to puberty is, strictly speaking, the preadolescent period, but in common usage the term *preadolescent* is confined to the three or four transition years immediately preceding puberty. The fact that most girls mature about two years earlier than most boys accounts in part for the relative lack of understanding between boys and girls which is frequently noted in the late elementary and junior high school period.

As all transition periods are times of adjustment, the preadolescent period is apt to be stormy for most youngsters. The teacher who realizes that the inexplicable and often annoying behavior of preadolescent children is only a passing phase will be able to ignore the teapot tempests and concentrate on the problems in which these youngsters really need help and guidance.

The In-between Nine-year-olds. Nine-year-olds are in or approaching the preadolescent period. Typically, they are closer in their thinking and activities to those one to two years older than to those one to two years younger.

The fourth grade is as transitional for the child as a student as the year from nine to ten is transitional for the child as a person. It may be difficult for some children to take the step up from the primary to the intermediate grades. Other children may show great improvement in their schoolwork. Children in the fourth grade are inclined to be individualists. Many of them are subject-minded. They "just hate" some subjects and "just love" others.

Perhaps the outstanding mental traits of the typical nine-year-old are the desire to accumulate facts and to perfect skills and the ability to concentrate for long periods on tasks in which he is interested. He is beginning to enjoy his mastery over the intellectual tools that he has been acquiring since he entered school.

Most fourth-graders are eager to get good marks, and failure is apt to be an emotionally upsetting experience. Some children may need a great deal of individual help to protect them from a sense of failure. Determining when to give help and when to delay it is sometimes a problem for the fourth-grade teacher.

Like the eight-year-old, the nine-year-old is eager to learn about people and places outside his own immediate environment. As a result, geography and history take on new meaning. There is also keen interest in the affairs and activities of his own community. This is the year during which trips to find out how things are done or made in business and industry fill a real need for the factual information that helps in expanding the child's horizons.

Expanding Mental Horizons. The earnestness with which fourth-graders concentrate on perfecting their skills in the use of intellectual tools largely disappears in the years immediately preceding puberty. That is because most preadolescents have acquired sufficient skill in the use of intellectual tools to use them with efficiency and dispatch. They are eager for factual information and like to know how things are made and how they work. This is the age period in which an introduction to elementary facts about the structure and functions of the body is of great help in health education because it supplies the reasons for much of what the youngsters are urged to do to keep healthy.

Preadolescents have a growing capacity for thought and reasoning and a fairly well-developed sense of justice. They are interested in social problems, and in discussing them show that they can see different sides of questions.

A feeling of loyalty to the ideals of their own country is strong in preadolescents. They worship heroes and are interested in the childhood and youth of great men and women and the qualities that contributed to their greatness. Many of them also develop hero worship for an adult or an older boy or girl of their acquaintance. Girls, especially, may express their deep attraction for another by saying or intimating that "they have a crush" on so and so.

Preadolescents are capable of self-criticism and are frequently critical of others. They are keenly observant and have their own ways of "sizing up" people. Sometimes they make quite frank and objective comparisons of their parents' or their family's way of doing things with those of their friends or neighbors. This is a healthy sign because it shows that these youngsters are beginning to realize that there are other ways of living besides those of their own family.

Differences in intellectual capacity and the possession of special abilities and talents become more readily identifiable in the junior high school grades. Recognition by the teacher of special interests and skills and the provision of satisfactory means of expressing them through challenging occupations are considered important for reasons of mental good health as well as for helping young people to find a vocation or to develop a satisfying hobby.

Emotional Expression. On entering the preadolescent period youngsters seem to go down a step or two from the level of emotional maturity they had reached earlier. With one foot on the last step of childhood, so to speak, and the other on the first step of youth, it is not surprising that preadolescents should occasionally show great variation in mood and behavior. Generally speaking, however, they are emotionally more stable than they were when they were younger. At least, they seem to recover from hurt or angry feelings more quickly.

Preadolescents are anxious to be among the chosen. Their feelings are easily hurt if they believe that they have been deliberately passed over when invitations to a party are issued, for example, or sides are being chosen in a game. Also they may feel that "nobody loves them" if they get the idea that others in the home or at school are getting more attention or more favors than they.

Both teachers and parents need to be sensitive to differences in children that may keep them from being accepted by the group. It is often possible to help such children by giving them opportunities to win admiration for some special talent or to make a contribution to the success of a group activity.

Preadolescents may be individualists so far as interests are concerned, but they seek uniformity as members of a group. In dress, manner, and talk they want to be like everyone else. Fairness plays a large part in their relationships with others. If they think that a criticism or a punishment is fair, they take it with good grace. If they think it is unfair, they are outspoken in their protests. Arguments over what is or is not fair in playing games are frequent.

Much of what is annoying in preadolescent behavior—disrespect for adult opinion, banding together in rebellion against authority, acting "fresh" or making "brutally frank" remarks, for example—may safely be ignored until good opportunities arise for discussing such behavior with the youngsters when they are in a reasonable mood. A sense of humor is a great asset to adults in overcoming exasperation in their dealings with preadolescents. It aids in avoiding issues which may be exceedingly difficult to meet without widening the gap of misunderstanding between the adult world and the preadolescent world. Preadolescents need adult support and will seek it if they are not antagonized by too rigid a show of authority or by frequent displays of emotional fireworks.

Social Behavior. Friendships play an important role in the preadolescent period. These children often have closer ties with their friends than with their families. Girls especially need "best friends" or pals with whom to "let off steam" and share secrets. There is much gossiping among girls and writing of secret notes to one another, both in school and out.

On the surface preadolescents are disdainful of the opposite sex. But in mixed groups, as in school, there is covert interest in the opposite sex as shown by giggling and preening by the girls and boisterousness or showing off by the boys. As girls mature earlier than boys, an overt interest in the opposite sex usually is shown first by the girls.

Preadolescents are ready and willing to assume responsibility both at home and in school. They like to discuss plans for work, especially if they have some assurance that their ideas and suggestions will be considered. They enjoy tasks and errands which make them feel important and trustworthy. However, routine chores for which they are made responsible may be forgotten in the press of their busy day, and frequent reminders may be necessary. These youngsters have so much to do themselves that it is hard for them to remember to do everything that other people expect of them.

Both boys and girls need to identify themselves with groups made up of youngsters of their own age and sex. That is why banding together in an organized group—the so-called "gang" or club—is very important during the preadolescent period. The preadolescent club is characterized by an air of secrecy because its members have a fondness for mystery and conspiracy. They take great glee in inventing passwords, handclasps, secret codes, and in establishing a hideout.

The intimate club or gang seems to meet a need so deep that the term "gang age" has been used to describe the stage of development in which it flourishes. Belonging to a gang or club brings with it a sense of solidarity and the feeling of prestige which is associated with the joy of being found socially acceptable. Joining such a group is often the first step away from the security of the home into the security which comes from having a congenial crowd to back one up.

Boys' gangs become undesirable only when the natural desire to be identified in group action has nothing wholesome and constructive to inspire it. If the principal incentive is escape from too rigid adult authority, the spirit of destructiveness may get the upper hand. But if the youngsters find understanding at home and in school and are given opportunities for safe and legitimate activities, the gang will satisfy the deep craving for fun and companionship characteristic of preadolescent youngsters.

Interest also is keen in clubs or groups under adult leadership, such as the Boy Scouts, the Girl Scouts, the Campfire Girls, and 4-H Clubs. Depending upon the facilities and leadership available in the community, membership in such groups is open to all youngsters upon reaching the ages at which they are eligible to join. Consequently there are no heart-burnings over being rejected, as there may be at being left out of clubs or gangs organized by the youngsters themselves. Under democratic leadership, the adult-directed group plans and carries out many different activities which furnish opportunities not only for acquiring individual status within the group but also for gaining the satisfaction of being of real service to the community.

Adolescence

The countdown years of preadolescence come to an end with the explosive changes that accompany puberty. The adolescent is growing and developing in every part of himself at a rate and in ways that are far from smooth, orderly, and predictable. It is not to be wondered at that perhaps the most outstanding characteristic of adolescents is their preoccupation with themselves. Even their appearance seems to fascinate them, and boys as well as girls are inclined to spend an inordinate amount of time gazing into the mirror.

Unevenness in Physical Growth as a Source of Anxiety. In many adolescents physical growth takes place so rapidly and unevenly that these youngsters may find that they are not nearly so skillful in handling their bodies as they used to be. Legs and arms lengthen so fast that their owners do not quite know what to do with them. Hands get big and clumsy. The girls begin to fill out, and their hips and thighs broaden. In boys the circumference of the chest markedly increases. Vertical growth in the trunk in both boys and girls is usually greatest after puberty. At this time boys' voices become deeper, and in some boys the voice "cracks." Both boys and girls may be troubled with poor complexions (see Acne in Chap. 15).

Adolescent youngsters need help in understanding that all such physical manifestations of rapid growth are normal and, above all, temporary. If their sense of humor is also maturing, they may be amused at their own clumsiness, even if it bothers them. This does not mean, however, that they will take kindly to being laughed at by others. One of the most common worries among high school boys and girls stems from the fear of making fools of themselves in public or of not being respected. Being laughed at is very hurtful to their self-esteem.

In every fairly large group of boys and girls there are bound to be some who are not growing and developing as they think they should. Their chief trouble seems to be caused by the habit of comparing themselves with others or with some preconceived image of physical perfection. The smaller-than-average boy, for example, may despair of growing up to match his picture of the perfect male—tall, strong, well-muscled. The widely publicized physical measurements considered desirable for young women set standards that most adolescent girls yearn to meet. It is all right to be tall, for example, but not too tall. Yet some girls shoot up with such bean-stalk rapidity that they fear they will not stop growing in time to be at least a little shorter than most young men. To be small is all right, too, but to be fat—that is a catastrophe! The tendency to make large gains of weight in the years immediately preceding and following puberty may, therefore, be a source of great worry for many adolescent girls. Unless these girls are reassured, they will be afraid that they are destined to be fat the rest of their lives.

The physical changes that accompany sexual development also may be a source of anxiety when their arrival is considered to be too far off schedule. Early signs of masculinity, such as changes in voice and growth of beard, and early signs of femininity, such as budding breasts, are so obvious that delay in their appearance may cause genuine anxiety in adolescents whose development is less advanced than that of their friends.

The menarche, that is, the beginning of the menstrual function, is probably the most dramatic event in a girl's maturation process. Its arrival much earlier or later than usual may seem to be a very serious matter to the adolescent and her parents. Here again this concern often involves a confusion between what is average and what is normal. The average age at menarche in the United States is about 13½ years. But this is by no means the normal or "ideal" age. The menarche may occur normally at any age from ten to seventeen. An adolescent girl dislikes being different, however, and she may need a great deal of reassurance, preferably from her doctor, if menstruation is delayed until after her fifteenth or sixteenth birthday.

Health as a Source of Anxiety. Another outstanding concern of most young people is the condition of their bodies. They like to think of themselves as being physically fit in every way, and it bothers them when some symptom, such as frequent headaches, or some sign, such as a skin blemish, or some habit which they think is bad, or some remark they have heard, or some article or book or advertisement they have read leads them to believe that something is wrong with their health. They are inclined, however, to keep their worries about their health to themselves. They don't talk about them very often with their parents. They may avoid going to a doctor because they are afraid that he might find something seriously wrong.

Young people may adopt a more commonsense attitude if they are sufficiently impressed in their study of health with what a doctor can do either in relieving their minds or in getting something constructive done if there is any actual cause for concern. The ideal physician for a young person to consult is, of course, the family doctor, but physicians serving the secondary schools usually have gained both skill in dealing with adolescents and knowledge of their specific needs.

Changes in Boy-girl Relationships. During adolescence relationships between boys and girls and between children and their parents undergo important changes. Ordinarily these changes gradually lead up to desired ends—courtship, marriage, self-support, the establishment of a home of one's own. While they are taking place, however, the emotional weather is likely to be stormy.

Boys and girls in their early teens tend to drift even further apart than in the years immediately preceding adolescence. This delay in learning to get along well with the opposite sex is caused largely by the fact that girls usually mature earlier than boys. What makes the problem more difficult is the fact that young people are thrown together in school on the basis of chronological age, which may not be at all in step with their physical, emotional, and social development. Many girls in early adolescence are unwilling to go out on dates with boys who, they think, are too young and childish, even though the boys are chronologically as old as they are. Unless these girls succeed in striking up friendships with older boys, they have to take out their yearnings in romantic daydreaming. At the same time boys who are left stranded by the girls they know and are just becoming interested in are left with the choice of dating a younger girl or of pretending that girls don't matter.

A more serious problem growing out of the uneven development of the two sexes is of special concern to girls who succeed in attracting boys who are older than they are. Actually these girls are seeking the companionship of boys whose level of growth and development is comparable to theirs. And in all ways except one the two probably have reached about the same level. That one way, however, is important, and it furnishes a valid reason for the concern of parents who don't like their daughters going out with older boys. Once boys do mature their sexual drive develops earlier than does that of girls. Boys develop more slowly in some respects, but not in this one. Here is an important fact for boys and girls to know and understand. Ignored—or not known about—by either boy or girl it can lead to unfortunate and unhappy experiences.

It is common knowledge that adolescent experiences with the opposite sex, such as dating, petting, and going steady, are a major source of family conflict. Such experiences, however, are normal preliminaries to the more serious business of courtship and marriage—part of the process of "getting to know you." It is imperative, however, for young people to know and to understand certain facts if the lessons experience teaches are to be happy rather than tragic ones.

Sex education is primarily the job of the parents and is best given in the home. Youngsters whose parents are themselves emotionally stable and are willing and able to discuss sex matters frankly have the best chance of developing wholesome attitudes toward sex. These youngsters also will be more likely to seek help with their sex problems from their parents or their doctor or clergyman. Some parents, however, find it difficult to give their children objective, matter-of-fact guidance in sex matters. At the end of this chapter several books and pamphlets are listed which will be helpful to parents in the sex education of their children.

Changes in Parent-child Relationships. The most common causes of friction between adolescents and their parents are the desire of the children for independence and the reluctance of parents to grant freedoms that they are not sure their children are ready to exercise. Wanting to be grown up and independent is perfectly normal and highly desirable. But running one's own life requires better judgment and a more mature sense of responsibility than most parents think young people possess. Indeed it means taking on more responsibility than the young people themselves want. This is evidenced by the quick changes of mood characteristic of the adolescent period. At one time a boy or girl may seem unaccountably childish and at another time exceptionally mature. Impatience with any sort of restrictions may at one time signal a child's craving for independence. Implied or expressed demands for reassurance that he is still a loved and valued member of the family may at another time show a longing for the safe and happy dependence of childhood.

Erratic behavior of this kind is puzzling unless parents and teachers understand that it is transitional. The tide of childhood is going out and the tide of maturity is coming in. The adolescent caught in the turning of the tide may often find himself "fishing in troubled waters." The adolescent can no longer act childish, because he is no longer a child. On the other hand, he cannot do many of the things that adults do, because he is not yet grown up. Lack of understanding and inconsistencies in dealing with him aggravate his bewilderment. At the very time when he shows signs of "feeling his oats," his parents may tighten up on the reins. He may be told an one occasion, "You're as big as a man, why don't you act like one?" and on another, "You're only a boy. What makes you think you can decide on such an important matter?"

Many of the problems of adolescence can be solved satisfactorily when parents and teachers cooperate in giving young people every opportunity to achieve success in their progress toward maturity. When early signs of independence appear, it is desirable to give youngsters as much leeway as possible in making their own decisions. The ability to manage one's own life with wisdom grows slowly, and boys and girls need the experience that only life can give. They need to feel what it is like to be on their own occasionally and to have only themselves to congratulate when things go right and only themselves to blame when things go wrong.

EMOTIONAL NEEDS OF ALL CHILDREN

Although children at different stages of development differ in their characteristics and interests, they are all alike in having certain basic emotional needs. Anything that prevents the satisfaction of these needs will have a harmful effect on the development of the child's personality. The basic emotional needs of children may be summarized briefly as follows:

1. *Every child needs the feeling of security that comes from being loved, being wanted, being understood.* This need must be met in the school as well as in the home. Children brought up in broken homes in which there has been no attempt to provide a satisfactory substitute for an absent parent, and unwanted (rejected) children deprived of the love of one or both parents, are those who are likely to live their early lives in the shadow of insecurity.

The personalities of parents and teachers also have a profound effect upon the developing personality of the child. Emotional instability is quite frequently mirrored in the behavior of children whose feelings of insecurity stem from not knowing where they stand with adults. In such cases, perhaps one or more adults in positions of authority may themselves be emotionally unstable and show their anxiety in their inconsistency in dealing with the child, for example, by punishing him for a certain misdemeanor on one occasion and overlooking it on another, or by adopting an attitude that differs from a previously expressed attitude, or by making promises or threats that cannot be carried out.

Most children are ready and willing to accept reasonable rules of conduct. An orderly, just code of rules, implemented with consistent rewards and punishments, helps to give them a sense of security. But they are bewildered or antagonized by too many rules, or by constantly changing rules, or by rules that seem to apply to them but not to others, or by impossibly high standards, or by too much disapproval and too little approval.

Children in school are bound to feel insecure—sometimes even humiliated and demeaned in their own eyes—if the methods of controlling them are determined by an arbitrary, rigid set of rules that does not take into account individual differences in family and cultural background, developmental level, physical and psychological makeup, and other factors.

2. *Every child needs to achieve enough success in dealing with the things and persons in his environment to build up a strong sense of personal worth.* The child begins to think of himself as a separate entity when he emerges from the complete dependence of infancy and realizes that certain things are expected of him. He finds that he cannot always be on the receiving line; he, too, must be a giver, and his success in giving helps to strengthen his ego—himself. He acquires his feeling of personal worth—his self-respect—from doing things that win expressions of approval from others and from his own conscience. Every child every day should have opportunities to win approval from both sources.

Religious experience often plays an important part in strengthening the child's sense of personal worth and in giving authority to the dictates of his conscience. During the adolescent period, especially, there is likely to be a resurgence of interest in spiritual needs.

To give opportunities for success in school, the capacities and the inadequacies of each child in the group should be taken into account and appropriate situations should be taken advantage of or created in which all children can capitalize on their abilities. Whatever immediate goal the teacher wants the children to reach should be attainable by sharing the work rather than by starring those who can do it best.

If the emphasis is placed on cooperation rather than on competition, the children will have many opportunities to find satisfaction and success in their relationships with their contemporaries. In the good-natured give-and-take of working and playing together, feelings of failure may disappear as children learn that other children, in general, are fairly easy to get along with—that one needn't be athletic or beautiful or especially gifted or rich or clever, for example, to be acceptable to one's group.

3. *Every child needs to acquire the ability to make necessary compromises with life.* Gradually, as the lessons of experience are learned, children discover that they are limited in what they can do. As a result they are bound to have disappointments and failures. Some of the limitations are man-made—the forces of custom, policy, law, and order in family, school, and society. Others arise from the child's own physiological and psychological makeup. Some children have physical or mental handicaps with which they must learn to live. All children are good at some things, not so good at others. Learning to accept necessary limitations gracefully and to work effectively within them is an important part of the child's education.

FOR REVIEW AND DISCUSSION

Cons. 1. Tell which of the following actions and feelings are chiefly related to the working of the conscious mind and which are chiefly related to the working of the unconscious mind:

Cons. a. Solving a mathematical problem

Unc. b. Taking a fancy to a person at first sight

Unc. c. Being afraid of the dark

Cons. d. Giving one's reasons for being in favor of an independent health course in high school

Unc. e. Fainting at the sight of blood

Unc. f. Having the name of a former teacher suddenly pop into your mind several days after trying to recall it

Cons. g. Taking part in a class discussion of the parts played by heredity and environment in the formation of personality

Unc. h. Feeling happy and gay or low in spirits for no particular reason

2. Which of the following statements about the development of conscience is most nearly accurate?

    a. Conscience is fully developed at birth.

    (b) Conscience develops through experiences that teach a child that some things are wrong and must not be done and that some things are right and must be done.

    c. Conscience is largely inherited but is modified by exchanges with the environment.

3. Select the correct ending for each of the following incomplete sentences:

    a. Adolescence is that period of life in which (1) a baby develops into a child, (2) a child becomes an adult, (3) an adult becomes a middle-aged person.

    b. The stage of development in which gangs flourish is (1) pre-adolescence, (2) adolescence, (3) maturity.

    c. The menarche is the period in a girl's life when (1) menstruation begins, (2) the adolescent growth spurt begins, (3) an interest in boys begins.

4. Have different teams of students describe in a report or in role playing the outstanding behavior characteristics of children at successive stages of development. After each presentation, have the rest of the class guess what age group was portrayed. Discuss the importance for a teacher of familiarity with the stage of mental, emotional, and social development reached by most of the children in her class.

SELECTED REFERENCES

Almy, Millie: *Ways of Studying Children; A Manual for Teachers,* Columbia University Press, New York, 1960. (A book for teachers giving suggestions on ways of understanding children as a basis for better teaching; includes a number of case histories.)

Breckenridge, Marian E., and E. L. Vincent: *Child Development; Physical and Psychological Growth through Adolescence,* 4th ed. (first given as reference in Chap. 3).

D'Evelyn, Katherine E.: *Meeting Children's Emotional Needs; A Guide for Teachers,* Prentice-Hall, Inc., New York, 1957.

Gallagher, James Roswell, and Herbert I. Harris: *Emotional Problems of Adolescents,* Oxford University Press, New York, 1958.

Gesell, Arnold L., and Frances L. Ilg: *The Child from Five to Ten* (first given as reference in Chap. 3).

Gesell, Arnold L., and others: *Youth: The Years from Ten to Sixteen* (first given as reference in Chap. 3).

Jersild, Arthur T.: *Child Psychology,* 5th ed., Prentice-Hall, Inc., Englewood Cliffs, N.J., 1960.

Jersild, Arthur T.: *Psychology of Adolescence,* The Macmillan Company, New York, 1957.

Lane, Howard, and Mary Beauchamp: *Understanding Human Development* (first given as reference in Chap. 3).

Martin, W. E., and C. B. Stendler: *Child Behavior and Development,* Harcourt, Brace and Company, Inc., New York, 1959.

Menninger, Karl A.: *The Human Mind,* Alfred A. Knopf, Inc., New York, 1945. (A well-known book that presents to the lay reader a psychiatrist's conception of the human mind and the factors that influence personality development.)

Strang, Ruth M.: *An Introduction to Child Study,* 4th ed., The Macmillan Company, New York, 1959.

Stuart, Harold C., and Dane G. Prugh: *The Healthy Child* (first given as reference in Chap. 3).

Sex Education

Baruch, Dorothy: *New Ways in Sex Education; A Guide for Parents and Teachers,* McGraw-Hill Book Company, New York, 1959.

Hymes, James L.: *How to Tell Your Child about Sex,* Public Affairs Pamphlet No. 149, Public Affairs Committee, New York.

Ilg, Frances L., and Louise Bates Ames: *Parents Ask,* Harper & Brothers, New York, 1962. (For parents; covers eating and sleeping routines, relationships within the family, physical growth, discipline, sex, morale and manners, school problems, and other difficulties which trouble the majority of parents.)

Joint Committee on Health Problems in Education of the National Education Association and the American Medical Association: A series of booklets in sex education prepared for the Committee by Marion O. Lerrigo and Helen Southard:

Parents Responsibility: For parents of children in the primary grades.

A Story about You: For children in grades 4 to 6 (age range from nine to twelve years).

Finding Yourself: For the junior high school age group (age range from twelve to fifteen years).

Approaching Adulthood: For young people from sixteen to twenty years.

Facts Aren't Enough: A sex education guide for parents, teachers, and youth leaders.

Landis, Paul H.: *Coming of Age; Problems of Teenagers,* Public Affairs Pamphlet No. 234, Public Affairs Committee, New York.

Wilkes, Edward T.: *Family Guide to Teenage Health,* Part IV, *Sex and Psychology* (first given as reference in Chap. 3).

Organizations

Child Study Association of America
National Association for Mental Health

Chapter 5   MATTERS OF INTELLIGENCE

Variations in Intelligence
Problems Related to Differences in Intellectual Ability
Identification, Please!
Providing Educational Opportunities for Gifted Children
Providing Educational Opportunities for Slow Learners
Mentally Handicapped Children in School

The exercise of intelligence is a function of the conscious mind. There is disagreement among scientists as to whether intelligence is a single ability or the sum of many different abilities. There is no doubt, however, that human beings are born with individual differences in intelligence. At birth these differences are only potentialities. They become real, measurable differences as children grow older, through the opportunities for accomplishment provided in the environment.

VARIATIONS IN INTELLIGENCE

Those who have made a study of the learning process agree that the most outstanding aspect of individual variations in intelligence is connected with the ability to acquire and to use facts. This ability is what makes it possible for a person to learn new things and to handle new situations.

Intelligence Tests as a Measuring Device

Intelligence tests are the yardsticks that have been devised for measuring how well the mind works. The norm of accomplishment in intelligence tests is determined by testing under similar conditions large groups of children of different ages so as to find out what mental tasks the majority of children of a given age can do. Thus a mental age of twelve means that the child tested can do most or all of the tasks that the majority of children of twelve can do. If a child of eight has a mental age of twelve and we wish to express his intellectual superiority in respect to his age group, we should say that he is older on the scale of intellectual growth than he is on the scale of chronological growth.

Normal Intelligence. Speaking in terms of intelligence quotients,[1] we may think that an IQ of 100 represents the normal level of intelligence at a given age of childhood—that which the average child of that age possesses. However, intelligence cannot be measured accurately enough to spot it exactly at a single point and so we say that normal intelligence ranges from an IQ of 90 to an IQ of 110.

Superior Intelligence. Going up the scale of intelligence from an IQ of 110, we come to very bright children with IQs of 120 and above. The lower limit of exceptional brightness, or giftedness, is usually placed at an IQ of 125 to 130. In any mixed group of 100 children, five or six are likely to be found with IQs of 120 or above, three with an IQ of 125 or above, and only one with an IQ of 130 or above.

Slow Learners. Going down the scale of intelligence from an IQ of 90, we come to the so-called "slow learners." It is common practice to classify students as slow learners when they score between 70 and 90 on repeated standardized intelligence tests. The mental ability of these children is high enough to justify keeping them in a regular classroom but low enough to give them trouble in keeping up with the average learning speed of the class. The magnitude of the problem for the teacher is highlighted by the fact that from 12 to 15 per cent of the child population falls in this category.[2]

Mental Retardation. Going down the scale of intelligence still further, we come to the children classed as mentally retarded. These children are now recognized as an important segment of the child population who need abundant help. For practical purposes, this group of children is subdivided into the following three subgroups, which altogether makes up about 3 per cent of the child population.

1. The *moderately retarded,* with IQs from about 50 to 70. These children are considered "educable," that is, they can do rudimentary academic work and, if they are given an education suitable to their needs, can hope to take a useful place in the world as adults.

2. The *severely retarded,* with IQs from about 30 to 50. These children are considered "trainable," that is, they can learn to care for them-

---

[1] A child's intelligence quotient (IQ) is expressed as the ratio between mental age (MA) and chronological age (CA), multiplied by 100 to eliminate decimals. For example, suppose three children aged fourteen, twelve, and ten, respectively, all do equally well on an intelligence test that the majority of twelve-year-old children can do. Then all three children are said to have a mental age of twelve. The IQ of the fourteen-year-old child is:

$$\frac{12 \text{ (MA)}}{14 \text{ (CA)}} = 0.86 \times 100 = 86$$

By the same computation, the IQ of the twelve-year-old is 100 and that of the ten-year-old is 120.

[2] *Focus on Children and Youth,* 1960 White House Conference, p. 275.

selves and may eventually be able to do some simple work under constant supervision.

3. The *extremely retarded*, with IQs below 30. These children are totally dependent and can do very little for themselves. Usually they are best cared for in a medical institution.

Usually mental retardation is either present at birth or begins during early childhood. Its cause in many cases is due to known brain abnormalities; in other cases its cause is obscure. The best known physical causes of mental retardation are discussed in Chap. 8.

Achievement Tests as a Measuring Device

Achievement tests, unlike intelligence tests, measure what a child *has* done rather than what he *can* do in various subjects, such as reading or spelling or arithmetic. Standard achievement tests often pick out gifted children very much better than school marks. In one study, for example, it was found that in almost every school grade there were children whose achievement in one or more subjects was rated by the teacher as average or below for the grade but whose achievement test scores showed them to be as much as two years above their grade norms in those same subjects.[3] One possible reason for this surprising finding is that few gifted children are as educationally advanced as their ability would warrant. In many cases boredom with school tasks develops when the mental nuts the child is called upon to crack are not tough enough for him. As a result the child falls into sloppy habits of work, which adversely affect his ability to achieve good marks.

Aptitude Tests as a Measuring Device

In addition to differences in general intelligence, children show differences in special gifts or aptitudes. Even among children of so-called normal intelligence, some are exceptionally "good" at music or art, for example, and others at working with tools or working with people. Children of high intelligence are seldom equally good in all school subjects and sometimes show definite specialization in their interests and abilities.

Numerous tests have been devised to distinguish children who exhibit special gifts or skills regardless of what their intelligence quotients may be. Such tests are important not only for the detection of creative abilities in science, mechanics, music, art, literature, leadership, and social relations, but also for helping all children to develop along the lines of their major strengths.

[3] Lewis M. Terman and M. H. Oden, *The Gifted Child Grows Up,* Stanford University Press, Stanford, Calif., 1947, p. 26.

Administering Tests

Administering standardized tests of general intelligence requires thorough training and experience. Teachers who have not had this preparation may call upon the services of a child guidance or child psychology clinic in the community if such services are not available through the school.[4] Standard tests of achievement can be administered by untrained teachers if directions are studied carefully and followed explicitly.

As for aptitude tests, there is a difference of opinion among psychologists as to the nature of special abilities and their relation to general intelligence. The question as to the best ways of measuring aptitude awaits to a considerable degree the settlement of such disagreements. Special abilities or talents are usually recognized through active performance, but sometimes a child expresses an interest which, if encouraged, leads to performance. Aptitude tests have been developed with a fair amount of success for identifying several abilities, for example, in music, mechanics, science, clerical work, and art. The value of these tests depends largely upon the background and training of those who interpret them.

Factors Influencing Intellectual Development

Several studies have shown that the ability to do well in school is not merely a matter of having average or above-average intelligence. Many different influences help or hinder a person in using the intelligence or the special abilities with which he is endowed. One person with an IQ below normal may function smoothly and efficiently. Another person with a high IQ may function so poorly that he might as well not have a "good brain."

Sometimes a child's physical condition may be to blame for his failure to use his intelligence to good advantage. That is why a physical factor like poor eyesight or poor hearing or a chronic infection or malnutrition or an endocrine disturbance is the first thing a physician looks for when a teacher reports that a child is obviously not using the intelligence he possesses. Frequently an emotional block of one kind or another profoundly influences the functioning of intelligence.

Environmental influences often have a marked effect on the school achievement of individual students. Children whose IQ is within normal limits may be low achievers because they come from poor or broken homes or culturally deprived neighborhoods. Children of unusual prom-

---

[4] Teachers may write to the U.S. Office of Education, Washington, D.C. 25, for special help or advice regarding the use of standardized intelligence tests if such help is not available in their school systems.

ise may come nowhere near to realizing their high potential of giftedness because there is no one at home or in school to give them understanding, friendly guidance, incentives for doing their best, and suitable material with which to work. Practically every study of giftedness has revealed the great waste caused by the failure to identify and encourage individuals who might have made significant contributions to society if they had been provided with opportunities to develop and use their gifts.

PROBLEMS RELATED TO DIFFERENCES IN INTELLECTUAL ABILITY

Every teacher knows that some students are comparatively rapid in learning and in applying what they learn; others are comparatively slow; still others—the majority—keep within the normal speed limits for their age. A great deal of attention has been given in recent years to problems presented to teachers by individual differences in the intellectual ability of their students. It is no easy matter for a teacher to meet in one class at the same time the educational needs of learners of high ability, learners of average ability, and learners of low ability. But what of the learners themselves? Being "outsize" in intellectual ability may be as emotionally upsetting as being outsize in physical size or shape. Let's first consider some of the problems with which intellectually gifted children may have to deal.

Problems of Intellectually Superior Children

The difficulties of many exceptionally bright youngsters seem to arise from the fact that they are inclined to be self-sufficient and unsociable. They may feel that their parents and teachers do not understand them. They often have trouble making friends. This is not surprising when we remember that it is natural to seek companionship on one's own intellectual level. Yet the children who are equal in mental age to the intellectually superior child are chronologically older—and hence physically bigger and stronger—and socially more mature. These older children may not like to be tagged around by a "smart-aleck kid." Even parents and teachers may be goaded into irritability by his exhibitions of superiority. If the superior child tries to associate with children who are his chronological equals, he is likely to be bored by them and they are likely to be antagonized by him. As a result the child is caught in a situation in which he feels that he is not wanted anywhere. And like all people who feel unwanted, he will develop emotional difficulties. Unless the situation is corrected in time, he may be driven further into himself and become a definitely asocial or even antisocial individual.

So far as scholastic achievement is concerned, a common complaint of students of high ability is that the work is too easy for them. Many a gifted child is an underachiever in school because the mental tasks he has been given to do furnish no challenge to his intelligence. Like the children in Kenneth Graham's *Dream Days*, he has scorned to excel in subjects "held to be necessary even for him whose ambitions soared no higher than to crack a whip in a circus ring. . . ." Or he may be interested in his work but may finish it quickly and then be left to twiddle his thumbs because there is nothing else to do.

Another cause of underachievement among intellectually talented youngsters is the attitude of average students toward superior academic achievement. As Ruth Strang[5] points out: "In some schools the morale is low; there is still an anti-intellectual attitude. The bright student who really enjoys reading and studying is looked down on; he is called a 'brain,' a 'square,' an 'egghead,' or some other name intended to discredit scholarship." The bright student who is afraid of being "different" may very well refuse to pay the price exacted by his classmates for getting higher grades than they do. "A shift in attitude among average students towards classmates who consistently receive high grades might alleviate one of the more stubborn causes of underachievement among the academically talented."

Great are the rewards of helping children of superior intelligence to solve their problems. Often the rapidity with which emotional and academic difficulties disappear when adequate outlets are supplied is quite surprising. These children will grow up into the leaders we so sadly need if their emotional problems do not set up a barrier against the full exercise of their intelligence.

Problems of Slow Learners

Students of average or high ability usually "get through school," as the saying goes, regardless of whether or not their academic performance comes up to expectation. But what of the slow learners whose academic path is too often studded with failure? These children are now dividing with the gifted the honor of being the object of special concern in efforts to provide all students with educational programs suited to their interests, needs, and abilities.

Judging children of below-average ability by the standards and accomplishments expected of children of average ability is a major cause of the problems of slow learners. Both classmates and teachers may contribute to their dilemma. Other children sometimes ridicule and show contempt for the not-so-bright child who cannot keep up with them in games and classwork. One teacher after another may call upon slow learners day after day to do work that is beyond their grasp; as a result these children may go on year after year without knowing the taste of success. To make up for his social and scholastic failure, the slow learner

[5] Ruth Strang, *Guideposts for the Gifted Children Themselves*, American Association for Gifted Children, New York, 1958.

may become aggressive, and his unacceptable behavior may alienate him even further from his peers. Or some slow-learning children—especially the girls—may withdraw unto themselves and give up trying to succeed in anything.

Teachers who can imagine what it feels like to "try, try again" without ever succeeding, can make school a rewarding educational experience, instead of a humiliating one, for slow-learning children.

IDENTIFICATION, PLEASE!

Before educational experiences can be geared to the abilities and needs of students of high ability and those of low ability, these students must be identified. Unless all children are routinely given intelligence tests before entering school, prime responsibility for identifying the exceptional children and the slow learners rests with the classroom teacher.

Identifying Superior Children

As the teacher observes the day-to-day performance of all children in the classroom, a child here or there may astonish her with his keen insight and reasoning ability. Perhaps he is the youngest child in the class, because studies have shown that usually the youngest children in a grade are the brightest. Some very bright children, however, move along from grade to grade at the regular pace. In such cases general excellence in schoolwork or consistently superior performance in areas of special interest may point to accelerated mental growth. The gifted child is the one who is most often able to supply the answers. He is eager to think things through and to extend his interests beyond the range of his immediate school tasks. Often the gifted child acquires an amount of special knoweldge that seems "simply uncanny" in some subject that has caught his fancy or fired his imagination.

Whenever possible, the delightful discovery of unusual mental ability in one or more children should be verified by the results of performance on standardized tests of general intelligence. Although current tests of general intelligence will not pick out all the intellectually gifted, they are probably the most effective single objective measure for use in corroborating or casting doubt on the observer's judgment.

Identifying Slow Learners

The one characteristic in which all slow learners are alike is a slow rate of academic learning plus poor retention. Other outstanding characteristics that the teacher may observe include difficulty in grasping abstract concepts, limited retention span, lack of curiosity, creativity, and critical thinking, and a small range in spoken and written vocabulary. Initial referral of the probable poor learner by the classroom teacher must, of course, be followed by a battery of tests, personality tests, and interest inventories, supplemented by information obtained from consultation of school records and from parent conferences.

PROVIDING EDUCATIONAL OPPORTUNITIES FOR GIFTED CHILDREN

Each community has the responsibility for planning an educational program that best covers and develops its human resources. In general what may be called the best medium for the cultivation of giftedness is an environment in which all children can reach the highest level of learning and accomplishment of which they are capable at each stage of their development. All children, no matter what their potentialities, are first of all children, each one setting his own pace and reacting in his own way to a number of situations.

Various plans for working with superior children are being tried in different school systems.

Acceleration

The oldest method used is acceleration. Acceleration means advancing an exceptionally bright child ahead of his group from one grade to the next after he has mastered the work in the grade from which he is moving. It allows a child to complete the standard amount of academic work in less than the usual time.

At present the wisdom of too-rapid acceleration, especially in the elementary school, is questioned by educators, largely because of the danger of social maladjustment. Bright children who are well developed physically, socially, and emotionally may get along well in a group in which the other members are one or two years older, but beyond that point social complications may arise. If acceleration seems to be the only answer to the problem, moderation is recommended, with special planning to make sure that there are no gaps in the child's experience.

Ability Grouping

Ability grouping is another device for meeting the educational needs of the brighter students. It may take the form of special schools, of special classes within a school, or of ability groups within the regular classroom. In some schools gifted children go to special classes for part of their work and remain in the regular classroom for the other part.

Curriculum Enrichment

A third method, which occupies the middle ground between acceleration and ability grouping, is curriculum enrichment. The enrichment for children of unusual promise differs only in degree and variety—not in kind—from that which all school children need. The dominant factor is the provision of a flexible program of challenging experiences and large areas of interest in which gifted children are encouraged to seek higher levels of creative expression and a greater appreciation of problems than is attainable by less able children in the group. Since elementary schools generally operate on a plan of self-contained classrooms, enrichment is the method open to most teachers for helping gifted children to find adequate means of expression and satisfactory outlets for their talents.

PROVIDING EDUCATIONAL OPPORTUNITIES FOR SLOW LEARNERS

The slow learner differs only in intellectual ability from other pupils; he has the same physical and psychological needs as other youngsters. Usually it is in school that he meets his major difficulties. The main point to remember is that he is slow but he *can* learn. Unfortunately, he knows the bitter taste of failure all too well. Patient, sympathetic teachers can give him a taste of success.

Perhaps the best clue to ways in which the slow learner may be guided to satisfactory achievement is to use his mental age, not his IQ, in determining his ability level. If a teacher knows the child's IQ—and most teachers do—she can easily find the child's mental age. To do this, multiply the child's chronological age by the IQ expressed as hundredths. For example, a six-year-old child whose score is 75 will have a mental age of only four years, six months ($0.75 \times 6 = 4.50$); he will not reach a mental age of six years until he is eight ($0.75 \times 8 = 6$). When he is twelve, his mental age will be nine. This twelve-year-old will have the mental ability to do fourth-grade work, whereas twelve- to fourteen-year-old children of average mental ability have the capacity to work at seventh-grade level. Even if slow learners work up to capacity, they can only be expected to achieve at between the seventh- to ninth-grade level in their senior year in high school.

How can the time slow learners spend in school be made years of worthwhile accomplishment rather than years of frustration? There are as many methods of helping the slow learners as there are of helping the intellectually superior children.

Retention

The oldest, largely outmoded method is retention. Keeping a slow-learning student in elementary school until he is working at the sixth-grade level may mean that he will not get into junior high until he is fifteen or sixteen years old. Consequently, he is quite likely to have social and emotional difficulties and to drop out of school as soon as he legally can. Children who fall far behind their grade, however, may benefit from retention for one or two years before entry into the tenth grade. In general, many authorities agree that slow learners should go into junior high school when they are no older than thirteen.

Deceleration

Making it possible for slow learners to advance at their own pace without falling too far behind their brighter contemporaries is a problem that is solved in various ways. One plan may be called *deceleration*, to contrast it with the acceleration method used for superior children. According to this plan, the slow learner may take as much as four years to complete the curriculum of three grades. This plan keeps the slow learner from experiencing the feeling of failure that arises when a grade has to be repeated.

Ability Grouping

To reduce the range of abilities in a class, the average and lower-than-average students may be placed in one group and the higher-than-average and gifted students in another. Generally the children in these two groups progress through the grade at their own pace and reach the junior high level at the same chronological age. In some large school systems the slow learners are placed in special classes throughout their school course. The trend in junior and senior high schools appears to be the grouping of slow learners together in some special classes or sections.

Providing Opportunities for Success

Modifications in curriculum and teaching techniques and standards of achievement are usually necessary in order to give slow learners success experiences to compensate for too frequent failures in academic subjects. In general the emphasis is on providing materials and learning experiences that have meaning for these youngsters in their everyday lives. Everyone—slow, average, or bright—for example, must master certain arithmetical skills in order to get along in adult life. It may be difficult for the slow learner to grasp the concepts involved, but through applying these concepts in concrete situations, he can develop the skills of making or counting change, for example, figuring baseball scores, and later on in high school planning budgets, doing the marketing, buying on the installment plan, figuring interest rates and income taxes. To put it in its simplest terms, the young slow learner may fail to comprehend the laws of computation or the rules of grammar, but he can learn *what* is correct through usage.

Most slow learners have reading difficulties, and in most school systems remedial work in reading is provided. The main difficulty as these youngsters grow older arises from the fact that they are not interested in the easy-to-read books written for much younger children. Fortunately, this difficulty is being overcome by the publication of books written at junior or senior high interest level but with a vocabulary at a lower-grade level.

It is generally agreed that the grading and promotional systems for slow learners should be adjusted to meet their need for some success experiences. If they are graded and promoted in terms of the standards set up for the average students, they fail continually even though they do their best. It is considered wiser for the teacher to give these students recognition for individual effort and to use their own previous records and accomplishments, rather than the norm for the whole class, in reporting their progress. Regular attendance, good effort, diligence, and reasonable accomplishment usually justify the granting of a high school diploma.

It is not uncommon for students classified as slow learners in school to do very well in adult life. After leaving school they nearly always lose their labels. Probably most of them will never again be thrown into a situation in which they must compete with others whose range of intellectual abilities and interests is greater than theirs. Usually they will enter fields of employment in which academic attainment is unimportant. Slow learners will be well equipped to carry a reasonable and important share of their responsibility as adult citizens if their educational program has been designed to develop their strengths and minimize their weaknesses.

MENTALLY HANDICAPPED CHILDREN IN SCHOOL

From the human point of view, it is as important to spot the mentally defective child in a group as it is to spot the superior child, the "intellectually average-minded," and the slow learner. Nothing can be done to improve the basic ability to acquire and use facts in mentally retarded children whose low intellectual capacity is due to some irreversible change in the central nervous system (see Physical Causes of Mental Retardation in Chap. 8). However, a great deal can be done to help such children use their existing capacities to the utmost by removing as many adverse environmental factors and emotional difficulties as possible. The provision of educational opportunities, vocational guidance, and training is an important part of the whole program for combatting mental retardation on a nationwide scale. (See the report of the President's Panel on Mental Retardation listed in Selected References at the end of this chapter.)

Enrollment in Special Classes

Educational authorities agree that mentally retarded children who have been given individual tests by competent testers and are found to be "educable" (IQs between approximately 50 and 70) should be enrolled in special classes. The education of these children is usually placed in the hands of teachers who have specialized in this professional field. The curriculum for the mentally handicapped, often quite different from that of the regular classroom, requires special teaching techniques and materials. However, these children need opportunities to join mentally normal children in play, in assembly programs, and in other group activities in which they are capable of taking part. Public recognition of the great need of these youngsters for social acceptance and adjustment has led in recent years to the gradual absorption by the public school of large numbers of retarded children who would once have been taught in segregated classes sponsored by welfare, church, and service organizations.

Identifying Retarded Children

Early and accurate diagnosis of retarded children is an important prerequisite to their proper care and education. Kindergarten and primary school teachers can be of very great help in identifying children who need specialized education and care. Teachers of older children are not likely to come into contact with youngsters who reach their mental ceiling anywhere from kindergarten to third grade unless they teach in a community where no provisions are made for taking mentally handicapped children out of the regular classroom. In increasing numbers of school systems, special classes for handicapped children are available. Any primary teacher who thinks that a child fits the classification of retarded should refer that child for psychological testing. The tests will determine whether the child is only a slow learner and should stay in the regular classroom or whether he should be placed in a special class for retarded children.

Parent Education

Mentally retarded children often have emotional problems that they are incapable of solving by themselves. All children need love and acceptance. Yet the mentally handicapped child may be resented and misunderstood by his family. Such a child must face not only the general problems of social adjustment but also the weight of his parents' disappointment. Recognizing that the mental health of children is strongly influenced by parental attitudes, programs of education and counseling have been established for the parents of mentally handicapped children in many community clinics or child guidance centers.

Work Training

Many children whose mental deficiency is not too severe may be prepared to earn a living. The establishment of sheltered workshops is helping to give more of these young people the encouragement, supervision, and patient training required to prepare them for gainful employment. Experience has shown that they can perform many simple but necessary tasks in industry, business, and the home. However, it is important to realize that these individuals must work under supervision and also must be protected from unfair treatment or exploitation. Knowing that their work is valuable to the organization will help greatly to bolster their morale.

The most important thing to remember about children who are mentally retarded is that they need to be treated sympathetically and realistically. There is nothing wrong with them that is any fault of theirs. They may not be quick-witted, but they have many qualities such as kindness, patience, and a capacity for love and goodness which persons of higher intelligence can profitably imitate. And when their education is completed it is important that they have opportunities to make the fullest and most satisfying contribution possible to the life of their community.

FOR REVIEW AND DISCUSSION

1. Tell the difference between the words or terms in each of the following pairs:

    a. Intelligence and aptitude
    b. Mental age and chronological age
    c. Intelligence tests and achievement tests
    d. A slow learner and a moderately retarded child

2. Determine the intelligence quotient of an eight-year-old child whose mental age is ten. What place would this child occupy on the scale of intelligence? What are some of the problems he may encounter? What are some of the ways in which his teachers can encourage him to reach his intellectual potential?

3. Determine the mental age of a ten-year-old child whose IQ is 80. How would you classify this child in terms of his intellectual ability? What are some of the ways in which his teacher can help him to make the best use of his time in his class?

4. Which of the following statements are true and which are false? Reword each false statement so as to make it true.

    a. Intellectually gifted children always achieve high grades in school.
    b. A child does not have to possess a high degree of intelligence to be exceptionally gifted in a particular field of endeavor.
    c. Many different influences—physical, emotional, or environmental—may keep a child from using his intelligence to good advantage.
    d. The fear of being considered an "oddball" has kept many a bright student from doing his best in school.
    e. Children who cannot keep up with their classmates in school work or games are too "dumb" to care.
    f. Giving slow learners opportunities to succeed in academic work

through meaningful learning experiences should help to lower the percentage of high school dropouts.

7 g. Mentally retarded children classed as "educable" are most likely to become socially well adjusted if they are enrolled in special classes in the public schools.

SELECTED REFERENCES

American Educational Research Association: *Education of Exceptional Children*, National Education Association, Washington, D.C., 1959.

Bereday, George Z., and Joseph A. Lauwerys (eds.): *The Gifted Child*, 1962 Yearbook of Education, Harcourt, Brace & World, Inc., New York, 1962.

Conant, James Bryant: *Slums and Suburbs; A Commentary on Schools in Metropolitan Areas*, McGraw-Hill Book Company, New York, 1961. (Dr. Conant's report of observations he made during his study of the junior high schools in large areas. Among the problems covered are those of minority groups and the slow learner.)

Council for Exceptional Children, National Education Association, Washington, D.C.:

Early Admission for Mentally Advanced Children—A Review of Research and Practices, 1962.

Educable Retarded Children in Elementary Schools—Administration of Special Education in Small School Systems, 1961.

Personal and Social Adjustment of Gifted Adolescents, CEC Research Monograph, Series A, No. 4, 1962.

Procedures for Teaching Trainable Children, CEC Research Monograph, Series A, No. 2, 1960.

Kough, Jack, and Robert F. De Haan: *Teacher's Guidance Handbook*, Science Research Associates, Chicago, 1955–1956.

Vol. I: *Identifying Children with Special Needs*, Sec. II, Chaps. 3–12; Sec. II, Chap. 17.

Vol. II: *Helping Children with Special Needs*, Sect. II, Chaps. 2–11; Sec. II, Chap. 14.

Magary, James F., and John R. Eichorn (eds.): *The Exceptional Child*, Holt, Rinehart and Winston, Inc., New York, 1960.

Pollock, Morris P., and Miriam Pollock: *New Hope for the Retarded; Enriching the Lives of Exceptional Children*, Porter Sargent, Publishers, Boston, 1953.

Prescott, Daniel A.: *The Child in the Educative Process*, McGraw-Hill Book Company, New York, 1957.

A Proposed Program for National Action to Combat Mental Retardation, The President's Panel on Mental Retardation, Washington, D.C., 1962.

Strang, Ruth: *Helping Your Gifted Child,* E. P. Dutton & Co., Inc., New York, 1960. (A book for parents—also helpful to teachers.)

Woolcock, Cyril William: *Hunter College High School Program for Gifted Students,* Vantage Press, New York, 1962.

Organizations

American Association for Gifted Children

Council for Exceptional Children, National Education Association

National Association for Retarded Children

Chapter 6   SYSTEMS OF CONTROL

Ins and Outs of the Nervous System
The Endocrine System in Action
Teamwork for Meeting Emergencies
Psychogenic Reactions to Repressed Emotions

The child comes to school with a whole constellation of thoughts, feelings, and patterns of behavior which is uniquely his own. He also has a body that reacts to stimuli from both without and within, according to physiological laws that apply to everybody. The forces that condition both uniqueness of personality and physiological sameness are lodged in the central nervous system (the brain and spinal cord). For that reason teachers will find it helpful to have some background knowledge of this system as a basis for the intelligent observation of children as individuals and as members of a group.

INS AND OUTS OF THE NERVOUS SYSTEM

The nervous system consists of (1) the brain, (2) the spinal cord, and (3) the nerves. The brain and spinal cord together are called the *central nervous system.* The nerves connect the central nervous system with all other parts of the body much as incoming and outgoing wires connect "central" in a telephone system with all the telephones in a certain district.

The Seat of Thought and Voluntary Action

The part of the brain known as the *cerebral cortex* makes it possible for each person to think, to remember, to learn, to act voluntarily—in short, to be himself in thought, word, and deed. It is a corrugated layer of gray matter composed of nerve cells, which covers the two hemispheres of the *cerebrum,* or upper part of the brain, as bark covers the trunk of a tree. *Cortex* is the Latin word for "bark."

The cerebral cortex (Fig. 6-1) belongs to the division of the central nervous system which is sometimes called the outward-acting system because through it the individual governs his dealings with people and things in the world outside himself. Information received about the world from his special sense organs makes it possible for him to govern intelligently. And voluntary muscles supplied with motor nerves from the seat of government make it possible for him to act as he wills.

Department of Internal Affairs

That part of the central nervous system which manages the internal affairs of the body is the *autonomic* (self-controlling) *nervous system.* The inward-acting nervous system is another good name for it. It supplies nerves to the glands and to the involuntary muscles of the eyes, heart, lungs, digestive tract, kidneys, blood vessels, skin, and other organs. Autonomic impulses, which may be provoked by emotional as well as by physical stimuli, are responsible for the rate of the heartbeat; for the amount of digestive juices secreted by the stomach and small intestine and the amount of sweat secreted by the sweat glands; for the dilation and contraction of the pupils of the eyes and of the tiny blood vessels(arterioles) in the skin; and for a great many other actions. In short, the autonomic system takes the government of our bodies off our minds so that we do not need to bother about what goes on inside to regulate the work of the organs and to maintain the living conditions to which the cells are accustomed.

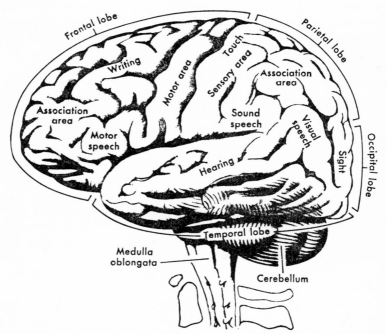

Fig. 6-1. A side view of the cerebral cortex showing the sensory areas, the motor area, and the association areas. The sensory areas are the centers in which impulses are received from the sense organs. The motor area is the center from which impulses go out to the voluntary muscles. In the association or "memory" areas, impulses received in the sensory areas are interpreted. Figure 17-9 shows the places in the motor area from which impulses go out to the muscles in different parts of the body.

Two in One

The autonomic nerve centers from which nerve fibers pass to the organs they influence have their places in the brain and spinal cord along with the groups of nerve centers that serve the will (see Fig. 6-2). We may visualize the two systems—the outward-acting, or voluntary, and the inward-acting, or involuntary—as occupying the same territory but located in different towns and cities (collections of nerve cells), connected with one another and with the rest of the body by an intricate network of streets, roads, and telephone wires (nerve fibers). Neither system operates as a completely isolated independent unit. That is why mind can affect body and body can affect mind.

The Psyche and the Soma

In medical parlance the life of the mind—emotional as well as intellectual, and conscious as well as unconscious—is referred to as the *psyche*. In Greek mythology, Psyche, meaning the soul, was personified as a lovely, butterfly-winged maiden, symbolic of immortality. The body, in medical language, is known as the *soma*, which is the Greek word for "body." Putting the two words together, we get "psychosomatic," which designates body–mind relationships. Bodily symptoms and signs of psychic origin are called psychogenic.

Blushing with shame or embarrassment, turning white with joy or rage, having a sinking feeling at the pit of the stomach from fright, watering at the mouth when an appetizing food is smelled are all psychogenic manifestations. That is, they are physical changes brought about by the effect of the psyche on the autonomic and endocrine systems. Since such changes occur automatically—when the proper psychic button is pushed —it is easy to see why a person may have all sorts of physical signs and symptoms without having anything organically wrong. Although thoughts and emotions have their home in the brain, they are not confined to home. Their echoes reverberate in every cell and tissue of the body. The reverse is also true. Physical sensations, as we all know, have a profound effect on our thoughts and feelings.

What Sensations Are and Why We Have Them

Sensations are conscious impressions produced by the reaction of sensory nerve endings (receptors) to stimuli to which they are sensitive. The simplest way to represent our sensory mechanism is, first, to draw a circle and place on its circumference (representing the outer, or peripheral, part of the body) dots to represent sensory receptors.[1] At its center we place a picture of the cerebral cortex to represent its sensory areas (see Fig. 6-3).

[1] For the sake of simplicity, only the receptors of the familiar five senses are represented here. There are other sensibilities, as will be explained later.

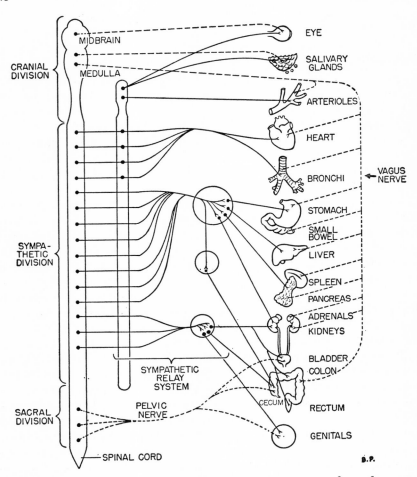

Fig. 6-2. The nerve fibers of the autonomic system pass out from the central nervous system in three regions: (*a*) the lowest portion of the brain (cranial division); (*b*) the lower end of the spinal cord (sacral division); and (*c*) the spinal cord between the cranial and sacral divisions (sympathetic division—solid lines in diagram). The two end divisions (cranial and sacral) together form what is called the parasympathetic division (broken lines in diagram). The vagus nerve and its branches carry the impulses from the cranial division to the organs of the trunk. In their influence upon any one organ, the parasympathetic division and the sympathetic division work against each other. For example, the sympathetic division supplies the nerve fibers over which impulses to contract the skin arterioles (vasoconstrictors) are transmitted, whereas the parasympathetic division supplies the nerve fibers that carry the impulses responsible for their dilation (vasodilators).

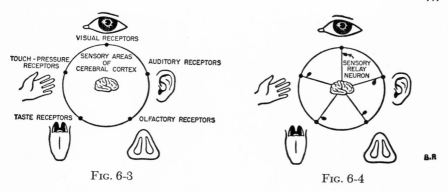

FIG. 6-3   FIG. 6-4

Next, we draw radii representing nerve fibers from the sensory receptors on the periphery to the cerebral cortex in the center, and somewhere
along each radius we place a dot to stand for a relay neuron (nerve cell)
(see Fig. 6-4).

Actually, this wheellike diagram is far too simple. It would resemble
a far more complicated web than any spider could ever spin if we at-
tempted to show the devious routes, the crossroads, the relay stations by
which nerve impulses from the sense organs finally reach the particular
areas in the cerebral cortex where they make sense.

The Stimulus. To make the sensory mechanism work, it is necessary to
apply the proper stimulus. Let us imagine that each of the dots on the
periphery of our circle is an electric push button. If we push the button
marked "auditory receptors" we hear something; if we push the button
marked "visual receptors" we see something; and so on. The push in each
case is the stimulus. It must be a different kind of push, or stimulus, for
each kind of receptor. For example, only light waves can stimulate visual
receptors; only sound waves can stimulate auditory receptors; only odors
can stimulate olfactory receptors. However, it does sometimes happen
that a receptor is excited by an unusual stimulus. When that happens the
sensation aroused is similar to that aroused by the usual stimulus. For
example, we "see stars" (light) when hit between the eyes.

The Nerve Impulse. The force started along a nerve fiber when the
proper stimulus is applied to its sensory ending, or receptor, is the nerve
impulse. The impulses carried by sensory nerve fibers leading from one
kind of receptors are practically the same as those carried by nerve fibers
leading from other kinds of receptors. An electric current makes a bell
ring or a light come on, according to the device to which it is connected
by wires. Just so, the nerve impulse gives us the sensation of sight or
hearing or some other sensation, according to the sensory area in the
brain to which it is connected by nerve fibers. That is, the starting point
of an impulse and its destination are what determine the character of a

sensation, not the impulse itself. Although all impulses in themselves are more or less alike, no one has yet explained exactly what they are. The nearest research scientists have come to defining a nerve impulse is to say that it is an excitation process associated with a series of electrical and chemical changes along its nerve-fiber route.

Somatic Sensibilities. So far we have been discussing the sensations which are so distinctive that they have been singled out and given special names. Four of these familiar quintuplets—sight, hearing, taste, and smell —still maintain their status as special senses. But in recent years touch and its refinements have been placed among the less distinct sensations designated as somatic, or body, sensibilities. These sensibilities make us aware, in varying degrees, of pressure, heat, cold, pain, and the movements and position of the limbs, trunk, and head. As their name implies, they are concerned with matters of vital interest to the body itself. When their receptors are stimulated, machinery is set in motion which brings about automatically the adjustments required, or calls our attention to conditions that only we, by thinking and acting voluntarily, can rectify.

Acting without Thinking

The adjustments that take place without our thinking about them are the simple, or unconditioned, reflexes. They are brought about by impulses that travel to nerve centers in the spinal cord or brain stem, and then out again over motor nerves to the gland or muscle that acts in response to them. They do not get to the boss—the cerebral cortex— because the personal attention of the boss is not necessary.

Ordinarily, we are not aware of the great majority of the simple reflexes that bring about desirable adjustments; for example, secretion of the digestive juices when food enters the mouth, and the widening or narrowing of the eye pupils according to the amount of light entering the eyes. But in the case of many reflexes we are aware of the action taken, even though we do not consciously initiate it. Often we think about it and, if necessary, take further conscious steps to remedy the situation. Without thinking, we snatch our hands from a hot stove. But some of the impulses started on their way by contact with the hot surface reach the cerebral cortex. As a result, we consciously feel the pain of the burn and run cold water over it. We may not be able to stop a sneeze. But we are aware of the premonitory tickle in the nose and reach for a handkerchief if we have learned regard for our fellowmen. We cannot stop a blush, the mechanics of which are handled autonomically. However, we are conscious both of the blush and of the embarrassment responsible. On the other hand, we may be completely unconscious of some other emotion or inner tension and yet be all too well acquainted with the violent headache or upset stomach caused by it.

Habit Acts

There are other things, like walking, dressing, and bathing, which we do almost without thinking, as we say, but which once gave our brains a lot of work. When definite nerve tracks and switches had been established for the impulses that initiate every move in these complicated acts, we could then devote our minds to higher things like deciding where to walk, or what to wear, or when to take a bath.

It is only necessary to watch a little child learning to string colored wooden beads to get an idea of the tremendous concentration required to master a performance which the child who has already mastered it does with the greatest ease. And once it has been mastered, what delightful ways of expressing himself are opened up! Be it reading or skating or stringing beads or walking or what not, it is only when the basic operation has become a habit act, or series of conditioned reflexes, that the child can proceed to the fairy tales or the figure eights or the soul-satisfying patterns or the desired destinations.

Thinking before Acting

The kind of mental activity through which we express ourselves—our own unique personalities—is the highest function of the mind. It requires our constant and direct personal attention. Thinking things through to arrive at decisions and performing the voluntary acts required to deal with new situations as they arise require the association of vast numbers of neurons in the cerebral cortex and often involve widely separated regions of the body.

THE ENDOCRINE SYSTEM IN ACTION

The autonomic nervous system has a partner in running the internal affairs of the body. This partner is the endocrine system, which is made up of glands especially designed for the business of producing and secreting chemical products known as *hormones*. The endocrine glands have no ducts, like the salivary and tear glands, for example, but deliver their secretion directly into the bloodstream. Hence another name for them is ductless glands.

Hormones are almost unbelievably powerful substances. Some hormones are present in the fluids of the body in strengths as low as one part in one billion. Yet they exert a profound influence on growth, physical appearance, body functions, and the mental and emotional behavior of every individual. This influence is expressed in many of the variations in body build and personality which teachers observe in school children.

Roll Call of the Endocrines

The best-known endocrine glands (Fig. 6-5) are (1) the pituitary, reposing snugly in a tiny ditch, or *fossa*, in a bone at the base of the

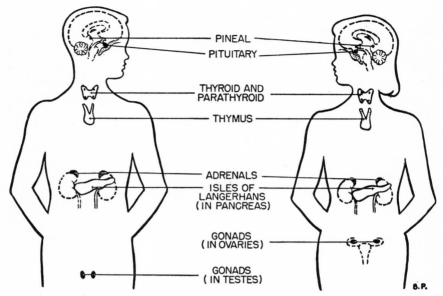

FIG. 6-5. Diagram showing the location of the endocrine glands.

skull and attached to the brain by a short stalk; (2) the thyroid, sprawling like the letter H across the front of the larynx and windpipe; (3) the adrenals, perched like triangular cocked hats over the rounded upper pole of each kidney; (4) the parathyroids, resembling minute reddish-brown beans marking the corners of an imaginary square on the back surface of the thyroid; (5) the islands of Langerhans, clusters of cells embedded in the connective tissue of the pancreas; and (6) the gonads, or sex glands. The ovaries are the female gonads, and the testes are the male gonads. Less well known are two glands whose functions have not yet been fully defined. Their names are the thymus and the pineal gland.

The thymus lies behind the breastbone and extends over the upper part of the heart. It has often been called the gland of childhood because it is largest at this period of life. It grows in size steadily from birth up to the time of puberty but shrinks rapidly thereafter. Beginning with the year 1961 research on the thymus has disclosed that the work of this gland is intimately linked with that of the lymph nodes and spleen in the production of lymphocytes (see Solving the Mystery of the Thymus, in Chap. 10).

The pineal gland is a tiny reddish-gray body about as big as a fat pumpkin seed which lies deep in the brain. It gets its name from the Latin word for pine cone because it somewhat resembles a pine cone in shape. In spite of intense scientific study over many years, the function of the pineal gland is still an unanswered riddle.

How Hormones Work

The function of the endocrine glands is to secrete individual hormones at the proper time and in suitable quantities to regulate and coordinate the work of other organs and tissues. Since hormones are poured into the bloodstream, which goes everywhere, there is not an organ or even part of an organ that escapes their influence. For this reason, hormones are utilized by and large to bring about desired responses from the body as a whole, or from a major portion of it, as in skeletal growth, in situations calling for unusual effort, and in preparation for the reproductive function.

Hormones work by influencing activities that are the natural functions of particular organs. Without organs with natural functions of their own, hormones could not act at all. To retard the activity of any organ, the endocrine gland involved sends a smaller amount of hormonal secretion to the organ, which must therefore plod along at its own slow pace. To speed up the activity of any organ, the endocrine gland involved increases its output of hormones.

The secretion of hormones is not constant. There are glands that secrete more or less continuously, it is true—for example, the thyroid, the adrenal cortex, and the anterior (front) portion of the pituitary during skeletal growth—but the amounts secreted vary according to need. Other glands secrete cyclically—for example, the ovarian gonads, or female sex glands, and the gonad-controlling portion of the pituitary. Still others secrete intermittently—for example, the islands of Langerhans after carbohydrate food has been eaten, and the adrenal medulla when there is urgent need for the release of sugar from the liver to meet some sudden demand for energy.

All for One; One for All

Like the old woman's pig that would not get over the stile until it was nipped by the dog, which had to be activated by a stick, which in turn was threatened by fire, and so on, the adequate functioning of one endocrine gland depends on the adequate functioning of a series of others. At this point it may be helpful to review briefly the principal business of the best-known glands, always keeping in mind that each one is part of a system and not simply one independent organ.

The pituitary has been called the master gland of the endocrine system because upon its activity the functions of most of the other endocrine glands depend. It has two main parts or lobes—the anterior, or front lobe, and the posterior, or back lobe. The anterior lobe is the most active. One of its best-known hormones is the growth hormone which controls the growth of the skeleton. Another which came into prominence in the 1950s is known by the letters ACTH (*adrenocoritcotropic hormone*).

ACTH, as its name implies, stimulates the adrenal cortex to increase the secretion of its hormones when needed in time of stress.

Each one of the two adrenals, like the pituitary, is a combination of two distinct glands—called the adrenal medulla and the adrenal cortex. The adrenal medulla is the inner dark-colored portion of the gland, and the adrenal cortex is its outer light-colored rim. The hormone secreted by the adrenal medulla is epinephrine; it heightens and prolongs the effect of sympathetic impulses in situations calling for sudden bursts of energy. The secretion of the adrenal cortex contains a large number of closely related hormones which are fatty compounds known as *steroids*. Some of the steroids are sex hormones similar to those produced by the gonads, or sex glands. Others are called into action to aid the body in dealing with stressful situations. The best-known steroid in this group is cortisone.

The hormone secreted by the thyroid gland is thyroxine, a chemical compound which is 65 per cent iodine. Practically all the iodine in food is absorbed from the blood by the thyroid. Thyroxine regulates the speed of energy metabolism, that is, the sum total of the processes by which the cells of the body transform food and oxygen into heat and energy.

The parathyroids secrete a hormone called parathormone. The function of this hormone is to keep the calcium content of the blood at a normal level.

The hormone secreted by the islands of Langerhans in the pancreas is insulin. This hormone aids the body cells in oxidizing glucose (sugar) to produce heat and energy. It also helps to change glucose into glycogen for storage in the liver. Glycogen is an insoluble starch sometimes called animal starch. Insulin also aids in changing glycogen back into glucose for use as fuel when extra energy is needed.

The hormone produced by the testes, or male gonads, is testosterone. Under its influence the boy becomes a man. His body fills out, his shoulders and chest broaden, his voice becomes deeper, and his beard begins to grow. The female gonads, or ovaries, produce two hormones—estrogen and progesterone. Under their influence the girl becomes a woman. Her body rounds out, her hips become broader, her breasts develop, and menstruation begins.

TEAMWORK FOR MEETING EMERGENCIES

The autonomic nervous system and the endocrine system working together are responsible for many different arrangements by which the body maintains the conditions necessary for ordinary, day-by-day effective living and by which the body prepares itself to meet emergencies that threaten health or even life itself. Although this work is carried on independently of the will and very often without our knowledge, it does produce reactions of which we are very much aware.

How the Body Is Cleared for Action

Many dramatic changes take place within the body to prepare it for action in situations that call for sudden bursts of energy. These changes are brought about by the teamwork of the sympathetic division of the autonomic nervous system and the adrenal medulla. When the sympathetic division gives the word "go" to the adrenal medulla, the latter starts secreting its hormone, epinephrine, into the bloodstream. The effect of this chemical is to put the body in a state of preparedness to take appropriate action in response to strong emotions like fear and anger. Surface blood vessels are tightened up to make extra blood available for the muscles; the force and frequency of the heartbeat are increased; the bronchial tubes are relaxed to ensure adequate ventilation of the lungs; glycogen stored in the liver is changed into glucose and released into the blood to provide extra energy; the pupils of the eyes are dilated, intestinal movements are stopped, and all sphincters in the digestive tract are closed. The ship of the body, so to speak, is cleared for whatever action seems appropriate—fighting or running away as the case may be.

What Happens When Action Is Not Taken

It is worth pointing out that the standards of civilized behavior which demand the suppression of motor responses to primitive emotions, like fear and anger, often have undesirable physical repercussions. Upset digestions and nervous exhaustion are part of the price paid for mobilizing the body's forces for fight or flight when no such action is called for or even possible. The secretion of epinephrine under emotional stress on signal from the sympathetic nervous system accounts for many of the signs and symptoms observed in persons known to be suffering from intense prolonged anxiety—for example, dilated pupils, cold wet hands, and excessive sweating in the armpits. These observations are the basis for the idea that a tie-up exists between long-continued anxiety or worry and such conditions as high blood pressure, gastric ulcer, asthma, and certain skin disorders.

Elementary school children are in the period of emotional and social development in which strong motor reactions to anger, fear, and frustration are natural and proper. Many teachers know this through their knowledge of child psychology or through their intuitive understanding of children's behavior. Yet getting mad and fighting with one another in the classroom or showing by hyperactivity or fidgetiness that some sort of emotional conflict is going on is not conducive to good working conditions. On the other hand, it is desirable to encourage acceptable forms of muscular response to strong emotion. Ordinarily this is accomplished during the school day by allowing periods for games and other motor activities during which children can work off the effects of the bodily changes provoked by their aggressive impulses.

PSYCHOGENIC REACTIONS TO REPRESSED EMOTIONS

It is not difficult to understand why emotions bottled up in the unconscious mind can bring about actual physical signs and symptoms when we stop to think of the effects upon the body of emotions we know about. Depending upon the emotion, we blush, turn pale, sweat, tremble, break out in gooseflesh—in short, show all the outward and visible signs of fear, anger, love, embarrassment, and so on which we cannot keep from showing whether we want to or not. These reactions are not conscious patterns of behavior. That is, we cannot start them or stop them because they are triggered by that part of the nervous system which is not subject to the will. Generally, however, they disappear when the cause of the emotion is removed.

But suppose strong feelings have been repressed, held down, by policeman conscience or by fear of punishment or by some other deterrent! Finding no other outlet, the impulses aroused by such bottled-up emotions are bound to cause psychogenic signs and symptoms of one kind or another.

Various behavior reactions which show that children are emotionally disturbed will be discussed in Chap. 9. Here some of the more common physical reactions to repressed emotions are briefly described.

Sometimes bodily manifestations are mechanisms used by the child to get satisfaction for some need inadequately met during earlier periods of his life, or to express resentment against his parents, or to punish himself for harboring hostile feelings. Many of them are connected with the mouth or the function of eating, for example, lack of appetite (see Loss of Appetite, in Chap. 13), vomiting (see Vomiting, in Chap. 13), finger sucking, nail-biting, overeating, and speech disorders (see Speech Difficulties, in Chap. 17). Others are related to bowel and bladder functions, for example, constipation (see Signs and Symptoms of Gastrointestinal Disorders, in Chap. 13) and urinary frequency (see The Kidneys and Their Work, in Chap. 13).

Disturbances of vision and hearing in the great majority of cases are due to some physical defect or condition (see Chaps. 16 and 17). Sometimes, however, they may arise because of a desire to close the eyes or the ears to some distasteful idea or unpleasant feeling associated with seeing or hearing. A child may have a reading difficulty, for example, because he associates his personal difficulties with his teacher with the subject matter of what he is required to read or because he wants to annoy his parents who have shown that they are anxious for him to learn to read. A child may fail to come when he is called or to answer when spoken to simply because he hears only what he wants to hear. If he doesn't hear, then he cannot blame himself or be blamed for his willfulness.

Restlessness is natural in children. They cannot be expected to sit still for any length of time. But there are some children who are extremely fidgety and "nervous." Excess motor activity when not due to some physical cause (chorea, for example) is, in most cases, a sign of frustration. Perhaps a child has had a long illness during which he has had to repress his desire to be active. After his recovery, his parents or teacher may try to restrict his activities unnecessarily. As a result the child feels frustrated and angry. Verbal expressions of his pent-up active impulses are objected to, and so he lets off steam by unpurposeful continual muscular movements. Children may be placed in many other situations in which they cannot express their anger or jealousy or resentment against too-exacting requirements in acceptable ways and so fall back on "the fidgets" as the solution.

In some children fidgetiness may be localized—that is, they may spasmodically blink their eyes or make queer grimaces with their mouths or twitch their noses. Such localized motions are called *habit tics*, or spasms, when no physical cause can be found. Their origin usually lies in some forgotten emotional experience in which the child was actually punished or feared punishment for something about which he felt guilty. If no notice is taken of a habit tic, it may clear up spontaneously. Usually, however, the child is ridiculed or urged to control it, with the result that he may begin to feel pleasure in possessing a trick so attention-attracting. It may then be hard for him to give it up.

FOR REVIEW AND DISCUSSION

1. Match the word or term in Group I with the definition or description in Group II that you associate with it.

Group I

a Brain and spinal cord
b Cerebral cortex
c Sensory areas of cerebral cortex
d Motor area of cerebral cortex
e Autonomic nervous system
f Endocrine glands

Group II

e Centers for the reception and transmission of impulses to involuntary muscles and glands
c Reception centers of impulses from the sense organs
f Manufacturing centers for hormones
d Transmission centers for impulses to voluntary muscles
a Headquarters of the nervous system
b The seat of the mind

2. Tell the differences between the words or terms in each of the following pairs:

   a. Psychosomatic and psychogenic
   b. Parasympathetic division (of autonomic nervous system) and sympathetic division
   c. Stimulus and nerve impulse
   d. Unconditioned reflexes and habit acts
   e. The adrenal medulla and the adrenal cortex
   f. Testosterone and estrogen

3. Select the correct ending for each of the following incomplete sentences:

   a. The hormone that enables the body to oxidize and store sugar is (1) cortisone, (2) insulin, (3) parathormone.
   b. The hormone that regulates the speed of energy metabolism is (1) thyroxine, (2) epinephrine, (3) ACTH.
   c. The team that gears the body for sudden bursts of energy consists of (1) the brain and the spinal cord, (2) the anterior pituitary and the islands of Langerhans, (3) the sympathetic division of the autonomic nervous system and the adrenal medulla.
   d. The emotions that are not likely to cause undesirable psychogenic reactions are those which have (1) led to aggressive action, (2) been repressed, (3) been released in a frank talk with a sympathetic friend or advisor.

SELECTED REFERENCES

American Medical Association: *The Nerves*, Part 3 of *The Wonderful Human Machine* series, The Association, Chicago. (The workings of the human body in words and pictures.)

Best, C. H., and N. B. Taylor: *The Human Body, Its Anatomy and Physiology* (first given as reference in Chap. 1). Part VIII, *The Nervous System*, Chaps. 33–37; Part IX, *Endocrine, or Ductless, Glands*, Chaps. 38–40.

Cannon, Walter B.: *The Wisdom of the Body*, W. W. Norton & Company, Inc., New York, 1939. (A classic by a distinguished physiologist on the relation of the autonomic nervous system and the endocrines to the self-regulation of physiological processes. Contains an excellent chapter on "The General Functions of the Two Grand Divisions of the Nervous System.")

Riedman, Sarah R.: *Our Hormones and How They Work*, Abelard-Schuman, Limited, New York, 1956.

Seyle, Hans: *The Stress of Life*, McGraw-Hill Book Company, New York, 1956. Paperbook edition, 1963. (A discussion of the stress mechanism and its implications and applications.)

Chapter 7   DEFENSE REACTIONS RESPONSIBLE FOR SIGNS AND SYMPTOMS

Types of Defensive Arrangements
Reactions to Infection
Allergic Reactions
Reactions to Internal Temperature Changes
The Mechanism of Pain

In most cases signs and symptoms are indications that the body is engaged in a struggle to defend itself from harmful influences or to adjust itself to adverse conditions that it cannot overcome. Symptoms are unpleasant sensations felt by the person affected. Signs are evidences of physical change that can be seen, heard, felt, or measured by someone else. A person whose signs and symptoms can be traced to a definite physical cause is said to have an *organic illness*. A person whose signs and symptoms have no detectable physical cause is said to have a *functional illness*. Roughly, the proportion of organic illness to functional illness is about half and half. In both types of illness the autonomic nervous system has a leading part in the production of signs and symptoms.

In organic illness or physical injury the autonomic nervous system acts upon impulses coming in from parts of the body that are in distress. In most cases the action taken is the instigation of remedial measures.

In functional illness, the impulses calling for action go out from the mind, or psyche, without prompting from outside. The action taken may exactly simulate that taken when some organic irritation is the exciting factor. To put it very simply indeed, a child may vomit because he has eaten green apples or because he doesn't want to go to school. In the first case the autonomic nervous system, acting in response to impulses from the stomach, initiates the appropriate action to help the stomach get rid of an irritating substance. In the other, the autonomic nervous system, acting in response to forceful impulses from the mind itself, helps the child to escape from a stressful situation.

TYPES OF DEFENSIVE ARRANGEMENTS

Some defensive arrangements are the familiar protective reflexes that enable us to meet the emergencies of everyday living. Sneezing, coughing, watering of the eyes, gagging, and vomiting, for example, take place immediately, without an act of the will, to force out irritating substances that might cause damage if they were not expelled.

Many different kinds of adjustments enable us both to cope with the vicissitudes of daily life and to mobilize defense forces of one kind or another. Among such adjustments is the stepping up of the tempo of breathing and the rate of the heartbeat when more oxygen is needed in vigorous exercise and fever. Another is the formation of a clot over a break in the skin to prevent the escape of an excessive amount of blood.

Related to protective adjustments of this kind are reactions to infection, allergic reactions, reactions to overproduction and underproduction of heat within the body, and reactions to injurious stimuli. As such reactions account for many of the signs and symptoms that teachers are asked to observe in children and report to the doctor or nurse, some explanation of them is given in this chapter.

REACTIONS TO INFECTION

The signs and symptoms of infection are the direct results of the interaction between living, multiplying microorganisms (microbes or germs) and the defense forces of the infected body. The scientific name for disease-producing microorganisms is *pathogens*.[1]

Classes of Pathogens

There are several different classes of pathogens. Some are one-celled plants; others are one-celled animals; still others occupy a sort of no-man's land between the living and the nonliving.

Bacteria. The largest class of pathogens consists of bacteria. These one-celled plants are the smallest members of the very large class of plants called *fungi*, which contain no chlorophyll. Chorophyll is the green coloring matter that permits green plants to use sunlight in manufacturing their own food out of inorganic, that is, nonliving, materials. As bacteria contain no chlorophyll, they must get their food ready-made from organic matter, living or dead. Pathogenic bacteria are classified according to their characteristic shapes as seen under a microscope.

THE COCCI. These bacteria are shaped like balls. The cocci (singular, *coccus*) get their name from a Greek word meaning "berry." The cocci that are important to medical science fall into five main groups:

1. *Streptococci*. These cocci grow in chains like strings of beads. The most dangerous streptococci belong to the species known as *Streptococcus hemolyticus* which produces a substance (hemolysin) that dissolves the red cells of the blood. In addition to an innumerable variety of local

[1] Many of the diseases listed in this section as examples of infections caused by pathogens in each class are described in appropriate chapters further on.

lesions, including boils and wound infections, the streptococci are responsible for epidemic diseases such as scarlet fever, streptococcal sore throat,
and erysipelas, as well as for other important infections such as septicemia
(blood poisoning) and puerperal fever. Doctors look upon the streptococcus as a potential Jack-of-all-trades, capable of attacking in many ways
(see Fig. 7-1).

2. *Pneumococci.* These cocci are lancet-shaped bacteria that usually
occur in pairs and are surrounded by definite capsules. They get their
name from the fact that they are responsible for about 90 per cent of all
cases of bacterial pneumonia. A great many specific types, or strains, of
pneumococci have been discovered. In addition to pneumonia, pneumococci may produce other infections, particularly sinus and middle-ear
infections (see Fig. 7-1).

3. *Staphylococci.* These cocci grow in clumps like bunches of grapes.
They often gang up with streptococci in causing various types of skin infections such as boils and carbuncles. Also, they are responsible for one
form of so-called food poisoning known as staphylococcal food poisoning.
The staphylococcus at its worst may cause septicemia if it gets into the
bloodstream or osteomyelitis (a bone infection) if it gets into a bone.

4. *Meningococci.* The meningococci usually square off in groups of four.

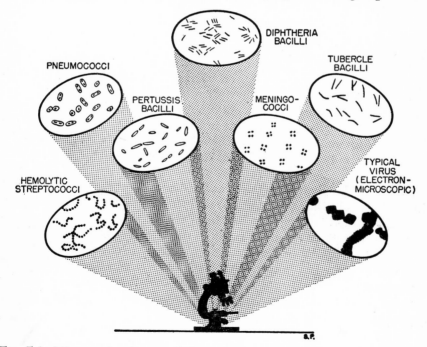

Fig. 7-1. Microscopic pictures of the principal causative agents of respiratory
infections.

They attack the meninges—that is, the membranes surrounding the brain and spinal cord—thus causing epidemic cerebrospinal meningitis (see Fig. 7-1).

5. *Gonococci.* The gonococci grow in groups of two and look somewhat like quotation marks. They cause the venereal disease known as gonorrhea.

THE BACILLI. These bacteria are shaped like rods or sticks. The bacilli (singular, *bacillus*) get their name from the Latin word for little stick or staff. So far as is known, they are the most common type of bacteria in existence. Among the best-known infections caused by bacilli are tuberculosis, diphtheria, typhoid fever, whooping cough, and tetanus (see Fig. 7-1).

THE SPIRILLA. These bacteria are shaped like curved rods. They vary from small comma-shaped forms to corkscrew-shaped forms made up of five, six, or more curves. The deadliest comma-shaped spirillum causes cholera.

Spirochetes. This family of pathogens belongs to a group intermediate between spirilla and protozoa. The spirochetes are slender, wavy, corkscrewlike microorganisms that move rapidly by sinuous, rotating movements. The best-known spirochete causes the venereal disease syphilis.

Fungi. The very large class of nongreen plants called fungi (singular, *fungus*) includes members ranging upward in size from the one-celled bacteria to the familiar yeasts and molds to the mushrooms and toadstools. Some microscopic fungi that depend upon living things directly for their food are capable of causing human or animal diseases. Ringworm is the most familiar skin infection caused by fungi. Certain kinds of airborne fungi cause infections of the lungs when inhaled.

Protozoa. Protozoa (singular, *protozoon*) belong to the lowest division of the animal kingdom. The ameba is a protozoon. One kind of ameba is responsible for amebic dysentery when it gets into the intestines. Malaria, of which there are several different forms, is the best-known protozoan disease.

Viruses. Today the word virus is as familiar to us as the word germ. Yet the existence of viruses was not known before the beginning of this century. Up to then investigators had been unable to see under the microscope the infectious agent of smallpox or of any other communicable disease not caused by bacteria, fungi, protozoa, or spirochetes. The mystery was solved when it was discovered that the causes of many plant, animal, and human diseases are so minute that they cannot be seen by means of ordinary microscopes. Now, however, some of the largest viruses can be seen by means of the electron microscope (see Fig. 7-1).

Another characteristic of viruses besides their small size is the simplicity of their structure. They are so simply built, in fact, that they lack wholly or in part the facilities for making the substances essential to their continued existence from the raw materials provided by their hosts. As a result, viruses must live right inside the cells of the host so that they can extract these substances from the cells which have the facilities for their manufacture. Most bacteria can be grown in the laboratory on a suitable culture medium containing no living cells. Not so the viruses! It is impossible to cultivate a single virus on anything but living tissue.

Human beings are subject to a great many different virus diseases, among them smallpox, yellow fever, measles, chicken pox, mumps, poliomyelitis, rabies, viral pneumonia, epidemic influenza, colds, and several kinds of encephalitis.

Rickettsia. Rickettsia are minute bacillus-like organisms which, like the viruses, can be cultivated only in tissue cultures containing living cells. They get their name from Howard Taylor Ricketts, the young American doctor who first described them in 1909.

Pathogens belonging to the rickettsial family are spread by insects and other arthropods (that is, a class of animals with many-jointed legs), including lice, ticks, fleas, and mites. The best-known rickettsial disease is typhus fever, and Rocky Mountain spotted fever is its first cousin.

General Lines of Defense

General lines of defense operate against all invading microorganisms. The first line is represented by the skin and by the mucous membrane which lines all hollow organs, tubes, and cavities that open to the outside of the body. If the skin remains unbroken, it keeps out most bacteria except those which may lodge in the opening of hair follicles or sweat-gland ducts. Any invaders that get by the outer barriers must then face destruction by the antiseptic or flushing action of various secretions, such as tears (in the eyes), mucus (in the nose), saliva (in the mouth), and gastric juice (in the stomach).

Once bacteria or viruses in sufficient numbers have succeeded in getting through the outer lines of defense into the blood and lymph streams and eventually into the tissues, they are confronted by a very powerful inner line of defense. This is the army of phagocytes (literally "cell-eaters") to which the white cells of the blood and many other cells widely distributed throughout the body belong (see The White Cells, in Chap. 10). White cells fight bacteria or any other foreign invaders by destroying them on the spot. The main object of the phagocytes in attacking bacterial invaders is to keep the infection localized. If this can be done, the whole body may be saved from bacterial invasion. The struggle between germs and phagocytes is marked by two signs that are familiar to us all. The first is inflammation, or the so-called inflammatory reaction, and the second is pus formation.

Inflammation. Inflammation is the typical first response of any part of the body attacked by bacteria or by any other physical or chemical agent that may cause injury, such as a blow or excessive heat or a strong acid or alkali. The capillaries (see The Circulatory System, in Chap. 10) in the region become irritated, and, as a result, their walls become more permeable. Thus fluid and white blood cells can escape from the bloodstream into the tissue spaces.

The classic signs of inflammation are the four "ors": *calor* (heat), *turgor* (swelling), *rubor* (redness), and *dolor* (pain). The heat and redness are caused by the rush of blood to the invaded area; the swelling, by the excess fluid in the tissue spaces; and the pain, by pressure on nerve endings in the neighborhood.

Inflammation is a defense reaction regulated by hormones secreted by the anterior pituitary and the adrenal cortex. In response to an SOS sent out by the autonomic nervous system, the anterior pituitary steps up its production of ACTH. This hormone in turn stimulates the adrenal cortex to increase the production of cortisone and other steroids that help the body to deal with inflammation.

The lay observer can see the objective signs of inflammation only if they are in an exposed region of the body, such as the eyes and the skin of the face, arms, and hands. Complaints of pain, of course, can be heard by all. Severe or extensive inflammation is also accompanied by fever, in most cases, and by other signs and symptoms of acute illness.

The noun ending "itis" attached to the name of any part of the body denotes inflammation of that part. Appendic*itis*, ot*itis* media, conjunctiv-

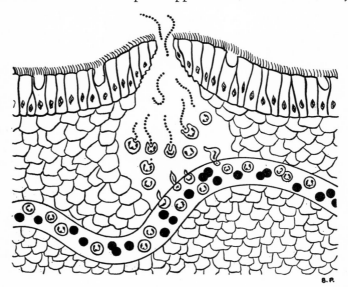

Fig. 7-2. The drama of phagocytosis. The invading army of bacteria (streptococci), entering through a beachhead in the skin, encounter the defending army of white blood cells passing through the capillary walls.

itis, bronch*itis,* and neur*itis,* for example, mean respectively inflammation of the appendix, of the middle ear, of the conjunctiva of the eye, of the bronchial tubes, and of the nerves. Since inflammation is only a sign that *something is wrong,* the use of a term denoting inflammation of a part is not, strictly speaking, a diagnosis. Only the physician or surgeon is competent to tell what is causing the inflammation.

Pus Formation. Pus is simply a collection of the dead bacteria and phagocytes that have lost their lives on the field of battle. It is white or yellowish-white because that is the color of the phagocytes.

The phagocytes devour bacteria after the fashion of amebas by means of the extension and retraction of their cytoplasm (the part of a cell outside the nucleus). The meeting of a phagocyte with a germ is not a chance encounter, nor does the phagocyte wander about seeking what it may devour. Apparently the aimless movements of phagocytes are directed by chemical attraction toward bacteria or other substances foreign to the body. Probably this accounts for the migration of large numbers of wandering phagocytes to points of infection or injury (see Fig. 7-2).

Pus is a danger signal because it nearly always indicates that an infective process is going on. We see it in infected pimples and cuts, and in discharges from the nose, ears, and throat. Many of the conditions described later on in connection with what may be observed about different parts of the body are characterized or accompanied by pus formation.

Specific Lines of Defense

Antigen-antibody Reactions. When specific bacteria or viruses or the powerful poisonous substances (toxins) they manufacture come in contact with body tissues, another defense mechanism comes into action. This is antibody formation (see Fig. 7-3). Any substance taken into the body which gives rise to the development of antibodies is called an *antigen.* Each complete antigen stimulates the production of an antibody that reacts to it alone. Hence antibody formation is a specific line of defense.

The antigen may be either the germs themselves or a toxin produced by them. If the germs act as the antigen, the antibodies unite with the germs and help to dissolve them or make them more vulnerable to attack by the phagocytes. If a bacterial toxin is the antigen, the antibody substance produced is an antitoxin that neutralizes the toxin.

Naturally Acquired Active Immunity. The ability to form antibodies that help the regular defense forces of the body to fight invading bacteria or viruses explains why one attack of certain communicable diseases protects the body against subsequent attacks. In many diseases—for example, typhoid fever, smallpox, scarlet fever, measles, chicken pox, mumps, and poliomyelitis—specific antibodies developed as the result of an attack stay in gamma globulin, one of the proteins in blood plasma (see **Blood** and Its Composition, in Chap. 10), and in most instances give long-lasting protection from that disease. Active immunity also may be acquired naturally by having certain infections in such a mild form that one does not know one has had them (inapparent infections) or by repeatedly taking in microorganisms in such minute doses that not even a mild infection develops.

Immunization. The foundations of the modern science of immunology were laid by Louis Pasteur. He discovered that doses of weakened chicken cholera bacteria failed to produce illness in chickens, but that chickens so treated were protected from virulent chicken cholera bacteria introduced at a later date. This discovery led the great French scientist to infer that vaccination against smallpox (introduced by Edward Jenner in 1796) works because microorganisms that are too weak to cause disease stimulate the body to set up specific resistance (immunity) against virulent microorganisms of the same species.

VACCINES. Pasteur gave the name "vaccines" to weakened, or attenuated, bacteria or viruses that are capable of setting up active immunity in previously susceptible animals. Later, the meaning of the word vaccine was extended to include killed or attenuated bacteria or viruses that have the ability to induce resistance against living virulent bacteria or viruses of the same species. Physicians still use the term vaccine to designate immunizing substances made of attenuated or killed bacteria or viruses. Examples of such vaccines are those for whooping cough, typhoid fever, measles, poliomyelitis, and smallpox.

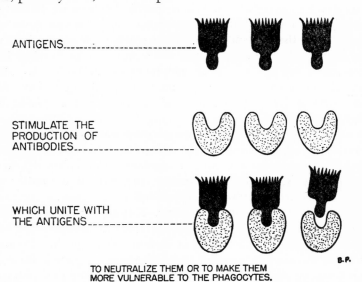

ANTIGENS

STIMULATE THE
PRODUCTION OF
ANTIBODIES

WHICH UNITE WITH
THE ANTIGENS

B.P.

TO NEUTRALIZE THEM OR TO MAKE THEM
MORE VULNERABLE TO THE PHAGOCYTES.

FIG. 7-3. A diagrammatic representation of the mechanism of antigen-antibody reactions.

TOXOIDS. Bacterial toxins also can be modified in such a way as to make them harmless and yet capable of arousing the body to produce antitoxin. A modified toxin is called a toxoid. The best known toxoids used in medical practice are diphtheria toxoid and tetanus toxoid.

Artificially Acquired Active Immunity. The injection of a vaccine or a toxoid stimulates the body to form antibodies which are carried in gamma globulin for varying lengths of time. This process produces what is known as artificially acquired active immunity. Usually the protection given in this way does not last so long as the protection given by an actual attack of the disease. For that reason, reinforcing, or booster, doses of the immunizing substance are necessary from time to time. (See Immunization Timetable, Appendix A.)

Passive Immunity. Temporary immunity from certain communicable diseases can be given by injecting antibodies obtained from the blood plasma of an actively immunized animal (immune serum) or from the blood plasma of human beings who have had an attack of the disease. Examples of antibody substances that are used to give temporary, or passive, immunity from a communicable disease are diphtheria antitoxin, obtained from a horse actively immunized from diphtheria, and gamma globulin obtained from pooled adult blood plasma. Immunizing substances of this kind give only temporary protection because the body quickly eliminates as foreign substances any antibodies that it has had no part in producing.

In using the protection of vaccines, toxoids, antitoxins, and other immunizing substances, physicians make use of one of the most extraordinary and ingenious natural defenses of the body—the production of antibodies. The use of such substances has led to our present control of diphtheria, smallpox, tetanus, polio, and other once-dreaded diseases.

ALLERGIC REACTIONS

It has been said that " 'allergy' is rapidly becoming a large wastepaper basket into which many diseases of unknown cause are being tossed—a catch-all phrase like 'eczema' or 'rheumatism.' " [2] "It must be an allergy" is a remark quite frequently made to explain the sudden appearance of some otherwise inexplicable skin rash or swelling. As a matter of fact, the skin and mucous membranes are the tissues most frequently involved in allergic reactions. The common manifestations of allergy are outlined in later chapters, but it may be helpful to get some idea of what is meant by allergy itself.

The word "allergy" comes from the Greek *allos* meaning "other," plus *ergon* meaning "work." It was proposed by C. von Pirquet in 1906 to

[2] John G. Downing, "Cutaneous Medicine," *New England Journal of Medicine*, Vol. 217, No. 24 (Dec. 11), 1947.

designate the change that is produced in the body as a result of coming in contact with a specific substance that it has found to be harmful. As a result of that first encounter, the body's relation to the substance becomes permanently changed. We have this broad conception of allergy in mind when we say that we are "allergic" to something or someone who has once annoyed or irritated us. And just as we set up ways of protecting ourselves from sources of annoyance or irritation, so the body has defense mechanisms for dealing with various substances that have once irritated or harmed it.

We have learned that one of these defense mechanisms is antibody formation in response to stimulation by antigens. Antigens and antibodies also play a part in allergic reactions. In such reactions the antigen is called an allergen. Allergens stimulate the manufacture of specific allergic antibodies, just as bacterial antigens stimulate the production of specific bacterial antibodies. Unlike disease-causing antigens, however, allergens are substances that are harmless for the majority of people. For the most part, they are protein substances which cause allergic reactions only in individuals who are sensitive to one or more particular proteins.

Shock Tissue

Allergic manifestations are usually localized. That is, a particular allergen sets off a reaction in one tissue or organ but not in others. The sensitive tissue is called the shock tissue. The shock tissue varies with each individual and may differ even in the same individual in response to different allergens. For example, in one person the shock tissue may be the mucous membrane of the nose (hay fever and allergic rhinitis); in another, the mucous membrane of the gastrointestinal tract (allergic stomach or intestinal upsets); in still another, the skin capillaries (hives and eczema).

Once allergic antibodies have been formed, the shock tissue becomes irritated every time they unite with the allergen that led to their creation. Instead of the silent combats that take place without our knowledge when the body is invaded by bacterial antigens against which it has developed antibodies, in allergic reactions the shock tissue—the field of battle, as it were—joins in the fray. And far from getting used to such encounters and ignoring them, the shock tissue, as if "remembering" former experiences, becomes much prompter and more violent in its expressions of resentment at each fresh meeting of the allergen and the allergic antibodies.

Types of Allergy

There are two principal types of allergy: (1) the familial type, and (2) the acquired or induced type.

In familial allergy, the shock tissue is inherited, that is, it "runs in the family." Examples of familial allergies are eczema, hay fever, bronchial asthma, allergic rhinitis, and some cases of urticaria (hives) and migraine (severe, one-sided headache). The allergens involved are usually those to which almost everyone is almost constantly exposed, such as common protein foods and plant pollens. Probably that is why allergy is most often defined as a condition of unusual or exaggerated sensitivity (hypersensitivity) to a substance harmless in similar amounts for most people.

Some forms of allergy are caused by substances with which most individuals seldom or never come in contact. Such uncommon substances include animal serums used in medical treatments, various drugs, products of bacterial growth, certain ingredients in cosmetics, and various materials used in industry. Allergy caused by some of these substances may be either familial or acquired, but usually it is acquired or induced. The defense mechanism involved is, in many instances, unknown; that is, no specific antibodies can be demonstrated. The reactions are so typical, however, that there is no doubt that they are allergies.

Sensitizing the Shock Tissue

Whether a predisposition to a certain form of allergy is inherited or hypersensitivity to a particular substance is acquired, no form of allergy ever develops unless previous contact with the allergen has occurred. That first contact results only in sensitizing the shock tissue. There is no sickness, no indication of what is going to happen the next time that particular allergen is encountered. A baby who has inherited a shock tissue sensitive to egg white, for example, will show no signs of distress when first given egg white. But after that first sensitizing dose, as it is called, all subsequent or exciting doses will result in allergic manifestations, the kind of manifestation depending upon the shock tissue inherited.

Finding the Offending Substance

Physicians now have various tests by which the offending substance, or substances, can be identified when some form of allergy is suspected.

Patch Tests. If the trouble seems to be a contact dermatitis, that is, a skin inflammation caused by sensitivity to one or more substances that come into contact with the skin (see Allergic Skin Reactions, in Chap. 15), the tests given will be patch tests, because in contact dermatitis the epidermis, or surface layer of the skin, is the shock tissue. In the patch test the suspected material is placed on the skin, covered with a small square of cellophane, and held down with a strip of adhesive, Scotch tape, or collodion. The reaction is read by the physician in two to four days.

Scratch Tests and Intradermal Tests. If suspicion lights on a food or foods or some other allergen that is brought to the shock tissue by the blood, the tests given will be scratch tests or intradermal tests. These tests are based on the fact that the allergic antibodies in the familial type of allergy (reagins) are skin-sensitizing antibodies. That is, when they are present in the blood they are also found attached to the skin. When the corresponding allergen is injected into the skin, fluid collects between the cells, giving rise to a wheal (see Formation of Wheals, in Chap. 15). In giving a scratch test, a specially prepared extract of the suspected substance is put into scratches made through the upper layers of the epidermis without drawing blood. In the intradermal test, a small amount of liquid extract of the suspected substance is injected between the layers of the skin. The appearance of a wheal and a surrounding area of redness indicates a positive reaction.

The Mechanism of Allergy

Although different individuals react to different substances in skin tests to find the allergens responsible for allergic conditions, the skin reactions themselves are alike. The lump or wheal raised on the skin after the injection of an extract of wheat in a person allergic to wheat, for example, will be no different from the wheal raised after the injection of a pollen extract in a person sensitive to that pollen. For this reason, scientists have long believed that there must be some substance released in the tissues which is common to all allergic reactions. It is now believed that histamine, which is a normal component of many tissues, is such a substance.

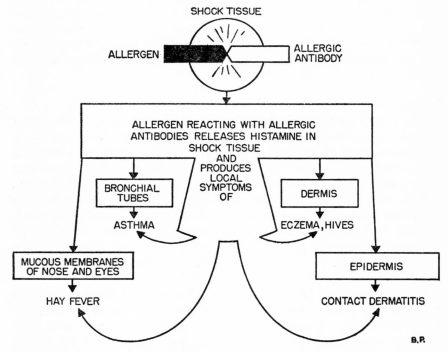

FIG. 7-4. A diagrammatic representation of the mechanism of allergic reactions.

According to the commonly accepted theory of allergy, the irritation of the shock tissue, which takes place when the allergen unites with its sensitizing antibody, results in the setting free of histamine (or a histaminelike substance). It is the liberated histamine that produces the manifestation of allergy.

The discovery of the role of histamine in allergic reactions naturally led to a search for substances that would neutralize or act as an antidote to histamine. A large number of drugs that act as histamine antagonists have been found. These "antihistamines," as they are called, do not cure any form of allergy but merely relieve its distressing symptoms—the intense itching of hives, for example, or the sneezing in hay fever.

Permanent cure of any allergic condition depends upon finding the offending allergen and then avoiding it or being protected from it. The means used to confer protection is to give the offending substance in very small amounts, which are gradually increased until the patient is able to tolerate it nearly as well as persons who are not allergic to it.

Emotional Influences

The emotions exert a strong influence on allergic disorders. Under the stress of worry, fear, anger, resentment, or excitement, an allergic attack may flare up in a susceptible person or an existing condition may become worse. Or persons not known to be allergic may develop symptoms of a severe physical allergy when emotionally disturbed. Sometimes the physical condition does not improve until the person is helped to iron out his emotional conflicts.

Bacterial Allergy

Several skin tests that have an allergic basis are used as aids in diagnosis or in finding out whether a person is susceptible to, or immune from, a specific communicable disease. The reason for this is that certain bacteria bring about the development of an allergy either to the protein in their bodies or to their secretions or toxins. This allergic reaction may take place instead of, or in addition to, the formation of protective bacterial antibodies. Tubercle bacilli are the best-known bacteria that bring about a changed response in a body that has once been invaded by them (see Tuberculosis, in Chap. 11).

Another manifestation of bacterial allergy is the hypersensitivity to bacterial residents of the skin which sometimes develops in chronic skin inflammations. In other words, skin that is chronically inflamed may become allergic to alien bacteria that it receives into residence. Although the bacteria may not produce open evidences of infection, they may slow up the progress of the skin to normality. That is why some chronic inflammations of the skin, eczema, for example, are often difficult to cure.

REACTIONS TO INTERNAL TEMPERATURE CHANGES

The temperature inside the body is due to the heat produced by the burning, or oxidation, of foodstuffs by the cells. Although there is a daily swing of a few tenths of a degree from a normal low in the small hours of the morning to a normal high in the afternoon, 98.6°F is generally accepted as normal mouth temperature.

How Body Temperature Is Regulated

A "thermostat" in the lower brain regulates body temperature. When too much heat is being produced in the body, as in strenuous exercise, the blood flowing through this thermostat is hotter than usual. This is a signal for sending the autonomic impulses to the small blood vessels in the skin which cause them to open up. As a result, the warmer blood of deeper regions is diverted through them and in its passage loses its excess heat through radiation, conduction, and convection.[3]

However, the air surrounding the body may already be so warm that not much heat from the skin can flow into it (conduction). Or the air may be so still that the heated air cannot be shifted away from the skin by means of air currents (convection). In these cases autonomic nerve impulses cause the sweat glands to pour out perspiration on the surface of the skin. The evaporation of the sweat aids in the removal of heat from the body.

In cold weather the temperature of the surrounding air is considerably lower than that of the skin. Then autonomic nerve impulses from the surface of the body cause the thermostat to send orders to shut down (constrict) the skin blood vessels. As a result, little or no blood can flow through them. Instead of being "red" with heat, the skin may become "blue" with cold and covered with gooseflesh (see Chilling, in Chap. 11). Also, the sweat glands are inhibited to prevent the flow of perspiration to the skin. Thus heat loss is reduced to a minimum. At the same time, body metabolism is speeded up so that additional heat is produced. If the amount of heat thus made available is still not enough, shivering sets in and perhaps the teeth chatter. Shivering is really forced exercise induced to increase muscular activity and thereby the production of additional heat.

Fever

Fever is a sign that the body is producing more heat than usual because of some unusual or abnormal stimulus. In the great majority of cases, the stimulus is the toxin produced by the pathogens responsible for an in-

---

[3] Radiation is the giving off of heat in all directions; conduction, the flow of heat from a warmer surface to a cooler one; convection, the transmission of heat by means of currents of air or water.

fection. Yet a person coming down with an infectious fever usually feels chilly and looks pale. This is explained by the fact that the toxin of the infecting organism at first touches off the same mechanism which in health prevents a fall in temperature when the body is exposed to cold; that is, the surface blood vessels are constricted and the heat production of the body is increased by shivering.

We all know that the fire in a furnace may be blazing merrily, but the building will be cold if the radiators in the different rooms are turned off. Just so, a person may have a high fever and yet shiver and complain of feeling cold because his skin radiators (surface blood vessels) are closed to the warm blood which in health keeps him comfortably warm by stimulating the heat receptors in his skin. Later on, in fever, heat impulses from the deeper structures of the body result in the opening up of the surface blood vessels, the blood flow through the skin increases, the skin becomes flushed, and the sick person feels hot. This is a sign that the balance between heat production and heat loss has been restored but has been set at a higher level than in health. In other words, the body's "thermostat" has been turned up a point or so.

Although fever rightly alarms us and we are glad when it starts to go down during an acute illness, it is actually a protective device. There is good reason to believe that its occurrence is an important aid to the body in fighting disease. The very fact of its presence, however, is an indication that the body is engaging in such a fight and needs the aid that only the physician is prepared to give.

Indications of Fever. The quickest and surest way of telling whether a child has a fever is to take his temperature with a clinical thermometer. In schools that have nursing service, the nurse usually does this when the teacher suspects that a child is feverish. Indications of fever may be pallor, chilliness, and shivering; or flushed skin and languor, drowsiness, or restlessness. Such signs and symptoms may or may not be accompanied by others, such as nausea or vomiting; headache, earache, or aching in the limbs and back; running nose, sore throat, sneezing, red watery eyes, or tight dry cough.

Some slowly developing infections may be accompanied by low-grade fever and other mild warnings before more alarming signs and symptoms develop. Rheumatic fever (see Chap. 10) and tuberculosis (see Chap. 11) are illnesses of this type.

THE MECHANISM OF PAIN

The stimulation of specific receptors called "pain receptors" arouses the sensation of pain. These end organs of pain are free nerve endings located in the skin, in blood vessels, in muscles and joints, in nerve sheaths, and in many other body organs. They are the most widely distributed receptors in the body.

It is generally agreed that a physical stimulus adequate to excite pain is one that threatens damage to the tissues. In other words, "where there is pain, there is injury." For this reason pain has been classified as a protective sensation, as opposed to sensations like sight and hearing which convey information. Pain gives warning of the injurious nature of a stimulus. It provokes reflex actions that are defensive or protective or result in withdrawal of the part from the stimulus. The classic example is the rapid withdrawal of a hand from a hot stove. If it is severe enough, pain inhibits all other reflexes and is imperative in its demand for attention. It is not protective, in the usual sense, because some injury has already been done before it is felt. Indeed it may actually be harmful, for example, in preventing full function of a part, as in a sprain, or in setting up a reflex that makes pain continue long after its original cause has disappeared. Under ordinary circumstances, however, pain is highly useful in calling attention to many conditions that might cause serious illness or death if allowed to progress.

Pain receptors do not respond to any one kind of stimulus as the other sensory receptors do. To produce the sensation of pain any type of stimulus—mechanical, chemical, or thermal (heat and cold)—will do, provided it is intense enough. No definite sensory centers for pain like those for sight and hearing have been located in the brain. Nevertheless, the brain interprets the sensation as coming from the part of the body which it associates with the particular nerve fibers affected. That is, it is trained to localize pain. This ability of the brain permits us to know that we have a pain in the stomach, or the foot, or the head, and so on. But what actually is causing the pain, unless it has a perfectly obvious cause, like a nail in the sole of a shoe, or a beesting, or a burn, is beyond us. Of course, this does not keep us from making guesses, which may or may not be correct.

Itching

The sensation of itching is caused by irritation of the touch-pressure or pain receptors in the skin. It has been called a low-grade form of pain. It draws attention to skin irritants and sets up the scratch reflex. The scratch reflex was designed to serve a useful purpose as a means of getting rid of causes of irritation. However, it has turned out to be something of a nuisance. Whenever intense itching impels us to scratch we remember that it is not good to scratch, since that act increases irritation of the skin and, in some conditions, leads to the spread of infectious material.

Itching is a common annoyance in a great many different varieties of skin irritations as well as in some systemic diseases. Children who complain frequently of itching or who show scratch marks should be referred for medical attention.

Referred Pain

The ramifications of the nervous system are so complex that pain impulses originating at one point are often felt at some other point. Any area from which pain originates has been called a "trigger point." The trigger point becomes a "miniature sending station" when stimulated by an anatomical or physiological change. Just as a man in California may tune in through a local hookup on music broadcast over a radio network from New York, so one area of the body may tune in through a local hookup with pain impulses broadcast over a nerve network from some other area. In whatever area pain impulses are aroused, either directly by contact with the stimulus or indirectly by referral from some other area, pain is felt.

The phenomenon of referred pain, as it is called, explains why any one organ, like the heart, or one part of the body, like the head, may be innocent of causing many feelings of discomfort blamed on it. For example, the cavity of the chest and the upper part of the abdomen, which is separated from the chest by only a thin sheet of muscle (the diaphragm), are packed tightly with organs. Any extra pressure, such as gas in the stomach or small intestine, may give rise to pain in the region of the heart with which the heart has nothing whatever to do.

Psychogenic Pain

Pain may be caused by psychic influences as well as by physical stimuli. If it seems strange to think that such an unpleasant symptom may in some cases have no physical basis, we have only to remember that emotion, when strong enough, can raise up many objective signs of distress—gooseflesh, sweating, pallor, and so on. When pain occurs without any discoverable physical stimulus, then it is ascribed to the influence of the psyche on the autonomic nervous system.

"Nervous headache" and "nervous indigestion" are two well-known terms which show that practically everyone has at least a vague understanding of the influence of emotional tension or worry in the causation of pain. The school child who persistently has "nine o'clock headache" has a pain no less real than has the child suffering from eye fatigue. And in both cases there is need to find the reason why.

Dealing with Complaints of Pain

In dealing with children it may be difficult to decide what complaints of pain warrant immediate medical investigation. As with many different signs and symptoms, pain as an indication of illness seldom occurs alone. It is so often associated with other indications of trouble that it is a common component of a symptom complex, that is, a combination of two or more signs and symptoms. That, in itself, may serve as a guide in deciding whether a child who complains of headache or stomach ache or leg ache, and so on, is in immediate need of medical attention. But whether other symptoms and signs are present or not, it is good sense to send children to the nurse or physician for any puzzling, unusual, severe, or persistent ache or pain. Only a physician has the training and experience required to detect signs hidden from a layman which help to supplement the evidence of pain and so point the way to a discovery of its cause.

FOR REVIEW AND DISCUSSION

1. Tell the difference between the words or terms in each of the following pairs:

   a. Signs and symptoms
   b. Organic illness and functional illness
   c. Cocci and bacilli
   d. Viruses and bacteria
   e. Vaccines and toxoids
   f. Active immunity and passive immunity
   g. Familial allergy and acquired allergy
   h. Chills and fever (give physiological distinction)
   i. Referred pain and psychogenic pain

2. What, if any, useful purpose is served by the following reactions:

Coughing	Shivering
Watering of the eyes	Fever
Inflammation	Pain
Sweating	Itching

3. In each of the following groupings of communicable diseases, there is one that does not belong in the group. Select the one that does not belong and tell why.

   a. Scarlet fever, pneumonia, tuberculosis, meningitis
   b. Diphtheria, syphilis, typhoid fever, whooping cough
   c. Poliomyelitis, measles, chicken pox, malaria

4. Select the correct ending for each of the following incomplete sentences:

   a. Antibodies differ from white blood cells in that antibodies (1) are formed by the body to fight specific diseases, (2) are not present in the blood, (3) are more resistant to bacteria than are white cells.
   b. Active immunity from a specific disease is acquired artificially by (1) having the disease, (2) receiving a shot of immune serum or gamma globulin, (3) being inoculated with a vaccine or toxoid.

SELECTED REFERENCES

American Academy of Pediatrics: *Report of the Committee on the Control of Infectious Diseases*, The Academy, Evanston, Ill., 1964.

American Medical Association: *Allergies*, The Association, Chicago. (A booklet explaining allergic reactions and various types of allergy.)

American Public Health Association: *Control of Communicable Diseases in Man*, 9th ed., The Association, New York, 1960. (A standard handbook listing diseases alphabetically and giving for each one the means of identification, occurrence, infectious agent (when known), reservoir and source of infection, mode of transmission, incubation period, susceptibility, resistance, and methods of control.)

Best, C. H., and N. B. Taylor: *The Human Body* (first given as reference in Chap. 1). Part III, *The Fluids of the Body*, Chap. 11. (Defensive mechanisms against disease, chemotherapy, antibiotics, surgical shock, anaphylaxis, and allergy.)

Feinberg, Samuel M.: *Living with Your Allergy*, J. B. Lippincott Company, Philadelphia, 1958.

Grant, Madeleine P.: *Louis Pasteur: Fighting Hero of Science*, McGraw-Hill Book Company, New York, 1959. (A book that will help both teachers and their students to understand the value of Pasteur's work as it developed from the study of crystals to the discovery of the principle of vaccination.)

Grenowicz, Antoni: *Bela Schick and the World of Children*, Abelard-Schuman, Limited, New York, 1955. (A story about the man who developed the Schick test for susceptibility to diphtheria.)

Selye, Hans: *The Stress of Life* (first given as reference in Chap. 6). Book II, *The Dissection of Stress*.

Swartz, Harry F.: *The Allergic Child*, Frederick Ungar Publishing Co., New York, 1959.

Swartz, Harry F.: *Allergy: What It Is and What to Do about It*, rev. ed., Faber & Faber Ltd., London, 1963.

Williams, Greer: *The Virus Hunters*, Alfred A. Knopf, Inc., New York, 1959. (Interesting account of many different accomplishments in the field of research in virology.)

Chapter 8   ORGANIC DISORDERS OF THE NERVOUS AND ENDOCRINE SYSTEMS

Infections of the Central Nervous System
Disorders of the Brain
When Endocrine Glands Go Wrong

In general, there are two causes for disorders of the nervous system. One is organic, the other functional. Organic disorders may be caused by infection or injury or by some defect of the brain. In functional disorders nothing organically wrong in the nervous system can be found. A person suffering from a disorder of this kind is said to be mentally ill. Various types of mental illness will be discussed in the next chapter.

INFECTIONS OF THE CENTRAL NERVOUS SYSTEM

With the exception of poliomyelitis, infections of the central nervous system are rare in school children. And with widespread immunization polio is also becoming a rare disease. Descriptions of several infections which attack the brain or spinal cord or both are given here for teachers or school nurses who may be concerned about them because of cases occurring in the school or community, or because methods of control depend upon knowing how they are spread and what measures are available for their prevention.

Poliomyelitis

Poliomyelitis (commonly called *polio*), or infantile paralysis, is an infection caused by a virus of at least three distinct types known as poliovirus Types I, II, and III. The paralytic effects of polio occur in about 40 to 60 per cent of the cases in which poliovirus invades the central nervous system.

Inapparent and Abortive Polio. In the great majority of infections with poliovirus, the central nervous system is not involved. The largest group of infections of this kind is made up of inapparent or "silent" infections. Available evidence indicates that these symptomless infections occur in most individuals at some time during life. Another group of polio infections in which the central nervous system is apparently not involved occurs mainly during epidemics and is classified as abortive.

Abortive infections are characterized by a brief febrile illness accompanied by lack of appetite, nausea and vomiting, headache, sore throat, and vague abdominal pains. Recognition of abortive poliomyelitis is considered important because bed rest during the fever and for some days afterward may be a factor in preventing viral invasion of the nervous system.

Paralytic and Nonparalytic Polio. In infections in which the central nervous system is involved, poliovirus attacks motor neurons, that is, nerve cells responsible for bringing about motion in the muscles to which their fibers run. In paralytic cases destruction of motor neurons results in paralysis of the muscle fibers controlled by the destroyed neurons. Individual muscles or scattered groups of muscles are involved, according to the area in the central nervous system attacked by the virus. The destruction of motor cells in one area may result in the paralysis of fibers scattered throughout several muscles without affecting other fibers in the same muscles. In that case, there may be weakness rather than complete paralysis of certain muscles. Mild paralysis is often followed by complete recovery.

The most severe form of paralytic polio (bulbar poliomyelitis) results when the medulla oblongata (the lowest portion of the brain) and the neck region of the spinal cord are involved. Since the respiratory center (see Nervous Control of Respiration, in Chap. 11) is located in the medulla, the breathing muscles may be paralyzed. Respirators of different types, including those sometimes called "iron lungs," are used to keep the patient breathing.

There is some evidence to show that immunizations from other diseases and operations performed on the nose, mouth, and throat during a polio epidemic may increase the danger of developing paralytic polio. For this reason, doctors used to advise the postponement of such procedures during polio epidemics, as they represented an unnecessary added risk. Even today, in certain cases, a physician may decide to postpone them if polio appears in the community.

In nonparalytic cases, the virus reaches the central nervous system and yet does not progress far enough in its depredations to cause paralysis. In most of these mild infections, there are no visible aftereffects. Some cases, however, may result in muscle weakness which goes unnoticed until minor deformities appear.

Early Signs and Symptoms. Signs and symptoms that may indicate the onset of polio are fever, drowsiness, headache, malaise (feeling ill), mild stiffness and pain in the muscles of the neck and back, nausea and vomiting, restlessness, irritability, diarrhea or constipation, sore throat, and chilliness. Naturally, all these signs and symptoms do not occur in the same individual, and many of them are typical of the onset of other communicable diseases of childhood. Diagnosis early in the disease, before paralysis has appeared or in nonparalytic cases, depends upon the results of specific diagnostic tests. Laboratory examinations of the feces and of the spinal fluid are helpful in reaching a diagnosis.

Improvements in Treatment. Physical therapy[1] under medical supervision after the acute phase of paralytic polio has passed is helpful in aiding stricken muscles to regain their use through exercise, reeducation, and training. How successful this treatment will be depends upon the number of nerve cells destroyed or damaged by the virus. In recent years there has been great improvement in techniques and devices for restoring function to paralyzed muscles, for example, muscle transplants, early splinting of the extremities using rubber bands to assist motion, and prosthetic devices to aid in moving paralyzed upper limbs. Great strides have also been taken in teaching patients whose breathing muscles have been affected to overcome dependence on iron lungs.

Mode of Infection. Poliovirus enters the body by way of the mouth or nose and multiplies in the intestines. It passes from the intestinal tract into the bloodstream. The virus invades the central nervous system by way of the bloodstream unless enough antibodies have been formed to destroy it before it gets there. As poliovirus is present both in the throat and in the intestinal tract of persons harboring it, both the nose and throat discharges and the intestinal discharges of infected persons (frequently those not suffering from a recognized attack) are sources of infection. Infection takes place most frequently through intimate contact between a susceptible individual and a person harboring the virus. If one member of a family group has polio, the others often are infected. These "contacts" may have slight febrile illnesses or show no indication of illness whatever. Mildly ill or apparently healthy carriers of the virus are supposed to play a major part in the spread of the infection. That is why it is best during epidemics to keep children away from people with whom they have not been associated right along.

Apparently the period during which individuals stricken with polio can communicate the disease to others is covered by the latter part of the incubation period and the first week of the acute illness. The incubation period is usually from seven to fourteen days but may be less than seven days and as long as thirty days.

Specific Control by Immunization. Natural immunity from polio is conferred on the vast fortunate majority by infections so mild that they pass unnoticed. But a small unfortunate minority must pay the price of paralysis for immunity gained naturally. The target toward which research workers aimed for well over fifty years was the development of a

---

[1] Physical therapy, as defined by the American Physiotherapy Association, is "the treatment of disability, injury, and disease by nonmedical means, comprising the use of massage, exercise, and the physical, chemical, and other properties of heat, light, water and electricity. . . ."

practical and safe vaccine capable of producing artificially, and without incurring the risk of paralysis, the immunity which nature produces in the course of polio infection.

The discovery made in 1949 by Dr. John F. Enders and his associates that poliovirus could be grown in the laboratory on non-nervous tissue made it possible to grow large quantities of virus of all three types for immunological studies. The object of these studies was to find a way to prevent the paralytic effects of polio infection by creating an antibody barrier in the bloodstream to intercept the virus before it could invade the central nervous system.

The first approach was passive immunization, that is, the injection of already formed polio antibodies to combat the virus before the body's own antibody-producing machinery was set in motion. The second approach was active immunization by the injection of a vaccine that would stimulate in the immunized person the formation of antibodies against all three types of poliovirus. Both of these approaches were explored by investigators whose work was financed to a large extent by the National Foundation for Infantile Paralysis (now the National Foundation) out of March of Dime funds.

Passive Immunization. In the polio epidemic seasons of 1951–1952, investigators made controlled field studies on the prevention of paralytic polio by gamma globulin. Since about 80 per cent of adults are immune from polio, largely as a result of inapparent infections, the gamma globulin obtained from pooled adult blood is sure to contain polio antibodies. Evaluation of the data collected indicates that gamma globulin is useful as a temporary protective measure against paralytic polio if injected within two days after exposure. It is now considered to be of little practical value in epidemics, however, because the virus may already be widely spread among household and other close contacts before the first case is recognized.

Active Immunization with Killed-virus Vaccine. The first successful vaccine for active immunization was developed by Dr. Jonas E. Salk and his collaborators in the Virus Research Laboratory, Department of Bacteriology, University of Pittsburgh School of Medicine. This vaccine contains poliovirus of all three types grown on minced monkey kidney tissue and killed with a solution of formaldehyde, commonly referred to as Formalin. Every particle of the disease-producing property of the virus in the vaccine is destroyed without destroying completely its capacity to induce the formation of antibodies.

After exhaustive tests made in experimental animals to prove that the vaccine was safe and effective, it was cautiously tried on human volunteers. The success of these preliminary trials led to the large-scale field trial of the Salk vaccine in 1954. The study population was made up of more than 1,800,000 first-, second-, and third-grade children in 217 study areas in forty-four states. The report on the safety and effectiveness of the Salk vaccine was given on April 2, 1955, by Dr. Thomas Francis, Jr., Director of the Poliomyelitis Vaccine Evaluation Center at the University of Michigan. The report indicated that the vaccine used in the field trial was safe and from 80 to 90 per cent effective in preventing paralytic polio.

After the field trial of 1954 the potency of the Salk vaccine was increased, and its efficiency estimated as between 90 and 95 per cent when the full course of inoculations has been administered. Hence the inactivated vaccine greatly reduces the risk of paralytic polio. It does not, however, prevent the multiplication of poliovirus in the intestinal tract or prevent the excretion of poliovirus in the intestinal discharges of those infected. Consequently, a person who is himself immune can become infected with poliovirus and transmit it to others.

The medically approved series of inoculations with Salk vaccine is given in the Immunization Timetable, Appendix A. Although the recommended thoroughgoing routine immunization of all persons in susceptible age groups was by no means carried out in the six years following the introduction of the Salk vaccine, there is no question that the use of this vaccine greatly reduced the incidence of paralytic polio (see Table 8-1) in the United States during that period.

Table 8-1

ANNUAL INCIDENCE OF REPORTED CASES OF POLIO
IN THE UNITED STATES BY PARALYTIC STATUS

Year	Number of Reported Cases			
	Paralytic	Nonparalytic	Unspecified	Total
1955	13,850	12,453	2,682	28,985
1956	7,911	6,555	674	15,140
1957	2,499	2,826	160	5,485
1958	3,697	1,941	149	5,787
1959	6,289	2,045	91	8,425
1960	2,525	626	39	3,190
1961	988	305	19	1,312

Source: U.S. Department of Health, Education, and Welfare, Public Health Service, 1962.

Active Immunization with Oral Live-virus Vaccine. Intensive efforts to develop live-virus vaccines were begun in the 1940s. The underlying theory on which this research work was based was that a vaccine containing attenuated, or weakened, live polioviruses given orally (by mouth) and allowed to multiply in the intestinal tract would stimulate the antibody response achieved through natural infection and thus give greater, longer-lasting protection from paralytic polio than could be given by a killed-virus vaccine.

The leaders of the teams searching for a safe and effective live-virus vaccine were Dr. Herald B. Cox of the Lederle Laboratories of the American Cyanamid Company, Dr. Hilary Koprowski (formerly a member of Dr. Cox's team) of the Wistar Institute, University of Pennsylvania, and Dr. Albert B. Sabin of the University of Cincinnati's School of Medicine.

In developing live-virus vaccines these research teams grew especially selected attenuated polioviruses of all three types in monkey kidney tissue, the same culture medium as that used in preparing the Salk vaccine. A different vaccine was developed for each type. After extensive tests on animals had demonstrated the safety and effectiveness of live-virus vaccines, human trials on an increasingly broad scale were made, particularly in foreign countries. In the Soviet Union and allied countries, for example, nearly 88 million persons were immunized with Sabin live-virus vaccine (manufactured in Moscow) in 1960.

Before being approved for general use in the United States, live-virus vaccines had to meet the rigid requirements for safety and effectiveness set up by the Biologic Standards Division of the Public Health Service's National Institutes of Health. Sabin Type I vaccine was licensed in August, 1961; Sabin Type II in October, 1961; and Sabin Type III in April, 1962. Community-wide immunization with live-virus vaccines is now recommended for all infants between the ages of six weeks and three months and for all other persons in susceptible older age groups regardless of whether they have already been immunized with Salk vaccine. The recommended schedule of immunization with oral polio vaccine is given in the Immunization Timetable, Appendix A.

The principal advantages of live poliovirus vaccines have been summarized as follows:

1. *Ease of administration.* The vaccine for each type of poliovirus is given by mouth in syrup, sugar, or candy.

2. *Speed in acquiring immunity.* Oral vaccines produce very prompt antibody response. Protection against all three types of poliovirus is achieved shortly after immunization has been completed over a twelve-week period (administration of Type I vaccine followed after an interval of six weeks by administration of Type III, and, finally, after another six-week interval, by the administration of Type II).

3. *Eventual development of a kind of "herd immunity" which hopefully may lead to the eradication of poliomyelitis.* The attenuated polioviruses in live-virus vaccines, like naturally occurring (wild) polioviruses, multiply in the intestinal tract and are excreted in intestinal discharges. The families and playmates of children who have been immunized with live-virus vaccine also become immunized through intimate contact with them. Furthermore, the multiplication in the intestinal tract of attenu-

ated polioviruses is followed not only by the development of antibodies in the blood but also by a change in the intestinal tract which interferes with the subsequent multiplication of naturally occurring polioviruses. Consequently, when a large proportion of any population group has received the oral vaccines, the increased intestinal resistance to infection leads to a break in the chain of transmission of wild polioviruses. The hope of completely eradicating poliomyelitis, however, depends upon the continued immunization of infants with live-virus vaccines after mass community-wide programs have been completed.

A number of years may go by before the grim story of paralytic polio ends with its elimination. Furthermore, the National Foundation points out that there were tens of thousands of patients suffering from the aftereffects of paralytic polio at the beginning of the "vaccination era," and doubtless there will be many more victims before nationwide immunity has been achieved and maintained.

What the Teacher Can Do about Polio. With polio added to the ranks of diseases from which children can be protected by immunization, teachers can take an active part in the fight against this disease. In class discussions youngsters may have questions about immunization which teachers can use to satisfy curiosity and allay fears. Some parents may need reassurance about the safety of the vaccine before they are willing to have their children immunized. Older boys and girls, especially high school students, will profit from the study of polio in their health and science classes. They will be interested in the story of the development of killed-virus and live-virus vaccines and in keeping abreast of the news in many areas of polio research.

As the most optimistic estimates of the prospects for victory over polio by immunization indicate that cases will undoubtedly occur for some time to come, teachers should continue to keep on the lookout before school closes in the summer and after it opens in the fall for symptoms which may, or may not, indicate polio. Any child who seems ill in school should be taken home, and the parents should be impressed, without being unduly alarmed, with the importance of putting the child to bed, isolating him from others, and getting medical advice promptly.

Another important function of the teacher is the supervision of children who have returned to school after an attack. Often she can be very helpful in encouraging parents and children to return to the hospital or clinic for scheduled checkups. Many children returning to school will have recovered completely. However, children who have had polio should be guarded for some time against fatigue and overexertion, as muscle weakness is a common aftereffect. It is recommended that they be watched carefully for at least two years for postural irregularities and speech defects,

Some children who return to school after a bout with paralytic polio may be severely or moderately crippled. It is generally agreed that "learning to help himself is the crippled child's salvation." The helpful sympathetic teacher will be able to find many ways of giving unobtrusive assistance to the disabled child and of guiding other children in giving him help and encouragement.

Meningitis

The outer covering of the brain and spinal cord consists of three layers of membrane called collectively the *meninges*. Meningitis is a general term for inflammation of these membranes. It occurs when pathogens of any one of several different families pass from the bloodstream into the fluid which bathes the brain and spinal cord. By laboratory examination of a sample of cerebrospinal fluid, physicians can determine which form of meningitis—meningococcal, pneumococcal, streptococcal, fungal, or influenzal, for example—is causing the infection in suspected cases. Once the diagnosis is made, most patients can be cured with appropriate sulfa or antibiotic drugs if treatment is started early in the disease. That is why prompt recognition of infections of the meninges is extremely important.

Meningococcal Meningitis. This form of meningitis is caused by members of the genus of bacteria known as meningococci. Characteristically it occurs in epidemics at irregular intervals. Since it attacks the meninges of both the brain and the spinal cord, it is sometimes called epidemic cerebrospinal meningitis. The sulfa drugs and the antibiotics are now being used successfully to control outbreaks of this disease. In the epidemic waves, which last two or three years, the most severe infections occur among adults. In interepidemic periods sporadic attacks occur chiefly in children.

Susceptibility to clinical, or severe, meningococcal meningitis is very slight; that is, the attack rate among those exposed is low. However, there are many subclinical, or mild, cases. Slight attacks may be marked only by a mild sore throat with or without headache, malaise, low-grade fever, and pains in joints and muscles. Many people recover from a mild attack without knowing they have had the infection.

Infection with meningococci takes place by way of the nasopharynx (see The Respiratory System in Chap. 11). The microorganisms live in the throats of apparently healthy people and are largely responsible for the spread of the disease during epidemic periods.

It is impossible to isolate carriers during epidemics because of their great number. Giving sulfadiazine in small doses for two or three days to all persons closely associated with one another (as in schools or camps) who have been exposed to a known case of epidemic cerebrospinal meningitis eliminates the meningococci from the nose and throat of carriers and usually stops the epidemic.[2]

Mosquito-borne Encephalitis

This name is given to a group of acute inflammatory diseases involving parts of the brain, spinal cord, and meninges which are transmitted by the bite of infective mosquitoes. Each disease in the group is caused by a specific virus. The three members of the group occurring in the United States and Canada are the Eastern equine type (eastern United States and Canada), the Western equine type (western United States and Canada), and the St. Louis type (most parts of the United States except the Northeast). Mosquito-borne encephalitis may resemble a great variety of other infections involving the central nervous system, and its specific identification requires laboratory examination of blood-serum specimens. Attacks vary greatly in severity, ranging from a mild, short-lasting illness to a very serious illness which may end fatally. Severe infections usually have an acute onset with high fever, stupor, and disorientation. Upon recovery permanent aftereffects are rare except in infants.

Mosquito-borne encephalitis is erroneously referred to as "sleeping sickness," the scientific name for which is *encephalitis lethargica*. The cause of this type of encephalitis is unknown. (It is not the same disease as African sleeping sickness caused by trypanosomes spread by the bite of the tsetse fly.) Encephalitis lethargica occurred frequently just before and after the year 1920, but apparently it has now disappeared from the world.

One or more species of mosquitoes are responsible for the spread of each type of mosquito-borne encephalitis. Mosquitoes usually acquire the infection from wild birds but occasionally from a mammal, such as a horse. The virus cannot be found in human blood after the onset of the disease, and probably there is never enough present to infect a mosquito.

Mosquito-borne encephalitis is commonly limited to areas of high temperatures where there are many mosquitoes. Outbreaks may occur in the temperate latitudes during the summer and early fall in years of high temperatures when mosquitoes are especially prevalent.

A great deal of local publicity is usually given to outbreaks of this disease. Teachers can be of great service in educating students and their parents as to its mode of transmission and the methods of controlling its spread. These methods include measures taken by the community to eliminate mosquito-breeding places, the spraying of homes with ap-

---

[2] Information concerning meningococcal meningitis is given in Sec. 1 of Appendix B. For general measures that should be taken in schools during epidemics of communicable disease spread by discharges from the respiratory tract, see The School and Respiratory Disease Control in Chap. 11.

proved insecticides to kill mosquitoes, and avoidance of exposure to mosquitoes during hours of biting, or the use of chemical repellents to discourage them from biting.

Tetanus

Tetanus (lockjaw) is caused by a toxin produced by a bacillus (*Clostridium tetani*) which multiplies rapidly in the absence of oxygen. Favorable conditions for the growth of tetanus bacilli occur when these organisms are driven into the tissues where they are sealed away from the air. Consequently, any deep wound with a narrow or sealed opening or any deep lacerated wound in which chips of glass, wood splinters, or grains of dirt have become embedded carries with it the danger of tetanus.

Tetanus toxin, produced by the bacilli living and growing within the tissues, has an affinity for the central nervous system. Having reached there, it exerts an action that produces painful muscular contractions, primarily of the jaw and neck muscles. In its efforts to counteract or neutralize the toxin, the body produces antitoxin. The incubation period elapsing between the time of infection and the development of the first symptoms is commonly from four days to three weeks, depending somewhat upon the character, extent, and location of the wound.

Tetanus bacilli are present in the feces of some domestic animals, especially horses. They are common inhabitants of the superficial layers of the soil in many localities, especially in the earth of cultivated and manured fields and gardens. They exist in soil and street dust in the spore state. Spores are the seedlike forms taken on by certain bacteria when conditions are unfavorable for their growth. Tetanus spores may lie dormant for many years and then germinate into living, virulent bacilli when they get into a wound where living conditions are favorable. That is why it is so important in first-aid education to emphasize the necessity for getting immediate medical care for any irregularly torn or deep wound. It also should be pointed out, however, that burns and trivial or unnoticed wounds may furnish a portal of entry for tetanus bacilli.

Active immunization with tetanus toxoid gives solid and satisfactory protection. It has the advantage of removing the risk of tetanus in injuries usually considered too slight to require protective measures. As young children in the rough-and-tumble stage are likely to incur injuries of this kind, it is considered advisable to begin the active immunization of all children with tetanus toxoid in infancy in combination with diphtheria toxoid and pertussis vaccine (see the Immunization Timetable, Appendix A). A reinforcing (booster) injection of tetanus toxoid also is given to a previously actively immunized person who has received a wound that carries with it the danger of tetanus.

Tetanus antitoxin produced by immunizing horses is used in the treatment of tetanus to supplement the antitoxin already being produced in the body of a person sick with tetanus. If a person who has not previously been actively immunized receives an injury carrying the risk of tetanus, the physician may decide to give an injection of antitoxin. Before using tetanus antitoxin for passive immunization, however, it is usually considered advisable to administer a skin test for sensitivity to horse serum.

Rabies

Rabies is primarily a disease of a large group of wild and domestic animals including dogs, cats, foxes, coyotes, wolves, skunks, and raccoons. Rabies-infected bats also have recently been recognized in the United States.

Rabies is caused by a virus that is present in the saliva of the infected animal. When a person is bitten by a rabid animal, virus-bearing saliva enters the body through the break in the skin. Rarely it may enter the body through any fresh break in the skin licked by a rabid animal. The virus seems to take the same route as tetanus toxin along the nerve trunks to the spinal cord and brain. Bites on surfaces covered by clothing are the least dangerous, and bites on the head, arms, and hands are the most dangerous.

The incubation period is variable, depending upon the severity of the bite and its location; it usually ranges from two to six weeks, but may be longer. Rabies does not develop in everyone bitten by a rabid animal; the virus may never get to the brain. But if it does get there the disease is almost invariably fatal. That is why everyone who has been bitten by an animal known or suspected of being rabid should be actively immunized from rabies with antirabic vaccine. If a biting animal is not captured and rabies is known to be present in a locality, vaccination should be started immediately. The vaccine is administered usually for fourteen consecutive days—sometimes longer in severe or multiple bites. Vaccination is often supplemented by antirabies serum containing already formed antibodies. In case of multiple bites, or bites on the face, head, or neck, antirabies serum may be given before the full course of antirabic vaccine is started.

The Biting Animal. A pet dog that has rabies usually shows a change in behavior. It may become greatly excited and vicious (furious rabies) or it may become unusually affectionate and very quiet and sleepy (dumb rabies). A stray dog or other animal that has bitten one or more persons should always be suspect. It is important to stress the fact that any pet animal that shows suspicious signs of rabies should immediately be taken to a veterinarian for observation. If such a pet animal or a stray animal has bitten one or more persons, it should not be killed except when necessary to keep others from being bitten. It should be captured, if possible. Then it should be shut up, preferably by a veterinarian or in an approved dog pound, and observed for ten days. If it remains healthy up to the end of that time, it does not have rabies. If it dies, immediate laboratory examination of its brain will show whether death was caused by rabies.

Healthy pet dogs and cats can be vaccinated against rabies. It is a great comfort to owners to know that their pets have been protected from this deadly disease and cannot transmit it to humans.

First Aid for Animal Bites. Wounds inflicted by animals should be cleansed immediately and thoroughly with soap and water or a detergent solution. The victim should then have prompt medical care so that required further treatment of the wound may be given and an investigation made to determine whether antirabic vaccine should be started.

DISORDERS OF THE BRAIN

When we remember that intelligence, thought, behavior, and all forms of voluntary and involuntary action are controlled by the central nervous system, we can readily understand that any disturbance at the seat of government is bound to be reflected in one or more deviations from normal in muscular action or in mental life or behavior.

Deviations of this kind include lack of nerve-muscle coordination, shown by such signs as dizziness, tremors, and twitching and spasm of the face and eyelids; rigidity or partial or complete paralysis of muscles; confused states, convulsions, drowsiness, and unlocalized headaches; and even changes in personality and character. Any one or more of such signs and symptoms may occur in infections or injuries of the brain or spinal cord or both, or in some disturbance of brain-cell activity.

Teachers may seldom or never have occasion to be the first to observe and call attention to conditions caused by actual destruction of tissue or by erratic functioning of various groups of brain cells. However, they may find it useful to have some knowledge of the more common brain disorders which may affect school-age children. Furthermore, there is much that teachers can do to help children suffering from such conditions when these youngsters are integrated into the regular classroom. They can also help to encourage in other children a humanitarian, accepting attitude toward handicapped individuals which they may carry into adulthood.

Epilepsy

Few disabilities are so misunderstood as epilepsy. The outcome of this ignorance is the wall of public prejudice faced by everyone known to be epileptic. It has been pointed out that the public's false concept is the greatest handicap that most epileptics must face. Teachers can perform a great service by helping to destroy this false image of epilepsy in the minds of their students.

Epilepsy is as old as man. From the beginning of recorded history it has been regarded as "an omen, a curse, the work of spirits, something fallen upon man, something that seized him from without." Even in modern times when belief in the supernatural causes of disease has practically died out in civilized societies, the attitude toward epileptics has changed little. Yet the great majority of persons subject to epileptic seizures are in every other respect perfectly normal human beings. Many of them are exceptionally talented or above average in intelligence. Indeed, epilepsy has not proved to be a barrier to outstanding achievement and distinction. Many celebrated personages in the past have been epileptics—among them, Julius Caesar, Lord Byron, Algernon Charles Swinburne, Guy de Maupassant, Paganini, and Vincent van Gogh—and there are famous people with epilepsy living today.

Epilepsy is not a rare disease, but it is difficult to determine its prevalence accurately largely because fear of disclosure is so great that the condition is kept secret by those who can do so. For this reason, typical health-survey methods do not uncover most cases of epilepsy. Its approximate prevalence in the United States is 1 per cent of the population. The estimated number of cases among children and youth is 300,000.

Causes and Types. Epilepsy manifests itself in widely different ways. "Seizure" is the word used in referring to its outward manifestations. Seizures and the form they take depend upon an underlying difficulty in the brain associated with an abnormal electrical activity (dysrhythmia).

The most useful instrument used in diagnosis is the electroencephalograph (*electro* meaning "electric"; *encephalo* meaning "brain"; and *graph* meaning "writing") which makes a written record of the brain's electrical activity. This record is called an electroencephalogram (EEG for short). An EEG consists of a series of little waves, called brain waves. The waves form typical patterns known as brain-wave patterns. In most persons subject to epilepsy the brain-wave patterns are different from those of people who do not have epilepsy.

The etiology (cause) of epilepsy is associated with three contributing factors—a hereditary factor, an acquired factor, and a precipitating factor. All three may enter into the causal chain of events. Persons who have epileptic seizures usually show the first symptoms in childhood.

In at least three out of ten cases, epileptics show evidence of brain damage due to head injury, infection, fever, tumor, a circulatory disorder, or some other abnormal condition in the brain. Many authorities believe that most if not all epilepsy results from such causes. But brain damage responsible for epilepsy is commonly slight and frequently cannot be identified. Such cases are called idiopathic (origin unknown), and seizures in this group may simply be attributed to disturbances in brain-cell metabolism. Emotional upsets or a sudden severe emotional shock may be a factor in bringing on seizures.

Most authorities agree that too much emphasis has been laid on the role of heredity in predisposing a person to epilepsy. The figures most frequently quoted indicate that an epileptic with a normal spouse will, on the average, have one chance in forty of having an epileptic child, while this chance is about one in two hundred when neither parent is epileptic. There are, however, no significant data that would enable an investigator to calculate specifically the chance of epilepsy develop-ing in the offspring of any marriage. Cases of epilepsy in which hereditary factors predominate actually respond better to treatment and have fewer seizures and fewer behavior difficulties.

The two best-known types of seizures are grand mal (great illness) and petit mal (little illness). There are, however, other epileptic disorders that may be manifested only in disturbances in learning and conduct. Grand mal seizures are convulsions that occur when an excessive release of electrical energy is generalized in the brain. In petit mal seizures the electrical disturbance is also generalized but is cut short before a convul-sion develops. The most common symptom of both types is loss or im-pairment of consciousness.

In petit mal interruptions in consciousness lasting for a fraction of a second to several minutes may take place many times a day or when some critical situation arises. A child suffering from petit mal may "blank out" when a direction is being given by his parents or teacher or during play or conversation. As the child may only blink a few times, look blank, and then keep on with what he was doing at the time, these seizures are often overlooked. Since he does not know what was said or done during his blank periods, the child may gain the reputation among adults of being inattentive or disobedient, and among his playmates of being stupid.

Teachers who have been especially tried by a child's inattentiveness or disobedience have, in some cases, been responsible for the discovery of previously unsuspected petit mal by reporting their observations to the school nurse or physician or to the child's parents. The confusion caused in the child's mind by frequent petit mal seizures usually clears up quickly when proper treatment is given.

The epileptic seizure, characterized by convulsions as well as loss of consciousness, is most commonly associated in the popular mind with epilepsy. Grand mal is frequently preceded by a warning called an "aura." The aura may consist of a feeling of unusual depression or ex-hilaration, smelling strange odors or seeing strange sights, pain in the limbs or stomach, trembling, or the impression that air is blowing on some part of the body and passing upward toward the head. A child subject to grand mal seizures should be watched for such premonitory symptoms. He may learn to report them immediately when he understands what they signify. When the aura occurs, the child should sit down or lie down in a safe place.

At the beginning of the actual attack, the epileptic becomes very pale, often cries or screams, and then loses consciousness. His body first becomes stiff, then his arms, legs, and head contract spasmodically in a series of jerks or convulsions. He ceases to breathe momentarily, and his face becomes blue. Often he froths at the mouth. The convulsive stage usually lasts for only a few minutes and is followed by a return of breathing and a normal color.

During the convulsive stage, the person rolls his eyes and clamps his teeth shut. He may bite his tongue or cheeks, with the result that the froth on his lips becomes bloodstained. Urination and a bowel movement may occur involuntarily. This stage lasts for several minutes, after which the person slowly regains consciousness or falls into a deep sleep resembling unconsciousness.

An epileptic seizure seems very alarming to those who witness it. However, the person feels no pain and rarely hurts himself seriously unless he is in a precarious position at the beginning of the seizure. No attempt should be made to restrain the convulsive movements of a child in an epileptic fit. The most that should be done is to keep him from injuring himself. Placing a pencil wrapped in cloth between his teeth will keep him from biting or chewing his tongue. Putting something soft under him like a folded coat or a blanket will help to prevent injury which may be sustained in thrashing about during the convulsive stage.

In the third, or "afterstage" the child should be kept quiet until he has fully regained consciousness or has awakened from sleep. He should be placed on his side, and his chin kept forward to aid breathing. Usually the child returns to normal within half an hour.

Medicines called anticonvulsants are proving to be very successful in controlling epileptic seizures of the grand mal type. Half the cases can be made completely free of seizures, and in an additional 30 or 35 per cent seizures can be reduced in severity or frequency.

The Epileptic Child in School. School authorities in most places now agree that, with reasonable seizure control available, there is no justification for the exclusion of the epileptic child from the regular classroom. The child should be institutionalized, or taught at home or in special classes, only if seizures are so frequent or so severe that their occurrence in the classroom seriously interrupts the work of the other children or are of such a character that attendance in regular class is harmful for the child.

Like other handicapped children, the epileptic child should lead as normal a life as possible. Segregation in most cases is not necessary and is apt to be harmful. An occasional epileptic seizure handled in a calm, informed way by a classroom teacher is a beneficial experience for other children. Indeed, the teacher may profitably discuss the whole problem of epilepsy with her students and help them to understand that an epileptic child, like the diabetic or the cardiac child, is in most cases no different from other children, except for his malady, and should be treated accordingly. She may broaden the discussion to help her children develop proper attitudes toward all sick or handicapped individuals.

Cerebral Palsy

Cerebral palsy is a sign that certain areas of the brain which govern muscular action have been put out of commission. In the great majority of cases some developmental defect in the brain before birth, or an intracranial hemorrhage occurring at the time of birth (birth injury) is responsible for this condition. When the areas of the brain involved in the ability to acquire and use facts are not affected, the child's intelligence is not impaired.

One common type of cerebral palsy is characterized by tense, contracted muscles (spasticity). The muscles tend to react far more strongly to stimuli than is necessary to bring about desired movements of the limbs. Spasticity is caused by damage to the motor area of the cortex. Another common type of cerebral palsy is athetosis. This type is characterized by involuntary or unorganized muscular movements. Usually it is caused by damage to the brain stem (a cerebral area below the cortex).

There are several other less common varieties of cerebral palsy. In one variety the child may have trouble maintaining his equilibrium (ataxia). He walks uncertainly or staggers and has great trouble in climbing stairs. In another variety the child may have constant regular trembling of the extremities, and in still another, a special kind of muscle rigidity "in which the muscles feel like soft lead." In the last two varieties (tremor and rigidity) large areas of the brain may be involved, with the result that intelligence is affected. However, few children with cerebral palsy have these involvements.

There are more victims of cerebral palsy than is generally realized. The estimated number in the United States under the age of twenty-one is from 200,000 to 300,000.[3] According to Dr. Winthrop M. Phelps, an authority on cerebral palsy, six out of every seven children born with cerebral palsy survive. Of these, two are feeble-minded and require institutional care. Of the remaining four who are presumed to be mentally normal, one is so severely crippled that he is classified as "homebound,"

[3] "Impairments among Young People," *Statistical Bulletin*, Metropolitan Life Insurance Company, Vol. 36, No. 8 (August) 1955. This range is based upon estimates made by Dr. Winthrop M. Phelps and confirmed by subsequent surveys of the incidence of cerebral palsy in a number of states and cities.

and one is handicapped to such a slight degree that he can compete on an equal basis with completely normal children. The remaining two are the ones "who present the greatest problems in physical and academic education."

With proper treatment and training, moderately disabled but mentally normal cerebral palsy sufferers can be greatly improved. In many cases they can attend regular school after everything possible has been done for them in therapeutic nursing schools or in other treatment-training centers. The teacher who has one of these children in her class can do a great deal to make his school life successful and happy. She can help him to win acceptance in his relationships with the other children and can do everything possible to raise his general morale and strengthen his will to achieve without seeming to give him undue attention.

Aphasia

This condition is the result of injury or disease of the brain centers that are concerned with the power of expression by speech, writing, or signs, or the ability to comprehend written or spoken language.

In recent years many people suffering from aphasia have been helped in special aphasia classes. Therapy is based on training the areas in the undamaged side of the cerebral cortex to take over the functions of those that have been put out of commission.

Aphasia occurs most frequently in adults as a result of disease or injury, but many children show a form of it. Such children may be very slow in learning to talk, although they are mentally alert. Or they may have great difficulty in acquiring any of the language skills. Of course, there are many possible causes for slowness in learning to speak, read, and write, but there is at least the possibility that a child who has this difficulty may have been born with some weakness in the language sphere. Since there are remedial measures that are helpful in many cases, a child who seems more than usually slow in acquiring the language skills should be referred to a physician, who may advise examination by a specialist.

Aphasia may be characterized by any one of four disabilities.

1. The power to express ideas in words may be almost completely lost. If the defect is less severe, words may be mispronounced, but the ability to construct sentences is not impaired. Persons with this type of aphasia have related difficulties in reading and writing.

2. The ability to speak is not lost, but the words come out in a jargon, or jumble, which is difficult to understand. Sometimes the speech is slurred. A person with this type of aphasia may be able to write but not to read coherently what he has written.

3. The ability to speak is not lost, but there is great difficulty in find-

ing the right words to express meanings or to name objects. Persons with this type of aphasia often substitute a descriptive phrase for the word they cannot recall. Best and Taylor give this example: "A painter when asked to name a series of colors could not say 'violet' but instead explained that "it was made with black, red, and a bit of blue.' " [4] It is difficult for these people to write coherently and carry out simple mathematical calculations.

4. The ability to speak, name objects, understand individual words, or pick out details in pictures, is not lost, but the general meaning of what is said or seen is not comprehended.

Physical Causes of Mental Retardation

Mental defectiveness in children may have its origin in conditions existing before or after birth. In about 50 per cent of all cases no specific cause can be found. The known causes of such conditions may be summarized as follows:

Head Injuries. Injury to the head occurring in prenatal life or at the time of birth or during childhood can leave a permanent effect on the development of the brain and of mental abilities. Any child who has received a severe blow on the head or has fallen on his head or has lost consciousness or has seemed dazed for even a very short time following a head injury should have medical attention at once.

Infections. The developing brain of an unborn child may be damaged by an infection transmitted to it by its mother. Rubella (German measles) and syphilis are the two infections that are definitely known to be transmissible from mother to unborn child.

Rubella during the first three months of pregnancy produces mental retardation, epilepsy, reading disability, or some other defect of personality development in about 10 per cent of the children. This knowledge has led to plans for seeing that every girl has German measles before puberty so as to protect any children she may have from this avoidable hazard.

Congenital brain damage caused by syphilis can be completely prevented because early diagnosis of syphilis in a pregnant woman followed by treatment protects the unborn child.

A number of general infections suffered during childhood have been known to produce permanent brain damage in some children. Fortunately, active immunization is available for some of these infections (whooping cough, influenza, and measles), and effective drug treatment for a few others can prevent brain damage.

Severe Malnutrition. Evidence to support the supposition that mental retardation in children can result from severe and specific nutritional

[4] Charles H. Best and Norman B. Taylor, *The Physiological Basis of Medical Practice* (6th ed., p. 1048). Williams and Wilkins, Baltimore, 1955.

deficiencies in the mother during pregnancy is not conclusive. It comes principally from animal experimentation and from observations of human beings during periods of famine. What evidence has been gathered so far has led to the suggestion "that if nutritional levels of proteins and vitamins in American women were higher than at present, some cases of mental retardation, epilepsy, reading disability, and other conditions would be prevented." [5]

There is no certainty that prolonged or repeated nutritional deficiencies in childhood can affect mental development. It is generally believed, however, that such deficiencies may cause considerable damage.

Genetic Influences. Mental defectiveness, when not due to environmental accidents (injuries or infections) before, during, or after birth, is often due to the fact that the child in question possesses a double dose of a particular defective gene which has been carried in hidden form by both his parents, or it may be due to the action of multiple genes. Most genes exert their influence through controlling one or more of the multitude of complex reactions on which our development and continued function depend (see Chromosomes and Genes, in Chap. 1).

Present prospects of identifying and remedying hereditary defects responsible for the less severe types of mental retardation are not bright. For many years to come most of the efforts in this field will probably be directed toward educating these children up to the limits of their capabilities (see Mentally Handicapped Children in School, in Chap. 5).

Expanding knowledge of genetics is, however, showing results in pinpointing the precise nature of several of the more extreme types of inherited mental defectiveness.

1. *Cretinism.* This condition is caused by the complete absence or extreme deficiency of the hormone (thyroxine) secreted by the thyroid gland. The cretin is a misshapen little creature with greatly retarded mental development. In regions of the world where there is a lack of iodine in the diet (see Goiter later in this chapter) the most common cause of cretinism is iodine deficiency in both mother and child because the thyroid must have iodine in order to produce thyroxine. With the widespread use of iodized salt instead of ordinary table salt all over the world, cretinism caused by iodine deficiency is being wiped out. But some children (fortunately very few) will still be born with cretinism either because the thyroid gland is totally absent at birth or because it is unable to synthesize thyroxine as a result of genetic (inherited) deficiencies. In both cases, recognition of the condition in the early months of life and administration of adequate amounts of thyroxine will permit the child to develop normally.

[5] *Mental Disorders,* American Public Health Association, New York, 1962, p. 43.

2. *Phenylketonuria.* This inherited disease causes a usually severe type of mental defectiveness. In a child born with phenylketonuria, the metabolism of one of the essential amino acids in protein (phenylalanine) is faulty. As a result, toxic by-products of phenylalanine accumulate in the blood and tissues in large quantities and affect the development and functioning of the brain. Mental defectiveness can be prevented by the early detection of a child born with this disease and by placing him on a diet very low in phenylalanine. Fortunately, a simple blood test is now available for detecting this disease soon after birth. The prevalence of phenylketonuria (PKU) is very low; it varies from 1 in 20,000 babies to 1 in 40,000.

3. *Galactosemia.* This disease causes profoundly retarded mental development due to an inherited defect that makes it impossible for a newborn child to change galactose (one of the two simple sugars in milk sugar) into glucose. Glucose is the body's principal source of energy (see Carbohydrates, in Chap. 12). The affected child literally starves in the midst of plenty. At the same time, the accumulation in the blood and tissues of the galactose that the child cannot use has a variety of harmful effects involving the eyes, the kidneys, and the brain. All the ill effects of this inherited defect disappear if the child is placed on a diet free of milk sugar. Again, early detection is of the utmost importance.

WHEN ENDOCRINE GLANDS GO WRONG

The effects of the hormones secreted by the endocrine glands are so interrelated that an extremely complicated sequence of events takes place when one gland does not function properly. Even physicians who specialize in endocrinology are cautious about diagnosing and treating endocrine disturbances. Temporary imbalances may occur, especially in children, which clear up spontaneously, that is, without special treatment. On the other hand, over- or underactivity of the endocrines does produce decided deviations from the normal, and teachers should have at least a speaking acquaintance with some of the possible effects of endocrine imbalance.

Variations in Body Build and Appearance

Hyperfunction (overactivity) and hypofunction (underactivity) of the endocrine glands controlling growth are associated with a number of variations in body build, appearance, and in some cases, mental development.

In reading the following summary of the anomalies of growth and development associated with the underactivity or overactivity of specific endocrine glands, it is important to keep in mind that the activities of the endocrines are so interrelated that more than one gland may be involved in producing the effects described.

Hyperfunction of the Anterior Pituitary. When the anterior pituitary is producing somewhat too much of its growth hormone the child is relatively tall for his age with the greatest length in the arms and legs, owing to accelerated growth of the long bones; also there is rugged development of the face, hands, and feet.

If far too much growth hormone is secreted before the fusion of the epiphyses (see How Bones Grow, in Chap. 3), the child will shoot up at a very rapid rate and reach a terminal height far above normal. This condition is known as *gigantism*. A human giant may become more than nine feet tall.

If excessive activity of the pituitary takes place after the fusion of the epiphyses, that is, after a person is fully grown, skeletal overgrowth occurs only in certain parts of the body. The condition in which parts of the skeleton and not the skeleton as a whole become enlarged is known as *acromegaly*. The bones of the face, hands, and feet often become markedly enlarged.

Hypofunction of the Anterior Pituitary. If the anterior pituitary is only somewhat underactive, the child is relatively slight in stature, reflecting the comparative delicacy of the skeleton and slower skeletal growth, especially in the long bones.

If the underactivity of the anterior pituitary is excessive, *dwarfism* is the result. The dwarf, or midget as he is commonly called, has normal skeletal proportions but is usually about one-half normal size. Some famous midgets have been much smaller.

Hyperfunction of the Thyroid. When the thyroid produces too much of its hormone (thyroxine) during the growth years, the rate of energy metabolism is speeded up above normal. As a result, the child is relatively tall and slender in stature, with slender hands and feet and delicately formed facial features owing to an acceleration of linear skeletal growth and a slowing down of lateral skeletal growth.

The hyperfunction that produces excessive loss of weight and marked restlessness and agitation in adults is very uncommon in childhood. It becomes more common in adolescence, but even then its incidence is undoubtedly low. One of the drugs that may be used in treating an enlarged, excessively active thyroid is thiouracil. This drug and others similar to it block an overactive thyroid and slow down its activity.

Hypofunction of the Thyroid. Complete absence or extreme deficiency of thyroid secretion at birth results in cretinism. (See Cretinism earlier in this chapter.) Cretinism is such a widely known condition that it is nearly always recognized promptly and adequately treated with thyroid extract. Occasionally, however, an adolescent is seen whose cretinism has been inadequately treated. Because the opportunity to remedy it should never be missed, any young person who shows signs of this form of hypothyroidism should have immediate medical attention. Failure to achieve a rate of linear growth far lower than the limits of normal variation is the outstanding finding. In addition, the skin is dry and the hair coarse; there is a puffy appearance, and the behavior is lethargic.

If thyroid deficiency develops after puberty, a condition known as *myxedema* develops. This condition is marked by sluggish mentality, vacant facial expression, obesity, and rough, puffy, dry skin. Treatment with thyroid extract usually produces brilliant improvement, especially in young patients. The excessive fatness and the facial dullness disappear, and mental keenness returns.

So much publicity has been given to the dramatic effects of thyroid extract in treating cretinism and myxedema that some adolescents—and their parents—get the idea that taking "a little thyroid" would help to remedy the situation if they are too fat or bored and lethargic and not doing too well in school. This thinking fails to take into consideration the fact that many young adolescents put on excess fat as part of their normal growth and development and that there are myriad other causes besides hypothyroidism for failure in school. Only a physician can decide, after making a variety of tests, whether thyroid medication is needed in a particular case.

Influence of the Adrenal Cortex on Growth. The sex hormones of the adrenal cortex appear to be in some way associated with the activity of the gonads, or sex glands. When the adrenal cortex is overactive, male sex characteristics become much more pronounced. A boy or man tends to be extremely masculine in build—the so-called "he-man" type. A girl or woman usually has a somewhat masculine build, masculine voice, much body hair, and frequently an excess of hair on the face. The development of masculine physical and mental traits in a girl or woman after puberty is called *virilism*. So-called "bearded ladies" are probably victims of an extremely overactive adrenal cortex.

Underactivity of the adrenal cortex has an inhibiting influence on growth and development. The child may be underdeveloped and thin in appearance with poor chest development and breathing capacity.

Goiter

The thyroid depends upon an adequate amount of iodine in the diet for the manufacture of its secretion, thyroxine. If it does not get enough iodine, it may become large enough to be noticeable. This condition is known as simple goiter. It occurs chiefly in regions where the drinking water and the soil in which foodstuffs are grown are deficient in iodine. In our country the chief goiter belts are in the Great Lakes region. In places near the seacoast many common foods contain iodine in small quantities. Seafood is especially rich in it.

Using iodized salt instead of ordinary table salt is the simplest way to be sure of getting enough iodine. In recent years the use of supplemental iodine in localities where the diet is deficient in iodine is helping to wipe out simple goiter.

Adolescent Goiter. Enlargement of the thyroid gland known as adolescent goiter is a very common thyroid manifestation in adolescents. It appears as a swelling in the neck just below the Adam's apple. It is much more common in girls than in boys. The cause of adolescent goiter is unknown. In goiter regions it is usually due to insufficient iodine in the diet and can be treated with supplemental iodine. An adolescent with a noticeable enlargement of the thyroid gland who does not live in a goiter region should certainly not take iodine in any form without medical advice. If the enlargement is not due to iodine deficiency but to a more serious condition, iodine may make matters worse instead of better. In some cases, it may mask the seriousness of the condition until it is too late for the physician to treat it successfully.

Diabetes

Diabetes is a disease of metabolism in which the body's ability to use sugar is affected. Normally the body is able to oxidize (burn) and store sugar because of the presence in the blood of insulin, the secretion of the islands of Langerhans in the pancreas. Diabetes develops when the flow of insulin from these insulin-secreting cells is lessened or completely stopped.

What causes the islands of Langerhans to fall down on the job of producing insulin is not yet known with certainty. These groups of cells are part of the whole endocrine system and are influenced by disturbances in other parts of the system. A hereditary factor is undoubtedly involved, because statistical studies have shown time and again that diabetes is most likely to occur in people who have diabetic relatives. Overweight in middle age is also an important predisposing factor.

Signs and Symptoms. When the tissues can neither use nor store sugar, signs and symptoms of diabetes appear. Sugar accumulates in the blood, and this causes thirst. Drinking large amounts of water to quench the thirst results in frequent urination. An excessive amount of sugar is present in the urine because that is the way in which the body gets rid of the sugar it cannot use. The inability to use sugar means that the body is robbed of this important source of energy. As a result, there is constant hunger and a loss of weight and strength. These are the most striking symptoms found in severe, untreated cases. Other symptoms may be tiring easily, itching, and slow healing of infections and wounds. The earliest manifestation may simply be not feeling so well as usual.

Doctors have several tests for detecting diabetes—even in its earliest stage. The first is urinalysis. The finding of sugar in the urine is strong— but not conclusive—evidence of diabetes. Usually it is checked by determining the sugar content of the blood (blood-sugar test) and in many cases by a glucose tolerance test which measures the body's ability to handle sugar.

Diabetes in Children. Diabetes is primarily a disease of middle and old age rather than of youth. But when juvenile diabetes does occur, it is usually severe and, if untreated, progresses rapidly. A diagnosis of diabetes in a child was equivalent to a sentence of early death in the days before 1922, when Sir Frederick Banting and his coworkers suc- ceeded in extracting insulin from the pancreas of animals in a form that could be used in treating human beings. Since then insulin has been per- fected and is now prepared in several quick-acting and slow-acting forms. Insulin in any form, however, is not a cure for diabetes. It simply sup- plies the diabetic with a hormone essential to life of which his body is making too little or none.

Oral Medicines. Insulin must be injected by hypodermic needle; it cannot be taken by mouth because the digestive juices destroy it before it can get into the blood. Since 1957 several chemical compounds have been discovered which can be taken by mouth and which are proving effective in the treatment of mild diabetes in the middle and older age groups. Two of these compounds come from the same chemical family as that to which the sulfa drugs belong. They are tolbutamide (trade- marked Orinase) and chlorpropamide (trade-marked Diabinese). A third of the oral medicines comes from another chemical group. Its name is phenformin (trade-marked DBI). Others are being developed which may prove useful.

In general, the oral drugs are rarely of value in juvenile diabetes, ex- cept for DBI, which is proving useful in combination with insulin in certain cases. The major action of these drugs is to stimulate the still active insulin-producing islet cells of the pancreas to secrete larger quantities of this essential hormone. The reason for their limited value in juvenile diabetes is that in almost all persons in whom diabetes de- velops before their twenties, there is a striking loss of islet tissue; con- sequently, either no insulin or exceedingly little is produced by the pancreas.

Living with Diabetes. It is a great blow to a youngster to know that he has a chronic disorder with which (so far as is now known) he will have to live for the rest of his life. It is especially hard for adolescents to accept this fact. Adolescents who have diabetes do not differ from others of their age in not liking to think that there is something wrong with their bodies. They resent any restrictions or rules that seem to single them out as being different. To children who develop diabetes in their early years, the condition holds less mystery and fear. If they acquire an understanding of it, feel that they know how to manage it, and have learned to accept rules and reasonable discipline and authority, they will cause their physicians less difficulty in their adolescent years.

If a youngster has diabetes it is important for teachers to know it so that they can cooperate intelligently with the child, his parents, and his physician. The teacher can help the child to understand that he cannot live in *exactly* the same way as other children but that he can *nearly* do so if he follows his physician's directions. Adolescents especially should have considerable knowledge of the disease so that the reasons for the doctor's rules and restrictions will be clear. Girls should be reassured that marriage and children can be a part of the "normal life" now possible for most diabetics whose disease is under control.

The physician tells the diabetic child, as well as his parents, "all about diabetes" so that the child may show the self-restraint and intelligence upon which good control of his disease and the prevention of complications depend. The "three R's" of the child's education in living with his diabetes are diet, insulin, and exercise. The kinds and amounts of each that seem best are worked out by the doctor with the child's help.

The diabetic child learns how to inject insulin and how to test his urine for sugar at the times set by the doctor. He is also given the information that will help him to keep out of trouble. The two chief dangers are diabetic coma and insulin reaction. These seldom occur in the child who conscientiously follows the program the doctor outlines for him.

Diabetic coma is due to poisons from acids formed in the body when sugar is not being burned. As coma may come on surreptitiously like a thief in the night, this is a condition that the diabetic child must understand thoroughly and learn how to avoid. *Even slight deviations from normal health,* such as a mild cold or other infection, while not a cause for alarm, should be treated with respect. This means that when the child has an acute illness the parents will want to keep him home for bed rest and medical care until he is fully recovered.

Insulin reaction takes place when there is too little sugar in the blood as a result of (1) too much insulin, (2) too little food or delay in eating after taking insulin, or (3) unaccustomed or unusual exercise. Hunger, trembling, sweating, and nervousness are the beginning signs when regular insulin is being used. If one of the long-acting forms of insulin is being taken, headache, nausea, drowsiness, and a sick feeling, hunger, and sweating occur. The treatment is to take sugar immediately. Diabetic children who are taking insulin should always carry two lumps of sugar to be eaten in case symptoms of insulin reaction develop.

FOR REVIEW AND DISCUSSION

1. Select the heading listed in the box which is related to one or more of the phrases in the list below the box.

1 Poliomyelitis	7 Epilepsy
2 Tetanus bacilli	8 Cerebral palsy
3 Meningococcal meningitis	9 Aphasia
4 Rabies	10 Rubella
5 Encephalitis	11 Phenylketonuria
6 Diabetes	12 Gigantism

3 Is largely spread by carriers in epidemic periods.

10 May produce mental retardation in the offspring if it occurs in the first three months of pregnancy.

9 Results from injury or disease of the speech areas of the cerebral cortex.

7 Can be controlled in many cases by anticonvulsants.

5 Can be kept from spreading in epidemic form by measures directed against its mosquito carriers.

1 Is caused by a virus of three distinct types which attack motor neurons.

2 Multiply in wounds sealed away from the air.

4 Is caused by a virus present in the saliva of an infected animal.

1 Can be eradicated by vaccinating all infants in each succeeding generation.

8 Usually results from an injury to the brain at or before birth.

12 Results from excessive overproduction of a pituitary hormone before the fusion of the epiphyses.

6 Is a metabolic disease in which the body is unable to oxidize or store sugar.

2 May exist for many years in the spore state in soil and street dust.

4 Can be prevented by vaccination after a bite from a mad animal.

7 Is classified by abnormal brain-wave patterns.

11 Is a congenital disease that can be detected soon after birth by a urine test.

6 Can usually be kept under good control by a well-balanced combination of insulin, diet, and exercise.

2. In the following groupings of disorders, there is one in each group that does not belong. Select the one that is out of place and tell why.

   a. Rabies, tetanus, cretinism, encephalitis
   b. Myxedema, gigantism, acromegaly, galactosemia
   c. Goiter, cerebral palsy, aphasia, epilepsy

3. Suppose you had a crippled child in your class, or a child suffering from epilepsy. Plan what you would say to the other children to help them to understand the handicapped child's problem and to cultivate the right attitude toward all handicapped children.

SELECTED REFERENCES

American Medical Association: *What You Should Know about Diabetes,* The Association, Chicago.

American Public Health Association: *Mental Disorders: A Guide to Control Methods,* The Association, New York, 1962. Chap. 3, *Mental Disorders of Known Etiology.*

Baker, Harry J.: *Introduction to Exceptional Children,* The Macmillan Company, New York, 1953. (A text for teachers on the characteristics and problems of all types of children. Physical handicaps and mental growth and development are among the topics covered.)

Burton, Mary L. H.: *Your Child or Mine: The Story of the Cerebral-palsied Child,* Coward-McCann, Inc., New York, 1949.

Childhood Aphasia: Proceedings of the Institute on Childhood Aphasia, September, 1960, at Stanford University School of Medicine, sponsored by the California Society for Crippled Children and Adults.

Conklin, Groff: *Diabetics Unknown,* Public Affairs Pamphlet No. 312, Public Affairs Committee, Inc., New York.

Killilea, Marie: *Karen,* Prentice-Hall, Inc., New York, 1952. (A story about a child with cerebral palsy.)

Lewis, Richard S.: *The Brain-Injured Child,* The National Society for Crippled Children and Adults, Chicago. (An interesting pamphlet primarily for parents describing the brain-injured child and the nature of his perceptive handicaps.)

Livingston, S.: *Living with Epileptic Seizures,* Charles C Thomas, Publishers, Springfield, Ill., 1963. (An excellent reference book which answers many questions about epilepsy and the management and education of epileptic children.)

National Committee for Research in Neurological Disorders: *Exploring the Brain of Man,* The Medical School, University of Minnesota, Minneapolis, Minn. (A booklet reporting progress on research in the prevention and cure of neurological and sensory disorders.)

Putnam, Tracy J.: *Epilepsy; What It Is, What to Do about It,* J. B. Lippincott Company, Philadelphia, 1958. (A comprehensive explanation of the disease with a helpful guide on what to do for an epileptic during a seizure.)

Siegel, Ernest: *Helping the Brain-injured Child,* New York Association for Brain-injured Children, New York, 1961.

Sterling, Dorothy, and Philip Sterling: *Polio Pioneers; The Story of the*

Fight against Polio, Doubleday & Company, Inc., Garden City, 1955.

Strother, Charles R.: *Discovering, Evaluating and Programming for the Neurologically Handicapped Child,* with special attention to the child with minimal brain damage, National Society for Crippled Children and Adults, Chicago, 1963. (A pamphlet for the parent and the classroom teacher describing characteristics of brain-injured children and what is involved in designing an adequate educational program.)

Yahraes, Herbert: *Now—A Brighter Future for the Epileptic,* Public Affairs Pamphlet No. 98, Public Affairs Committee, Inc., New York.

Organizations

American Diabetes Association
National Association for Retarded Children
National Epilepsy League
National Foundation (formerly National Foundation for Infantile Paralysis)
National Society for Crippled Children and Adults
New York Association for Brain-injured Children

Chapter 9   EMOTIONALLY DISTURBED CHILDREN AND YOUTH

Behavior Reactions to Environmental Stress
Forms of Mental Illness
Progress in the Treatment of Mental Illness
Identifying Children with Emotional and Social
  Problems
Meeting the Need for Guidance in School-age
  Children

Some children, as we saw in the last chapter, are mentally handicapped because of clearly defined physical causes or structural damage to the brain. In this chapter we are concerned with children and youth who develop illness of the mind for which no organic cause can be found. Generally speaking, the behavior of these children shows that they have failed to make a satisfactory compromise between the emotional needs and demands of their personalities and the requirements of life as they must live it.

Most young people can usually handle their emotions in ways that do not interfere with their family relationships, their friendships, their work or study, or with their ability to do what they are capable of doing. But it sometimes happens that a young person gets into emotional difficulties that he cannot handle easily or quickly. Such a person may then become mentally ill. Illness of the mind ranges all the way from mild and temporary upsets to severe, long-lasting personality disorders.

It is important, however, to make a distinction between normal behavior and behavior that indicates that a child is so emotionally disturbed that he needs help. A child who hits back when hit by one of his pals is "normally aggressive." A child who withdraws from his playmates for a while when his feelings are hurt shows a perfectly "normal" response. But children who are always "picking a fight" or bullying others; children who are markedly shy or constantly withdrawing from their group are showing exaggerated responses that are clear cries for help. In fact, any response or mood that is not appropriate to the incident, or that exceeds "normal response" in degree, is a danger signal. Prolonged abnormal reactions are not easily adjusted, and these children need prompt help.

BEHAVIOR REACTIONS TO ENVIRONMENTAL STRESS

Some understanding of the ways in which children and youth react emotionally to the environment will help to explain what lies back of various forms of mental illness. There are innumerable life situations in which strong instinctual drives within the unconscious mind come up against inhibitions and frustrations emanating from the world outside (see under Psychological Makeup in Chap. 4). The hostile impulses arising when such brakes are applied come in conflict with the friendly impulses arising from the child's love and respect for those who show their love and respect for him. The inevitable outcome of this conflict is a feeling of guilt that is often a source of much anxiety.

The solution of the difficulty raised by hostile impulses which make the child feel guilty must be found in one of two ways. Either the child must repress them or he must redirect them into acceptable channels.

Unconscious Conflict

The most frequent way in which the child solves his emotional problems is repression. That is, he succeeds wholly or in part in banishing from conciousness those impulses which, in his experience, are condemned and forbidden. However, many of these impulses continue to lead an active existence in the unconscious mind, where they constantly seek for expression. Opposing them are the ego (the self) and the conscience. As a result, there is continual conflict between repressed desires and impulses and the ego ideals, social taboos, and standards of conduct derived from the interaction of the child and his environment. This inner conflict, together with the struggle between the personality and the outside world to which everyone must adjust, continues throughout life. It is important to remember that the battleground of this conflict is in the unconscious. The individual is not aware of what is going on. However, he does consciously experience the symptoms of anxiety generated by it.

Individuals vary greatly in their capacity to resist anxiety. One person may have a strong enough sense of personal worth and integrity to keep from being overwhelmed either by powerful instinctual drives and repressed impulses or by the "thousand several tongues" of conscience condemning him "for a villain." Such a person seems able to let off emotional steam in satisfactory, useful pursuits and to stand up under any or all of "the slings and arrows of outrageous fortune." Another with a less well integrated personality structure may be able to jog along comfortably even when the going is not too good but breaks down in the face of extraordinary or greatly prolonged emotional stress. Still another may be so lacking in ego strength that he is unable to make a satisfactory compromise even under reasonably favorable circumstances.

Hostile Feelings

As we have seen, guilt arises when the child's ego and conscience tell him that he ought to be ashamed of himself for harboring hostile feelings toward those upon whom he is dependent for security and love. When he does things like lying, stealing, or other acts of which he knows his parents disapprove, he feels guilty because parental disapproval has tagged them in his mind as hostile acts. When he is punished for his wrongdoing, the punishment becomes associated with the sense of guilt he already harbors. Hence, there is built up in his mind the idea that punishment—suffering—atones for guilt.

The idea that there must be punishment for every misdeed is deeply ingrained in our society. Even when acts or thoughts that are considered wrong remain undiscovered, practically everyone is bothered with the vague guilty feeling that punishment is merited.

In childhood, naughtiness brings concrete retribution like a spanking or the withholding of some pleasure or privilege. The suffering caused by the punishment brings with it the satisfaction of making up for the naughtiness. With the pangs of his guilty conscience relieved, the child can once more feel at peace with his parents.

Gradually the child learns to accept the rules of conduct of his social code. If they are reasonable and fair and opportunities are given to express his hostilities and antagonisms constructively, he learns how to deal efficiently with his hostile impulses.

However, if he is made to feel insecure because of a rigid or erratic system of discipline or a lack of true love and understanding in the home, or because of differences between the standards of behavior required at home and in school, or for some other reason, he may develop the guilty feeling that almost everything he does will meet with disapproval if it is found out. Hostile impulses seem as wicked to him as bad behavior would be. That is, he feels as guilty for harboring such impulses as if he had actually done the things that would bring punishment. The anxiety generated in this conflict, of which the child is completely unaware, is almost sure to lead to neurotic trends unless its cause is discovered and removed. Perhaps the child may be oversubmissive or overdependent or unusually demonstrative to atone for the guilt he unconsciously feels. Or he may behave badly in order to get the punishment that will relieve his guilty feelings. Or he may frequently show symptoms of illness to get the sympathy and attention he craves or to make himself suffer for his hostile impulses.

Overdirection

As they grow older children need freedom, within reasonable limits, to make their own decisions, and time in which to do what they want to do. Unfortunately, many solicitous or domineering or insecure parents try to limit the activities and conversation of their children long after the need for freedom to express themselves in their own way has been established. As a result, difficulties arise which cause the child to be labeled a "problem child." Perhaps the child's feelings of resentment and frustration are expressed in a form of obstreperousness technically called "negativism." The child has received so much direction that he refuses to obey any commands, whether they are reasonable or not. Or he may go to the other extreme and become abjectly submissive.

When overly aggressive, defiant, chronically disobedient children who are suffering from an overdose of protection or overdirection understand that they are free to act and speak or be silent as they choose, without penalty of any kind, in conference with a psychiatrist or guidance counselor, they often relax and pour out their troubles. This emotional catharsis not only is usually a great relief to the child but also may indicate the correct solution to the child's problems. Quite frequently, it is one or both parents who need treatment more than the child does. Children labeled as problem children are often essentially good children who are reacting in completely normal ways to overdirection or nagging.

Frustration

All behavior patterns develop in the interactions of the child with his environment. Among the most important environmental influences are the requirements of the society in which he lives. No one—child or adult—is able to accept completely and gracefully all the frustrations and inconveniences imposed by these requirements. If a requirement is too severe, or if it interferes with his personal desires for no good reason that he can see or understand, it is perfectly natural to seek ways of circumventing it. Practically everyone does it, no matter how well adjusted he may seem to himself or others.

Psychologists tell us that there are two main forms of evasion—attack and withdrawal. By attacking a natural force or social regulation that frustrates his desires or by finding ways to escape from it, the individual may avoid the necessity for accepting it or adjusting himself to it. The motive for both attacking and withdrawing behavior is the same, and streaks of both are often found in the same individual. Some persons, however, learn to depend more upon one than upon the other.

Evasion by Attack. It is easy to see that evasion by attack may be a potent constructive force. Civilization could not have progressed if everyone had meekly accepted, or adjusted to, things as they were at any particular stage. A large part of human history is a record of circumventing natural restrictions like those of distance on going places and of unaided vision on seeing things. Social and economic change has its roots in discontent with the existing order. And practically every individual has some unfavorable conditions in his own life which he must attack in order to get ahead. However, evasion by attack may be destructive if it keeps a child from eventually making inner peace with himself, his parents, his teachers, and the forces of law and order.

In dealing with aggressiveness in children, it is important to make distinctions both in degree and kind. "Being bad"—disorderly, disobedient, boastful, noisy, curious about sex, and so on—is natural in the period of child development characterized by the impulse to experiment, to investigate, to show off, to determine just how far it is possible to go before parental ire or pedagogical wrath is aroused. On the other hand, consistently defiant attitudes or extreme expressions of hostility or antagonism usually indicate some form of emotional or social maladjustment. Very often the pattern of aggressive behavior which the child presents to the world is a cover-up for feelings of inadequacy or guilt that he is afraid or ashamed of expressing.

The Teacher and the Aggressive Child. A teacher does not have to be an old-fashioned martinet to be annoyed by bullying, defiance, quarrelsomeness, truancy, failure to submit to school routine, and other forms of attacking behavior that interfere with her teaching and wreck her efforts to create a friendly, helpful classroom atmosphere. If she shows her annoyance, however, and responds to attack by counterattack—ridicules or punishes or penalizes the child in retaliation for the flouting of her authority—she simply drives in deeper the feelings of fear, or resentment, or insecurity, or guilt, which are making the child misbehave. On the other hand, if she recognizes that the attacking behavior is not the tug-of-war between child and teacher that it appears to be but is rather the outward sign of some unsatisfied emotional need or inner conflict, she will appreciate the importance of detecting and seeking help in correcting its underlying cause.

Evasion by Withdrawal. Evasion by withdrawal also has its constructive and its destructive aspects. There is no one who has not found ways of escaping at times from the troubles and cares of everyday life. Daydreams, sleep, literature, music, and drama, for example, provide natural and necessary channels of escape. In many cases, however, the retreat from reality becomes so pronounced that it interferes with the ability to meet the requirements and responsibilities of social living. Some individuals upon reaching maturity are able to make constructive use of their habits of withdrawal and escape. The ability to shut out the outer "working-day world" and labor undisturbed in the inner workshop of the mind has resulted in many great scientific discoveries and inventions and many great accomplishments in the fields of literature, art, and religion. Sometimes, however, the habit of withdrawing from active participation in normal social living because of some deep-seated anxiety leads to mental illnesses of varying degrees of severity.

It is just as important in dealing with shy, overdependent children as in dealing with the aggressive ones to make distinctions between what is normal and what, under the circumstances, may be a serious deviation from normality. In the adolescent period, for example, it is natural for boys and girls to have occasional spells of dreaminess. This is the spring of life, in which there is poetic license for being fanciful and starry-eyed. In younger children, however, aggressiveness and other forms of attacking behavior are more natural than dreaminess and other forms of withdrawing behavior.

Many different experiences may lead a child to develop overdependence. Perhaps the parents are overprotective or afraid of what might happen to their child in rough play with other children. Or they may be too anxious to hear good reports of their child—"He is such a little gentleman." "She is such a nice girl." Such parental attitudes may lead a child to shun physical competition with schoolmates, to withdraw more and more into himself, and to find compensation in daydreams or in a reputation for studiousness and excellence in schoolwork. As a result, the child may be unfitted to meet the hard facts of existence and be deprived of the independence he needs to stand on his own feet.

Possibly, a child's views of the world or his manners or his ambitions may be radically different from those of one or both parents. The parents may be trying to make him conform to their conception of the ideal child, or reproaching him for disappointing them, or disagreeing with each other as to the best way of coping with him. In that case the child may be finding necessary solace in a dream world created by and for him, where he can be and think and do as he likes.

Another possibility is that unfortunate experiences of one kind or another in early childhood have given a child the feeling that he is weak or bad or that nobody loves him. To earn the affection and security he craves, he may have developed the pattern of behavior which he knows, from his own observation and experience, adults approve of. Yet without knowing it he may deeply resent this dependence. In that case, the conflict between his love for those who protect and discipline him and his desire to be free may make him feel fearful and guilty. And so the child forms the habit of retreating into a dream world or a storybook world where he can attain his desire with no strings of doubt or fear attached.

The Teacher and the Overdependent Child. The child who habitually resorts to withdrawing behavior in response to feelings of guilt or frustration or inadequacy may have a much easier time of it in childhood than the child who uses methods of attack, but he is more likely to develop pronounced neurotic tendencies later on. The submissive, shy, timid, solitary, dreamy child usually behaves well and gives his parents and teachers little trouble. His apparently inadequate equipment for dealing with life often arouses the sympathy and protective feelings of those in authority.

If his respectful behavior and his diligence in school tasks win him the favor of his teachers, the habit of withdrawal tends to become entrenched, just as meeting attack with counterattack tends to entrench the habit of defiance.

The "teacher's pet" type of child may have heartburnings over his unpopularity with his schoolmates and secretly admire the "big bad boys," but he can take comfort in the snug warm feeling of being cherished and protected by those who matter most in the ordering of his life. His worst troubles come when he is thrown on his own—when there is no loving parent or sympathetic teacher to turn to in stressful life situations.

FORMS OF MENTAL ILLNESS

Many mental disorders, as we have seen, have physical causes. Such causes include brain tumors and injuries of the brain, infections, acute poisonings, genetic diseases produced by abnormal genes, severe nutritional deficiencies, certain general systemic diseases, and, among older people, changes in the brain due to the aging process. Measures for the detection, prevention, and treatment of organic causes of mental illness must be part of the total program for the mental health of children. There remains the stubborn fact, however, that it is at present impossible to find physical bases for more than half the illnesses characterized by mental disturbances.

The two most common forms of mental illness of this kind are the psychoses and the neuroses. The psychoses, in general, involve marked disruption of personality. In some forms, particularly schizophrenia, there is abandonment of reality. Schizophrenics seem to live outside the world as we see it, in an inner world of their own. Neurotics are much closer to normal in their continuing awareness of reality, no matter how poor an adjustment they make to it. In spite of their basic anxiety, they are able to accept and react to explanations of the underlying causes of their illness.

Neurosis and schizophrenia sometimes occur in childhood and youth. In addition, children may suffer from a variety of behavior disorders and a number of conditions indicative of emotional disturbances such as bed wetting, stuttering, school phobia, compulsive eating, nervous loss of appetite, and learning difficulties.

Some emotional disturbances may well be the prolongation of the normal process through which children must pass in the course of growing up. Spontaneous recovery may occur with maturation. On the other hand, emotional disturbances in childhood may be the precursors of neurosis or psychosis in adult life.

Neurotic Patterns

A neurotic pattern often begins to develop in childhood when the ego is weak and its ideals, largely a product of parental prohibitions and demands, are threatened by strong instinctual drives or repressed impulses. A neurosis may be defined as a device used to bring about a compromise between irreconcilable drives which call for opposing courses of action. Since the mechanisms unconsciously used not only bring about the compromise but also disguise its purpose, the neurotic person does not know what is making him ill.

All of us as we go through life experience anxiety when we meet circumstances that make us feel afraid or guilty or frustrated or angry. Even those of us who react adequately to most situations are familiar with many of the physical symptoms of anxiety which, as we have learned, are the result of the influence of emotions on the autonomic nervous system. We think of these symptoms as perfectly natural when the emotional stimulus is known. If it scares us to make a speech, for example, it does not surprise us to have the heart beat more rapidly and the mouth feel dry when we are called on for "a few words." The same mechanism operates when a bad headache or a spell of indigestion keeps a person from doing something he dreads doing, or expresses the outrage he unconsciously feels when powerful impulses must be suppressed.

In childhood, physical responses to anxiety, such as an attack of nausea or vomiting or a headache or stomachache, or a reversion to some form of behavior that he has given up—for example, finger sucking or bed wetting or temper tantrums—are relatively common. These are neurotic manifestations which usually clear up as the child's ego becomes stronger and he gains experience in handling the frustrations and instinctual drives which have produced his anxiety. However, if he fails to receive any real understanding or constructive help, he may use childish devices all his life long to escape from painful life situations.

Psychoneurotic Reactions

Full-blown neuroses are known as psychoneuroses. In these disorders the individual either shows symptoms indicating anxiety or adopts psychological mechanisms to deal with or allay it.

Anxiety Reactions. Some unfortunate people live in a state of almost perpetual anxiety. Except in cases in which the anxiety has some physical cause, such as hyperthyroidism, the origin of the anxiety is usually due to a psychological wrestling match with powerful instinctual drives arising from the unconscious which make the individual want to feel and act in ways that he has come to think of as not "nice" either from his own or from society's point of view. Never having learned in the process of growing up that aggressive and sexual impulses are normal and natural and can be successfully managed and directed, the anxious person feels threatened in real or imaginary situations that involve the risk of losing the esteem of others, for example, or of failing to measure up to his own impossibly high ideals.

Long-continued threats may be real or imaginary, but the anxious person often meets both in an ineffectual or indecisive way that he usually calls a "worry." When the average mentally healthy person is faced with some difficult problem he usually faces it squarely, thinks it over carefully, and then decides how it may be solved. Even if the problem seems insoluble, a normal person will tackle it anyway. He may fail, but at least he will have acted as well as he possibly could under the circumstances. Once having made his decision, he will give the matter no further thought. The anxious person recognizes the problem; he may think about it; but he cannot decide what to do. When forced into making a decision, he continues to worry about whether his final judgment was right.

Some anxious people are never entirely free from symptoms and have severe acute flare-ups in times of stress. Others have comparatively free intervals sandwiched between their attacks of anxiety.

Severe Anxiety Reactions. In a severe anxiety reaction, the individual experiences extreme apprehension bordering on panic. He has the feelings of helplessness and utter dependence that a young child feels when confronted with the unknown. His physical symptoms are the same as those everyone experiences when obliged to cope with threatened danger from without (see Teamwork for Meeting Emergencies in Chap. 6). In his case, however, the threat of danger he feels in the conscious part of his mind arises from the unconscious part.

Chronic Anxiety States. Many people have symptoms expressing anxiety which are considerably milder than those experienced in severe anxiety reactions. Under ordinary circumstances they can attend to their personal affairs and carry on their work. Often they do not even know that they are suffering from anxiety. Although they feel more or less constantly tired, unhappy, worried, apprehensive, confused, ill, or at odds with life, they do not realize that some underlying emotional disturbance may be to blame. Often they go from doctor to doctor or from quack to quack or try every brand of patent medicine guaranteed to alleviate their symptoms, or they change jobs frequently, or they seek peace of mind in change of scene.

Obsessive-compulsive Reactions. One of the most devious pathways that anxiety finds for itself is the formation of obsessive and compulsive symptoms. An obsession is the feeling that one is compelled to go through with some frequently repeated ritualistic act. Ceremonial handwashing is probably the most frequent symptom in people suffering from an obsessive-compulsive reaction. A person suffering from the compulsion to wash his hands whenever he has touched something knows that it is silly, but he cannot stop doing it. The obsessive thought or compulsive act is often the result of a long-lasting anxiety process and has become so firmly embedded that it is practically impossible to uproot.

Phobia Reactions. Another strange manifestation of anxiety is a phobia. A phobia is an irrational and persistent fear. Familiar examples are fear of enclosed or open places, fear of certain animals, and fear of running water. Usually a phobia symbolizes a fear experienced so long ago that it is lost to conscious memory but is retained in the unconscious mind.

A phobia that has attracted a good deal of attention recently is school phobia. This is defined as "a partial or total disability to attend school because of an irrational dread of some aspect of the school situation." The basic fear is not that of going to school but rather that of leaving home. School phobia, therefore, is classified as a separation anxiety. A child suffering from school phobia usually belongs to a family in which the mother, especially, exhibits fear of separation at least as much if not more so than does the child. Such a mother is oversolicitous and concerned about her child and increases his dread by communicating her own anxiety to him during the process of separation. Usually there is a precipitating factor such as an unpleasant experience in school, illness in the child or his mother, the birth of a brother or sister, or an increase of tension in parental relationships. Elementary school children suffering from school phobia usually do not display more severe symptoms of anxiety. School phobia in junior and senior high school students, however, may be a manifestation of a severe personality disturbance.

Psychosomatic Conditions. The physical symptoms into which anxiety is often "converted," or changed, are a kind of language used by the body to express pent-up emotions. Many of our most common expressions show that we have some understanding of this language. "He burns me up"; "This is more than I can stomach"; "That makes my blood run cold"; "He gives me a pain in the neck"; "She makes me sick"; "It really gets under my skin" are only a few of the examples in everyday speech which show that we realize that the soma (body) can speak for the psyche (mind).

Some people have the idea that the physical manifestations of anxiety —the chest pains, stomachaches, and headaches, for example—which are caused by anxiety are less real than those caused by physical disorders. Nothing can be further from the truth. People feel pain whether the cause is in the body or in the mind. The fact that a persistent headache or recurrent indigestion is caused by worry does not make the head hurt less or the stomach behave any better. A headache is a headache, whether caused by a bump on the head or by emotional tension.

Only a physician can tell whether the cause of any illness is physical or emotional. If he finds no apparent physical cause, he may be able, in talks with the patient, to find out what is causing his distress. This finding of itself may help the patient to get a better perspective on his difficulties.

But in many cases the trouble may be an emotional conflict or anxiety so deeply seated that it cannot be brought to light without psychiatric help.

Helping Children to Avoid the Neurotic Pattern. Teachers may seldom encounter full-blown neuroses in their students. However, neurotic trends are quite common in childhood. It is usually possible to arrest the development of such trends if the child's teachers and other adults intimately associated with him understand their significance and give him reassurance. All children should be helped to realize that it is natural to feel cross or resentful or fearful when confronted with disappointments or failures or strange or violent emotions. They should be encouraged to get rid of such feelings by talking them out to someone who understands. If a child who exhibits antagonistic tendencies is given opportunities through socially acceptable activities for gaining the attention and approbation or the sense of security that he needs, his teachers may help to keep him from growing up to be an "antisocial, egocentric, contentious, maladjusted adult." And if the shy, timid, dreamy, easily discouraged child is unobtrusively drawn out and given self-confidence through a series of small successes, his teachers may help to keep him from growing up into a neurotic, complaining, economically dependent adult.

In many cases of emotional distress in young people, healing has come through talking over and sharing problems with an understanding physician, clergyman, nurse, or teacher. We all know the relief obtained merely by getting our troubles off our chests. If hand in hand with this catharsis, or emotional release, go reassurance and the wise use of suggestion, the way is open for education or reeducation directed toward giving the disturbed youngster an understanding of how his emotions and poor mental habits are interfering with his health and behavior.

Children who have failed to get sympathetic help early enough to prevent the development of permanent neurotic trends and children who are seriously disturbed usually need study and treatment by specialists in psychotherapy. (See Psychotherapy, and Identifying Children with Emotional and Social Problems further on in this chapter.)

Psychotic Patterns

The psychoses are far more serious forms of mental illness than the neuroses. They account for the great majority of the mentally ill who require hospitalization for varying lengths of time.

There are many different forms of functional psychosis, as serious mental illness without apparent organic cause is called. The two most common patterns of psychotic behavior are the manic-depressive and the schizophrenic.

Manic-depressive Illness. Happiness and unhappiness in the lives of most individuals are as fleeting as the play of sunshine and shadows when clouds form and disappear in the sky on a fair day. The terms in which we try to define these qualities are as elusive as the qualities themselves. All we know is that sometimes we're happy and sometimes we're blue. In some people, however, a peculiar combination of unpleasant events or a loss or reversal in fortune may bring about a prolonged state of deep blueness. In mentally healthy people this period of profound unhappiness is usually comparatively short. In others less stable mentally it may last much longer. Such a state is called a "depression." If there is a swing from depressed periods of greatly reduced activity to excited "manic" periods of greatly increased activity, the condition is called a manic-depressive psychosis.

Depressions in young people are uncommon and when they do occur they are normally short-lived. However, they should always receive professional attention, as they may be the harbingers of manic-depressive illness.

Schizoid States. There is no more puzzling problem in medicine than that of determining what factors in schizoid persons make the world as seen by most people so different to them. There are a very great many different varieties of schizoid states. It is only when an individual shows by his actions and words that he has left the practical world about him to live in a world of fantasy that he is considered to be psychotic. Psychoses that occur in dreamy people far outnumber any other one type of psychosis.

The best known mental illness of the withdrawing type of personality is schizophrenia. The term *dementia praecox* was first used to designate this psychosis because its onset so often occurs in adolescence (*praecox,* in Latin, means "early ripe," and *dementia* means "madness"). However, this name later was considered to be something of a misnomer. Dementia praecox does not always begin in youth and early maturity, and its victims do not always develop madness. Both to meet these objections and to describe the splitting of the personality that is characteristic of this psychosis, the term *schizophrenia* was introduced in 1924. This term is derived from two Greek words: *schizo-* from a word meaning "to divide or split," and *-phrenia* from a word meaning "the mind."

It should be emphasized again that all people indulge to some extent in daydreams and in other forms of escape from reality, but of these comparatively few retreat wholly or even in part into a dream world of their own. Some individuals with definite schizoid tendencies are able to make good adjustments and even to do highly useful work. It is not safe to assume, however, that children who show pronounced forms of withdrawing behavior will outgrow them or that they are of no significance.

Anyone who has indulged in daydreams—and who has not!—knows how rough the coming back to reality can be. Young inexperienced lotus-eaters who hug the cloak of fantasy that gives them some protection from the rigors of actuality feel more keenly than their weathered companions the discrepancy between the ideal and the real. Even if their tendency to dream never makes them lose touch with reality, they are bound to be unhappier than those whose ideals are not so far out of reach that they can be attained only in made-to-order fantasies.

PROGRESS IN THE TREATMENT OF MENTAL ILLNESS

We are all familiar with the age-old conception of serious mental illness as demonic possession. The neglect and even physical abuse of its victims, cruel as they were, seemed to be justified on the principle that demons would leave a body, as tenants would leave a house, which had been made untenable. Philippe Pinel's act in striking the chains from the limbs of the insane in the Salpêtrière in 1793 has become symbolic of the setting free of the minds of the sane from the prejudice and superstition that so long delayed advances in an understanding of mental illness.

We now know that mental illness in all its forms is real, treatable, and in many cases preventable. Removing through education the age-old stigma attached to it is one of the principal aims of the mental hygiene movement. Early diagnosis and treatment offer the best chance of avoiding much of the human suffering and economic cost of mental illness.

Psychotherapy

The process of guiding mentally ill persons back to mental health by psychological means is called *psychotherapy*. For the most part psychotherapy includes the entire collection of approaches by which the physician attempts to influence his patient toward more desirable ways of thinking, feeling, and acting. Common to all the approaches is the doctor-patient relationship. Any doctor can use supportive psychotherapy at any time in dealing with any patient, no matter what ails him. There is, however, one branch of medicine, known as *psychiatry*, which deals as a specialty with the prevention, recognition, and treatment of mental disorders. Through long training and extensive experience the psychiatrist has developed an understanding of certain symptoms in the life of the individual and of the complexities of mental life.

The primary object of psychotherapy in the treatment of the neuroses is to foster the disturbed individual's growth toward emotional maturity and to strengthen his self-mastery by helping him to become aware of and understand the unconscious conflict that is causing his symptoms. Evaluating the effectiveness of psychotherapy for the neuroses is difficult. Psychoneurotic symptoms in many persons disappear without any treatment. Not all persons under treatment recover; others under treatment seem to recover completely. The Program Area Committee on Mental Health of the American Public Health Association sums up the situation in this way:

Currently a number of investigating teams are struggling with systematic evaluations of psychotherapy. No adequate trials have been performed. In estimating the worth of psychotherapy for an individual or a community program it is important to recognize several goals. There can, in fact, be no treatment of mental disorders without some psychotherapy, that is, a relationship between a patient and physician, even when this relationship cannot reasonably be expected to terminate many emotional disorders. In practice the issue is not whether psychotherapy should be used, but what method, in which cases, and in what quantities.[1]

Methods of Psychotherapy. Psychotherapeutic treatment varies from a mild supportive approach to classical psychoanalysis. It may be carried on individually or in groups. In some cases a whole family takes part in group therapy sessions.

In the so-called "short-term supportive approach," the therapist directs the patient's talk and lets the patient express his feelings. In his treatment he emphasizes reassurance and guidance. He is no magician. He cannot make problems disappear; but he can try and often succeeds in helping the patient to understand the true nature of his problems and his unconscious motivations. This understanding may, of itself, bring relief of symptoms and give the patient a feeling of greater mastery over his impulses and his life situation.

In more severe types of mental illness, it may be very difficult to bring the source of trouble to the surface, especially if it is linked in consciousness with unhappy emotions (sorrow, shame, anger, fear, or guilt). In that case some form of so-called "deep psychotherapy" may be required. Deep psychotherapy involves probing into the vast psychic reservoir of buried memories and repressed impulses. In classical psychoanalysis, the method of deep psychotherapy introduced by Sigmund Freud, the chief technique used is that of free association in which material buried in the unconscious is made available to the conscious mind by the association of freely expressed thoughts and feelings and of the ideas and images in dreams. Psychoanalysis is very rarely suggested for young people.

Various forms of somatic (physical) treatment are now used as adjuncts of psychotherapy. These measures include electroconvulsive therapy and the use of tranquilizing and antidepressant drugs.

Electroconvulsive therapy is being widely used in the treatment of manic-depressive psychosis, schizophrenia, and a number of other conditions. The patient is sent into a state of physiologic shock by convulsions induced with electricity, from which he may emerge much improved for varying lengths of time.

The drugs known as tranquilizers and antidepressants are used for the

[1] *Mental Disorders: A Guide to Control Methods,* American Public Health Association, New York, September, 1962.

relief of symptoms in both the neuroses and the psychoses. Tranquilizers are used to calm patients during periods of excitement. They have proved to be a great help in carrying out the "open-door" policy (now followed in many hospitals), which is based on the realization that physical restraints and locked wards are unnecessary and that much of the antisocial and irresponsible behavior of mental patients disappears when they are treated as responsible human beings. Tranquilizers are helping also to reduce or to remove some of the barriers which make it difficult for the psychiatrist to reach and treat his patients' sick minds. Patients who respond well to tranquilizing drugs may be allowed to leave the hospital and continue any further treatment necessary in out-patient clinics or physicians' offices.

Physicians also are prescribing these drugs for mildly psychotic patients who do not require hospitalization, for neurotic patients, and even for mentally healthy persons to relieve tension in times of strain and stress. Medical authorities warn, however, that like other valuable drugs tranquilizers can be harmful as well as helpful. Even the mildest may cause toxic side effects. They should never be used unless a doctor prescribes them.

The use of new drugs in psychotherapy combined with the open-door policy has had the effect of reducing the length of treatment in mental hospitals for many patients. As a result an increasing number of patients who have learned to function reasonably well can now be treated at home or in a clinic or a doctor's office instead of having to spend years or even their whole lives in a hospital. This means that mental hospitals and the psychiatric department of general hospitals can admit and treat many more mentally ill persons than formerly. It also means added responsibilities for official and voluntary health agencies engaged in public health education and in the provision of home-care programs and psychiatric treatment centers.

Convalescent mental patients need to be welcomed back into their communities without being made to feel that there is any stigma attached to the fact that they have been mentally ill. Their families and their teachers or employers need to learn what they can do to smooth the pathway of return to home and school or work. They need the personal, competent aftercare that will help to prevent further breakdowns. Some of them may need to go back to the hospital for varying lengths of time. All of these needs and many others point up to the greatest need of all—the development of integrated community mental health services for convalescent mental patients as well as all others who require professional help.

IDENTIFYING CHILDREN WITH EMOTIONAL AND SOCIAL PROBLEMS

Probably no other single factor in helping emotionally disturbed children is as important as early detection of those who need professional help. Only two institutions in our society have contact with all children, the family and the school. Several studies have been made to determine the reliability of judgments of mental health made by teachers and mothers as a basis for referral to professional people trained to give psychological assistance to disturbed youngsters. The results, for the most part, show that teachers are in general valid observers and raters of children's emotional status. Mothers, too, came out well on the score of reliability. In one study of families with at least one child in the third grade, the results showed that "the greater the number of symptoms reported by the mother, the greater the likelihood that the child will be rated disturbed by the teacher." [2]

Self-appraisals and Sociometric Ratings

Increasing the use of data available to the teacher has the effect of increasing the breadth and depth of the teacher's understanding of the child. Other sources of data, besides the teacher's own observations and what she learns from parents, the school nurse, and other school personnel, are self-appraisals and sociometric ratings. In self-appraisal the answers given by students to questions designed to bring out what they themselves think of their own feelings and behavior and their relationships with, and their attitude toward, others may provide a sort of inventory of their emotional health.

No one, however, has the power of seeing himself as others see him. Sociometric testing serves to measure how children see other children. Each child in a group is requested to give, in strict confidence, his opinions as to which children in the group fit certain descriptions, for example: those who are always complaining; those who are most liked by everyone; those who always want to have their own way; those who are too shy to make friends easily; those who often get into fights; those who have trouble reciting; those you would like for best friends. A host of studies confirm the effectiveness of peer response in noting those children who are becoming or have become alienated from self or group. Teacher judgment, however, holds first place as the "most valid and reliable indicator of pupil adjustment and maladjustment."

Putting together her own observations and the data she collects from easily available sources can help the teacher to make more positive and earlier referrals of children who need help. All that she can say, however, is "On the basis of information I have at this time, it appears that a further look should be taken at this child to find out if my guess that he is emotionally disturbed is correct." The teacher in most schools refers the child to the school health service or the school guidance staff, who will determine the most appropriate follow-up procedure.

[2] Cited in *Reference Papers,* 1960 White House Conference on Children and Youth, pp. 237–238.

Points to Consider in Identifying Children Who Need Help

The attitude of teachers toward their children's behavior is important because attitudes determine reactions, and reactions in turn determine how behavior problems are handled. Although a teacher may realize that a child is emotionally disturbed, her own feelings may stand in the way of giving the right sort of help. It is extremely difficult to be objective about the behavior of others. That has always been the principal drawback in getting symptoms of maladjustment recognized for what they are. It is easy to feel personally affronted or disgusted by behavior we dislike —hard to realize that our feelings may lead us to make serious mistakes in interpreting and dealing with such behavior—still harder to admit that we may dislike a person because he possesses attributes that we dislike in ourselves.

Teachers who understand children know that all forms of behavior have underlying causes. If there is one sure thing that has been learned in the study of the mind, it is that no one lives in a vacuum. Every pattern of behavior in a child is the result of the reactions of that particular child to a series of particular environmental situations. Knowing this, the understanding teacher will not reject any child whose behavior differs markedly from that of the average healthy, well-adjusted child. This does not mean that she will condone his undesirable behavior. Rather she will seek to understand its significance so that her methods of dealing with him will serve to counteract rather than to entrench unsatisfactory ways of meeting life.

It has been pointed out that teachers have a unique opportunity to observe deviations from normal behavior in children which indicate that professional advice is needed. The most helpful observations are those in which specific descriptions are given of how the child acts in concrete situations. Instead of giving snap judgments, colored by what the teacher personally thinks about the child's behavior, it is better to record incidents that will give a clear picture of how the child is failing to react adequately to the requirements of social living. It takes practice to do this, because most of us are in the habit of interpreting and judging behavior, often without sufficient evidence, instead of recording simply what we hear and see.

In deciding what children need to be studied, it is important to keep in mind the stage of personality development through which all the children under observation are passing. As we have learned, children normally and characteristically have different emotional reactions at different periods in their lives. Although understanding teachers and parents know this, they are sometimes hard put to it not to show their embarrassment or anxiety when children fail to make a good impression on less understanding outsiders. Because of fear of criticism from "visiting firemen" or from relatives with antiquated notions of child upbringing, they may try to force the children into patterns of behavior for which they are not yet ready. At least part of the feelings of frustration or even of guilt which children suffer come from such attempts on the part of those who love and understand them.

Knowing that children go through various stages of personality development helps us to determine whether behavior at a certain age should be tolerated as "natural" or tackled as a problem. For example, lying, stealing, and temper tantrums are natural in young children but undesirable in older children. We may adopt as our definition of children who should be reported for study, then, those whose pattern of acting at a certain age is markedly different from that of the average child in that age period.

It is possible to give here only general descriptions of some of the characteristic ways of behaving which indicate that a child may need help in adjusting to his life situation (see Table 9-1).

Table 9-1

SOME COMMON INDICATIONS OF MALADJUSTMENT IN SCHOOL CHILDREN

Attacking behavior........	Temper outbursts Aggressiveness, defiant attitude, resistance to authority, disobedience Quarrelsomeness, fighting, boasting Rejection of school routine; wanting always to be the leader in school activities or to pursue own methods of work Contentiousness, poor sportsmanship Overactivity Delinquency, truancy
Withdrawing behavior.....	Shyness, timidity, cowardliness Unsocialness, solitariness, inability to make friends Dreaminess Extreme docility, overdependence on adults or on routine Sensitiveness to criticism, feelings easily hurt Fearfulness, suspiciousness Pedantry, overdiligence in schoolwork Inability to carry responsibility
Somatic manifestations.....	Nail-biting Finger sucking Pencil chewing Blinking Facial twitching Infantile speech Frequent use of toilet
Educational problems......	Difficulty with reading despite normal intelligence and vision Difficulties with arithmetic Lack of application Speech difficulties

The Different Child

In her initial contact with the children in a class, the teacher will notice whether there are any children who "stand out like sore thumbs" in appearance or behavior. Children of school age normally are conformists. They want to look and act as much as possible like the other children of their age and social status.

Of course, the teacher knows from her training and experience that there is a wide variation within normal limits in social behavior, intelligence, and appearance, just as there is in physical body measurements. Children intuitively know this, too. They will not reject another child simply because he is a little cleaner or neater, or a little dirtier or more slovenly, or a little more withdrawn or aggressive, or somewhat brighter or duller than the average. It is the Little Lord Fauntleroys and the Ugly Ducklings, the sissies and the bullies, the highly gifted or the extremely backward who frequently find themselves misfits in the school community. A child who is radically different from the others in his group may need special attention in order to keep him from becoming permanently stigmatized as an outsider during his school life.

The Suddenly Changed Child

As the teacher becomes acquainted with her students, she knows what to expect of them in appearance and behavior. She also knows the child's record of previous scholastic attainment and, in most schools, his health record. When a child who has always been clean and neat suddenly becomes slovenly and unkempt for several days; or a normally cooperative child suddenly becomes hostile or negativistic for any length of time; or a child who has done adequate schoolwork begins consistently to fail; or a child who has hitherto shared the enthusiasms, fads, and prejudices of his classmates suddenly shows little interest in school activities, there may be something wrong physically or some alteration in personality or in the home situation or in relationships in the child's life which ought to receive attention.

Sudden changes in the other direction—from bad behavior to good—also may have psychiatric significance unless the change is the result of the correction of some physical disability like poor eyesight or malnutrition. Although such a change may come as a relief to the teacher, it sometimes is a sign of an alteration in attitudes or in relationships which presages a more profound alteration in personality.

The Unhappy Child

Young people, like their elders, have fits of the "blues," but it is not natural for them to act "broody" for any length of time.

Sometimes, however, particularly during adolescence, a boy or girl may go through a prolonged period of depression. Any one or more of a great variety of factors in the environment or some inner duel between warring impulses may be responsible. Being like everyone else in appearance, in attitudes toward the other sex, in enthusiasms and "pet hates" is extremely important to adolescents. It may be that a despondent girl is not able, for some reason, to meet the standards of her school group. Perhaps she cannot dress like the other girls for economic reasons or parental foibles and feels sensitive about her appearance. Or special skills or talents may not give her the prestige they did earlier and will again later. A boy may be hiding rebellious impulses under his cloak of gloom. Perhaps he resents the fact that he is not allowed as much freedom as his companions. Or some physical disturbance of metabolic origin may be the trouble. Or he may be developing physically at a much slower or faster rate than the other boys of his group. Whatever may be the cause, these unhappy youngsters may develop a stubborn or sulky or morose manner, or consistently fall below their demonstrated ability in their schoolwork, or take no interest in school activities, with the result that their relations with their group deteriorate.

The chances are that they will recover spontaneously, but even so they need understanding, special guidance, and perhaps psychiatric attention. The teacher and the parents cannot know whether the depression is transitory in nature—"just one of those things"—or whether repeated episodes may be expected to occur.

Nothing will be gained by trying to kid a youngster out of a prolonged fit of blueness. An older, wiser person may talk himself hoarse about the advantages of distinction, of being different, or of making the best of things for the time being, without giving the slightest help to the unhappy girl or boy who is depressed because of repressed feelings of inferiority or guilt or insecurity. Making light of things, because they really do seem of little importance from the adult point of view, only aggravates the young person to whom they are of great importance.

The Solitary, Friendless Child

During elementary school age, particularly, children normally are friendly and gregarious. They want intensely to "belong," to be chosen when sides are being chosen in a game, to have chums or good pals. Hence, manifestations of pronounced withdrawal behavior should be viewed with suspicion. At best, they may clear up spontaneously; at worst, they may indicate emotional trends that may sweep the child from the safe harbor of actuality.

The withdrawn child is usually very timid. He may shun his classmates —refuse to take part in group games—have no close friends—sit dreamily staring into space when the others are playing or studying. He is likely to be docile and give the teacher no trouble except for his extreme sensitiveness. He may be easily embarrassed while reciting and stutter when asked to "speak up" or when his recitation is criticized. However, he may do well in his written work and test above average in intelligence.

It is a great mistake to allow the solitary, friendless, dependent child to drift further and further out of touch with the real world of social and economic competition in which he must eventually make a place for himself. He is already failing to meet the social requirements of his companions. He may long to "get in," to be acceptable to his group, but he gives the impression that he prefers to be "out." Left to himself he is often helpless to overcome this impression. He literally doesn't know how to break in, and so he doesn't try. But since he has to be "in" somewhere, he retreats more and more frequently into his own private world, and makes his bid for approval from the outside world of adults. The adults, however, cannot or will not go on indefinitely giving him sympathy and protection when he has reached the age at which society expects an individual to stand on his own feet. Also he is acquiring a taste for the delights to be found in getting what he wants in dreams without having to go to all the bother of working for it in a hard, cold world, which in his experience is as likely as not to reward his best efforts with failure.

The Accident-repeater Child

A history of repeated accidents indicates a need for studying a child and his environment. Perhaps he is simply having a run of bad luck. Or, he may have some physical defect like poor eyesight or poor hearing. Or, his history of repeated accidents may be explained by a tendency to be overactive and impulsive combined with a poor reaction to stress or by indifferent parental supervision or possibly by pent-up feelings of hostility and aggression.

Whatever may be at the bottom of repeated accidents, the child's teacher can be of real help in preventing the establishment of the accident habit by recognizing it as a symptom that should be brought to the attention of those responsible for the child's well-being.

The Young Social Rebel

As we have seen, aggressiveness is normal in school children in the elementary school period. This is largely because they want to feel important, to boss others, or at least to feel that they can do so. This is a period of intense likes and dislikes, and it is natural for children to pick on or gang up against those they dislike when they feel they can get away with it. This is especially true of children who have seen parents or teachers use bullying or tyrannical methods successfully to gain power over others, or who have never learned by experience the value of kindness and consideration in human relations.

Children whose social maladjustment is manifested in various forms of overaggressiveness usually need psychiatric help. Very often the parents as well as the children will require treatment.

Overdependence upon one or both parents or repressed feelings of guilt or inadequacy or unfortunate experiences with authority in the home usually lie back of personality disorders characterized by overaggressiveness. Perhaps a boy may be boastful and quarrelsome—always wanting to be the leader in every activity, constantly looking for ways of securing attention—because he is not so good as the other children in his schoolwork and in playing games and hence has failed to gain the approval of his schoolmates or his teacher. Making a nuisance of himself is his way of gaining prestige—of excelling in something. Asked why he acts as he does, he cannot possibly give the real reason because he doesn't know it himself.

Another child may be a troublemaker—a bully and poor sport with his classmates—a "tattletale" and "apple polisher" with his teachers—because he has learned that the easiest way to deal with authority is to placate it. But he must have some outlet for his outraged feelings, and so he takes out on his smaller or weaker classmates the impulses he is obliged to repress in the more complicated home situation, where the love of family he thinks he ought to feel conflicts with the hate he would be ashamed to admit even if he knew it existed.

Still another child may be a chronic truant, showing that he hates school by staying away whenever he gets the chance and by defying the teacher when he is present. Investigation may show that he has a stern, unbending father, or a domineering, selfish, exacting mother, or a bossy older brother or sister. The deep-seated resentment he feels is unconsciously transferred to his teacher, toward whom he can show his hostility without feeling guilty because he does not have to love as well as to obey her. In many cases of truancy or delinquency it has been shown that the children involved are letting off emotional steam in their relationship with persons or institutions which may be entirely blameless in their dealings with the children, but which have the misfortune to stand for authority.

The Adolescent Social Rebel

Consistently defiant attitudes and extreme egocentricity carried over from childhood into adolescence often have serious consequences. Adolescent social rebels present a very real threat to life and property in many urban and suburban areas. The origin of their antisocial attitudes and behavior lies primarily in the home, where most of the emotional difficulties of children develop. In practically all studies of delinquency, it has been found that there is little or no correlation between the socioeconomic status of the home and the development of delinquency. Antisocial tendencies may become rooted and flourish in any child from any home, where his needs for parental love, guidance, and supervision are not being met.

Obviously, parents cannot relegate their responsibilities to the school or to the police. But teachers can help to identify chronic aggressive reaction states and refer predelinquent children for psychiatric help before they get into serious trouble. The earlier the identification is made, the more successful the preventive efforts will be (see the Young Social Rebel earlier in this chapter).

Venereal Disease. Another serious social problem is the increase in venereal disease among adolescents in the United States. The American Social Health Association cites a rise among teen-agers of 130 per cent in reported cases from 1956 to 1960. The Public Health Service figures by age groups are shown in Table 9-2.

Table 9-2

REPORTED CASES OF VENEREAL DISEASE BY AGE GROUP
UNITED STATES, 1956–1960

Age groups	1956	1957	1958	1959	1960	Percent Increase 1956–1960
Primary and Secondary Syphilis						
0–9	11	33	23	39	20	+81.8
10–14	75	80	90	90	139	+85.3
15–19	1,093	1,192	1,228	1,620	2,577	+135.8
0–19	1,179	1,305	1,341	1,749	2,736	+132.1
All ages	6,399	6,581	7,134	9,798	16,144	+152.3
Gonorrhea						
0–9	1,222	1,628	1,164	1,325	1,619	+32.5
10–14	2,425	2,363	2,706	2,601	3,261	+34.5
15–19	44,264	43,705	48,723	50,088	53,649	+21.2
0–19	47,911	47,696	52,593	54,014	58,529	+22.2
All ages	224,687	214,872	232,818	240,265	258,933	+15.2

Source: *The Eradication of Syphilis,* A Task Force Report to the Surgeon General. U.S. Department of Health, Education, and Welfare, Public Health Service, 1962.

There is no single cause for these alarming increases. One factor is probably the false security offered by effective medical therapy. A lowering of moral and social values combined with more permissive attitudes toward sex undoubtedly contributes to increased promiscuity among teen-agers. Sex-oriented advertising aimed at capturing the teen-age market, estimated to have over 9 billion dollars to spend annually, has been cited as a factor. Most students of the problem believe that the major cause is the widespread lack among youngsters of forthright, accurate information on sex and the venereal diseases.

The home is, of course, the ideal and most effective place for the passing on of this information. (See Changes in Boy-girl Relationships in Chap. 4.) As is well known, however, home is often the last place children receive it. Therefore, the recommendation has been made that wherever possible "matter-of-fact" sex education and accurate information about VD should be given. Social studies and courses in health, biology and physiology, in history, and even in chemistry offer many opportunities for correlation. In some areas, unfortunately, laws prohibiting sex education and objections from parents prevent schools from offering the sane, unemotional sex teaching that could contribute to the control of VD.

Teen-age Pregnancies. Births out of wedlock are hardly new, but when the rate of such births more than doubles within a twenty-year period among teen-age girls, and the average age becomes younger, the problem requires attention from all community agencies. Like venereal disease, the problem is a symptom of serious social ills. Although no figures are available on the exact number of girls who drop out of high school because of pregnancy, the increasing incidence is of grave concern to educators.

Studies make it clear that these girls belong to no one group. They come from every walk of life, but certain factors are often present. Faulty child-parent relationships frequently enter the picture. Crowded living conditions, lack of good recreational facilities, and inadequate supervision by parents all undoubtedly contribute to illegitimacy. Adolescents themselves in the 1960 White House Conference on Children and Youth mentioned the influence of some of today's books, magazines, and TV programs.

The solution of the problem calls for the provision of community services based on the concept of the intrinsic worth of the individual—both mother and child. Following two studies of unmarried mothers in New York City, the Community Council of Greater New York included some specific suggestions for schools:

1. The broadening of family life education courses in junior and senior high schools, and the provision of neighborhood parent education courses as possible channels for reaching young girls and their parents.

2. Assumption by school personnel of more responsibility for counseling pregnant girls and referring them to appropriate community services, and modification of attitudes so as to break down the girl's fear of telling the school counselor about her condition.

Teen-age Drinking as a Social Problem

The use of alcoholic beverages is so much a part of present-day social life in this country that all teen-agers sooner or later are faced with the necessity of deciding for or against taking a drink. The American Medical

Association[3] estimates that the average teen-ager starts experimenting with drinking around seventeen years of age.

Young people cannot be expected to understand warnings, or to make sensible decisions, unless they know the facts about alcohol—what it is and how it affects body and mind. They must learn that alcohol is a potentially dangerous drug; that some people should *never* drink; but that others can use alcohol, always in moderation, without harm, *except when driving!*

In their teens, young people are particularly vulnerable to social pressure from their group. It is vital, therefore, that they learn to respect abstinence in others. Refusal to drink should always be a free choice—respected as such. They are more likely to learn acceptance of individual decisions if the school gives them the unbiased, scientific facts, good and bad, about alcohol and its history. High schools especially can include these facts in many courses—in general and social sciences, in biology, in physical education, and in health courses.

Teen-age Smoking as a Psychosocial Problem

Cigarette smoking has been increasing steadily in the United States since the beginning of this century. In the year 1900 the average number of cigarettes smoked per person was 49; in 1963 it was 3,958. Associated with this tremendous increase is the statistical and scientific evidence that links smoking to several serious disorders (see Chronic Diseases Associated with Cigarette Smoking, in Chap. 11). An evaluation of this evidence is contained in a report entitled *Smoking and Health* which was made in 1964 by a committee of ten medical and other pertinent authorities appointed in 1959 by the Surgeon General of the Public Health Service (see Selected References at the end of this chapter).

On the basis of its prolonged and detailed examination of the many converging lines of evidence on the ill effects of smoking on health, the committee delivered its now famous final judgment: *Cigarette smoking is a health hazard of sufficient importance in the United States to warrant appropriate remedial action.*

Of particular interest to teachers, school nurses, and all others concerned with the health education of young people are the reports of studies given in *Smoking and Health* which relate to the formation and continuation of the smoking habit. All available knowledge points toward the years from the early teens to the age of twenty as a significant period during which the majority of later smokers began to develop the active habit. At the twelfth-grade level, from 40 to 55 per cent of children have been found to be cigarette smokers.

Why do young people start smoking? Why does smoking become a

[3] Marvin A. Block, Chairman, Committee on Alcoholism, American Medical Association: "Teen-age Drinking: Whose Responsibility?" *Today's Health*, May, 1961.

habit? If a smoker discontinues the habit, what makes him stop? There is no single answer to any of these questions. There is overwhelming evidence, however, that smoking is to a large extent psychologically and socially determined. Social stimulation appears to play a major role in a young person's early and first experiments with smoking. The smoking patterns and attitudes among the adults in the family seem to have a strong influence on many youngsters. Striving for status in one's peer group—the adolescent desire to be like everyone else—the satisfaction of inner needs that vary singly and in combination from individual to individual—these are among the many psychosocial factors that may enter into the teen-age smoking problem.

Even less is known about why a youngster may stop smoking than about why he may begin. The longer a person smokes, however, the harder it is for him to stop. This fact taken together with the fact that the risks of smoking increase greatly with the duration of smoking makes it especially hazardous to begin the smoking habit early in life. Consequently school-age children, especially teen-agers, compose the most important target group for education designed to make smokers and potential smokers fully aware of the risks they run in beginning or in continuing to smoke cigarettes.

Teen-agers and Drug Addiction

Shortly after World War II, narcotics addiction among teen-agers, and even among the pre-teen ages, rose sharply in certain areas of the country.

Authorities in adolescent behavior believe that drug addiction, like other severe forms of aggressive behavior—stealing, reckless driving, and drinking—is one of the ways in which teen-agers react to tension created by home and community problems. This is substantiated by the fact that addiction among high school students seems to be highest in crowded neighborhoods or large cities where youngsters are not on good terms with the police and social conditions are poor. Broken homes and inadequate parent-child relationships are also a common finding. Other contributing factors are the urge to be "one of the gang," curiosity, imitation of an adult, and the "try anything once" attitude.

The slightest experimentation with narcotic drugs is highly dangerous. Youngsters can be made addicts within a few weeks or less. Before they have a chance to recognize the danger, they are "hooked," too sick physically and mentally to be able to stop. Moral sense is lessened or completely killed. The cost of illegally sold narcotic drugs is so high that girls often turn to prostitution, and boys to theft and other crimes to obtain the money needed for their necessary doses.

Heroin, by far the most dangerous narcotic drug, is made from opium. It is the principal cause of the serious drug-addiction problem uncovered among teen-agers in certain sections of our larger cities. It is so easy to become addicted to heroin that its use, even by physicians, is prohibited by law in the United States. Heroin is peddled illegally to addicts in capsule form called a "cap" or in package form, known as a "deck." Addicts are usually "mainliners," that is, they dissolve the drug in water and inject it directly into a vein.

Cocaine, made from the leaves of the South American coca plant, acts on the nervous system as a stimulant. First it produces feelings of power, joviality, alertness, and superiority. Later it causes nervousness, insomnia, and loss of efficiency. Cocaine addicts usually sniff it in the form of a white powder which they call "snow."

Marijuana, made from the dried leaves and flowers of fully matured hemp plants, is another dangerous narcotic drug. Its effects are produced principally by smoking marijuana cigarettes, which are most commonly known as "reefers." Smoking marijuana cigarettes produces a strange dreaming state of intoxication, especially among emotionally unstable individuals. Many crimes have been committed under its influence. Individuals react differently to its effects, however. Young people who are normally happy and well adjusted seem to get no pleasure from marijuana. Although not in itself habit-forming, smoking "reefers" is almost invariably the first step among teen-agers to the greater "thrill" of the deadly heroin habit.

Barbiturates, drugs made from barbituric acid, are the base for many sleeping pills sold legally on prescription under a variety of trade names. They are also sold illegally to drug addicts, who call them "goof balls," and use them to produce relaxation and sleep when they cannot get their normal supply of narcotics. The barbiturates are also habit-forming in themselves and addicts become mentally confused and unable to coordinate movement, much like alcoholics.

Amphetamines are benzedrine-like drugs which act as stimulants on the central nervous system. "Bennies" and "pep pills" are slang terms for these drugs. Physicians may prescribe amphetamines in small amounts when needed. Unfortunately, however, an increasing number of young people are using them on their own responsibility in order to keep awake while studying for examinations or to improve athletic performance. Even in moderately small doses, these so-called pep pills have in many instances resulted in habituation. Excessive nervousness, impairment of judgment, and even hallucinations are among the effects they may produce. Tragic highway accidents have followed their use.

Both the barbiturates ("goof balls") and the amphetamines (pep pills) are classed as *psychotoxic drugs.* Many authorities consider them to be a more widespread public danger than narcotic drugs because they are cheaper and more easily obtained. They believe that the rising traffic death tolls and the increases in juvenile delinquency and crimes of violence can be blamed in part on the uncontrolled use of psychotoxic drugs.

The School's Responsibility. The problem of finding, treating, and preventing narcotic drug addiction among young people is, like most other serious problems, complex. Its solution lies in giving people all the facts and then enlisting their cooperation in taking every action, national and local, needed to control it.

Next to parents, schools have the greatest responsibility toward children's mental and physical health. Education on the nature and effects of taking narcotics should be made part of school health education, preferably after discussion with parents, church groups, social agencies, or other community groups concerned. Many young addicts have claimed that they would never have taken their first "shot" if they had known "what it was all about."

Just as teachers and nurses watch for other signs of ill health, they should also be alert to indications of drug addiction. Such indications include watery eyes, frequent yawning and drowsiness, abnormal restlessness, poor appetite, burnt finger tips from cigarettes, body odor, long stays in washrooms, sleeves kept rolled down to hide arm puncture marks, and marked mental and physical deterioration. Other signs are the presence, in desks, washrooms, or other places, of articles associated with taking drugs—hypodermic needles or syringes, bent-handled teaspoons, medicine droppers, capsules or small packages of white powder, or the empty containers. Children known or suspected of taking drugs should be referred to the school physician as promptly as possible.

MEETING THE NEED FOR GUIDANCE IN SCHOOL-AGE CHILDREN

In recent years rapid progress has been made in the science of psychology, upon which the recognition and treatment of unhealthy emotional patterns are based. Unfortunately, however, the facilities for applying this science in the guidance of school children with behavior problems are at present very inadequate. A few school systems do have a bureau or department of child guidance, together with a mental hygiene clinic or child guidance center to which children requiring psychiatric study and treatment may be referred by the teacher, school nurse, or school physician. Lacking such an arrangement, it is possible in some of the larger cities to obtain psychiatric services for school children with behavior problems from child guidance or mental hygiene clinics in the community. Even where professional services are available, it is agreed that, for the best results, administrators, teachers, and parents must cooperate closely with the specialists in dealing with a particular child.

Important as it is to have specialists to treat the serious problems of emotional disturbance among school children, it is more important to use the time and skill of these specialists to help teachers and principals to understand the emotional health of all children so that, in the day-to-day contacts that the educational staff has with children, they may prevent serious disorders from developing.

One of the great advantages of clinic guidance is the opportunity it affords for getting at the source of the trouble in problems arising out of the home situation. Even if the teacher knows that defective parent-child relationships or unresolved conflicts of parents and their frustrations or economic difficulties are the cause of the child's behavior problem, the home and community environment is seldom within the sphere of her influence. In the clinic, parents are encouraged to talk over with professional interviewers their own problems and those of their children. The most recent trend is to involve the entire family in simultaneous treatment. Also an increasing number of clinics are assuming responsibility for helping to give school personnel, especially teachers and school nurses, an understanding of the problems of emotionally disturbed children so as to avoid conflicts in methods of handling that would confuse the children still further. It is sometimes possible to arrange conferences to give teachers, school nurses, and parents opportunities to sit down with specialists in the clinic and work together on plans for changing misunderstood, unhappy children into well-adjusted, happy children.

Far more important than the treatment of mental illness is its prevention. There is growing recognition of the need for specialists in child psychology to devote at least part of their time to helping teachers, principals, and school nurses to understand the significance of various forms of child behavior so that in their day-by-day contacts with children they may prevent serious disorders from developing. An orientation program of this kind is possible in schools with guidance staffs or mental health personnel, or both. As things stand at present, however, the personnel shortages in the mental health specialties are so acute that it is impossible even to staff adequately child guidance clinics, psychiatric hospitals, and other treatment centers. The great majority of teachers must depend on what they have learned about emotional development in childhood and upon their experience with child behavior to cooperate with parents, religious leaders, school nurses, and physicians in the friendly teamwork necessary to help children to escape mental illness.

Above all is the need for a climate in the school which permits healthy mental and emotional development in all children. The teacher herself is the key to this situation. Serenity, stability, understanding, patience, and tolerance are essential attributes in all teachers if the need for psychiatric study and treatment in childhood is to be reduced to a minimum.

FOR REVIEW AND DISCUSSION

1. Tell the difference between each of the following words or terms:

   a. Evasion by attack and evasion by withdrawal
   b. Neuroses and psychoses
   c. Obsession and phobia
   d. Psychoneurotic and psychosomatic
   e. Psychotherapy and psychology
   f. Sociometric testing and self-appraisal

2. Which of the following statements are false and which are true? Reword each false statement so as to make it true.

   a. Physical health and mental health are interdependent.
   F b. Anger is an antisocial emotion that children should learn always to repress.
   T c. Consistently good behavior nearly always signifies that a child is well adjusted.
   T d. Persons who have mild neuroses usually can attend to their personal affairs and do their work with reasonable success.
   T e. Physical symptoms caused by anxiety are consciously felt repercussions of unconscious conflict.
   F f. Behavior patterns caused by consciously felt anger or fear and behavior patterns caused by repressed hostility resemble each other.
   F g. A person suffering from a psychosis can usually cure himself.
   T h. It is unwise and may be dangerous to take a tranquilizing drug on one's own responsibility.
   T i. Teachers have proved that they can be relied upon to detect students who need professional help in solving emotional problems.
   F j. A teacher should be greatly relieved when a consistently aggressive child suddenly becomes docile and easy to manage.

3. Discuss these questions in class:

   a. Why is it important to help children understand that emotions like anger and fear are common to everyone in certain situations?
   b. How can we help children to acquire techniques for meeting difficulties ranging from minor disappointments to conditions that cannot be changed, such as irreversible mental retardation, intellectual superiority with its hazard of social maladjustment, and irremediable physical defects or handicaps?

SELECTED REFERENCES

Mental Illness and Health

American Public Health Association: *Mental Disorders: A Guide to Control Measures*, The Association, New York, 1962.

Atkin, Edith L.: *Aggressiveness in Children,* Child Study Association of America, Inc., New York. (Describes and discusses aggressiveness, what it means, and how to use it constructively.)

Beers, Clifford W.: *A Mind That Found Itself,* Doubleday & Company, Inc., New York, ed. 1953. (The fascinating autobiography of the founder of the modern mental-hygiene movement.)

English, O. Spurgeon, and Gerald H. J. Pearson: *Emotional Problems of Living; Avoiding the Neurotic Pattern,* W. W. Norton & Company, Inc., New York, 1955.

Gallagher, James Roswell, and Herbert I. Harris: *Emotional Problems of Adolescents,* Oxford University Press, New York, 1958.

Joint Commission on Mental Illness and Health, of the National Institute of Mental Health: *Action for Mental Health,* Basic Books, Inc., Publishers, New York, 1961.

Joint Commission on Mental Illness and Health, of the National Institute of Mental Health: *The Role of Schools in Mental Health,* a report by Wesley Ali Smith and George W. Goethols; Basic Books, Inc., Publishers, New York, 1962. (Includes a field study.)

Moak, Helen: *The Troubled Child,* Holt, Rinehart, and Winston, Inc., New York, 1958. (A book primarily for parents, but valuable for everyone working with children.)

Ogg, Elizabeth: *Psychotherapy: A Helping Process,* Public Affairs Pamphlet No. 329, Public Affairs Committee, Inc., New York.

Peck, Robert F., and James V. Mitchell, Jr.: *Mental Health,* Department of Classroom Teachers, American Educational Research Association of the National Education Association, Washington, D.C., 1962. (A pamphlet on the importance of mental health in the classroom. It reviews the world in which children live psychosocially, the mental health of children in the home and classroom, and the importance of the mental health of teachers.)

Rogers, Dorothy: *Mental Hygiene in Elementary Education,* Houghton-Mifflin Company, Boston, 1957. (A book for teachers on the mental health of the parent and mental health in the school; gives suggestions on ways of helping children.)

Juvenile Delinquency

Brecker, Ruth: *The Delinquent and the Law,* Public Affairs Pamphlet No. 337, Public Affairs Committee, Inc., New York.

Butcher, Ruth L., and Marion O. Robertson: *The Unmarried Mother,* Public Affairs Pamphlet No. 282, Public Affairs Committee, Inc., New York.

Hymes, James L., Jr.: *Behavior and Misbehavior, a Teacher's Guide to Action,* Prentice-Hall, Inc., New York, 1955.

Kough, Jack, and Robert F. De Haan: *Teacher's Guidance Handbook* (first given as reference in Chap. 5). Vol. I, *Identifying Children with Special Needs,* Sec. III, Chaps. 13–15; Vol. II, *Helping Children with Special Needs,* Sec. III, Chap. 12.

Kvaraceus, William C., and Walter B. Miller: *Juvenile Delinquency Project,* National Education Association, Washington, D.C., 1959. Part I, *Culture and the Individual;* Part II, *Principles and Practices.* (A report of research on the problem prepared especially for teachers.)

Neisser, Edith G., and Nina Ridenour: *Your Children and Their Gangs,* U.S. Department of Health, Education, and Welfare, Washington, D.C., 1960. (A booklet describing and discussing gang behavior among children and adolescents.)

Richman, T. Lefoy: *Venereal Disease: Old Plague—New Challenge,* Public Affairs Pamphlet No. 292, Public Affairs Committee, Inc., New York.

Strang, Ruth: *Facts about Juvenile Delinquency,* Science Research Associates, Chicago. (A guidance booklet.)

Alcoholism

American Medical Association: *How Teens Set the Stage for Alcoholism,* The Association, Chicago.

Cain, Arthur H.: *Young People and Drinking,* The John Day Company, Inc., New York, 1963. (A scientifically sound appraisal of the facts about alcohol written for young people, their parents, and teachers by an authority in the field of alcohol studies.)

McCarthy, Raymond G.: *Discussion Guides for Questions about Alcohol,* Yale Center of Alcohol Studies, New Haven, Conn., 1961. (A guide for teachers. Presents areas of student interest in alcohol and alcoholism; and offers subject matter for questions and discussion.)

McCarthy, Raymond G.: *Drinking and Intoxication—Selected Readings in Social Attitudes and Controls,* The Free Press of Glencoe, New York, 1959. (A collection of interesting readings which gives a cultural perspective on drinking problems among different people at different periods and on the efforts of various societies to control the use of alcoholic beverages.)

McCarthy, Raymond G.: *Facts about Alcohol,* Science Research Associates, Chicago. (A guidance booklet.)

Smoking

Smoking and Health, Report of the Advisory Committee to the Surgeon General of the Public Health Service, Public Health Service Publication No. 1103, 1964.

McGrady, Pat: *Cigarettes and Health,* Public Affairs Pamphlet No. 220, Public Affairs Committee, Inc., New York.

Drug Addiction

Murtagh, John M., and Sara Harris: *Who Live in Shadow*, McGraw-Hill Book Company, New York, 1960. (About narcotic addiction—its prevention and treatment.)

Nyswander, Marie: *The Drug Addict as a Patient*, Grune & Stratton, Inc., New York, 1956. (The author's experiences with teen-age drug users.)

Vogel, Victor H., and Virginia Vogel: *Facts about Narcotics*, Science Research Associates, Chicago. (A guidance booklet.)

Organizations

National Association for Mental Health
American Social Health Association

Chapter 10

CIRCULATION SURVEY

The Circulatory System
Signs and Symptoms Associated with Circulatory
   Disturbances
Young Hearts in Trouble
Dealing with Circulatory Emergencies
Blood and Its Composition
Blood Disorders
Diseases Spread by Blood-sucking Insects
The Circulation of Lymph

The more or less solid tissues of the body may be compared to an expanse of wet sand on the seashore. The grains of sand are the cells, and the sea water that moistens them is tissue fluid, or lymph. The cells are fixed in their places. They cannot forage for the supplies they need or conduct the waste materials that result from their activities to the appropriate dumping grounds for removal from the body. Two moving streams within the body—one swiftly flowing, the blood; the other sluggish, the lymph—serve continuously as carriers between the fixed secluded cells and the places in the body where provisions are stocked and wastes are removed. Only by understanding the significance of these remarkable fluids and the manner in which they are kept in circulation can teachers appreciate the meaning of much of what they observe in healthy children as well as in those in need of medical attention.

THE CIRCULATORY SYSTEM

The blood moves swiftly from the heart and back to it in a completely enclosed system composed of miles upon miles of tubular vessels. The sole function of the heart is to act as a pump to keep the blood in motion.

The Heart

The heart is a powerful, highly specialized muscle containing two chambers, a right and a left. Each chamber is equipped with valves to keep blood flowing through the heart in the right direction. These valves are located at the inlet and outlet of each of the heart chambers, and at the opening in the partition that separates each heart chamber into two compartments, an upper (auricle) and a lower (ventricle).

When the Heart Beats. At each beat or contraction of the heart (the systole), the inlet valves close and blood is driven through the outlet valve of the left ventricle into the great main arterial trunk of the body, and through the outlet valve of the right ventricle into the vessels that carry it to the lungs. The heart must then rest before it can contract again. The split second of rest between beats makes it possible for the healthy heart to keep up its work of driving out a heavy load of blood seventy times a minute or faster for seventy years or more without noticeable fatigue. During this period of relaxation (the diastole), the outlet valves of the heart chambers close and the inlet valves open, permitting blood to flow from the great veins into the right auricle from all the remote regions of the body and into the left auricle from the lungs.

The Circulatory Trees

The blood vessels are arranged in two distinct but continuous systems. Because of their elaborate branchings they are often compared to luxuri-

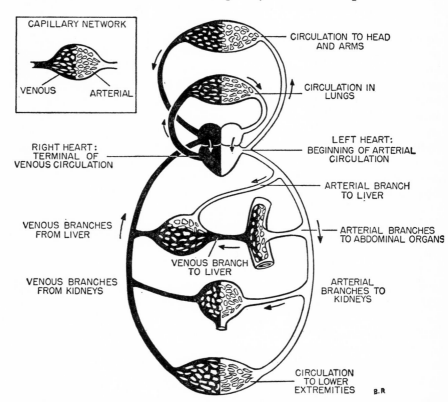

FIG. 10-1. Diagram of the circulatory system. Arterial blood is pumped from the left side of the heart into arteries, which lead into capillary networks. Venous blood is collected from the capillary networks and returned to the right side of the heart through veins. Then it is pumped to the lungs for oxygenation and returned to the left side of the heart.

antly growing trees. The arterial tree carries blood *away* from the heart. The venous tree carries blood *toward* the heart. The blood finds its way into the tree of veins from the tree of arteries through delicate networks of minute blood vessels called *capillaries* (see Fig. 10-1).

The General, or Systemic, Circulation. The grand trunk of the arterial tree is the aorta, into which blood is forced directly from the left ventricle of the heart. Its big branches run to the arms and legs, the head, and the organs of the abdomen—the stomach, intestines, liver, kidneys, and spleen. In these regions the large arteries in their branchings get smaller and smaller until finally they dwindle to the size of minute twigs. These twigs of the arterial tree are the arterioles.

Blood flows from the arterioles into the exceedingly thin-walled capillaries which wind in and out among the cells in all tissues. The capillary networks may be compared to a vast irrigation system of closed canals through the walls of which water, food, oxygen, and other materials for the cells are exchanged for the wastes produced by the cells. After passing slowly through the capillaries, the blood with its load of waste products flows into the first tiny branches, or twigs, of the tree of veins. These little veins, or venules, merge to form veins which become increasingly larger until finally they join the two grand trunks of the venous tree, through which the blood is returned to the right auricle of the heart. The venous trunk for the head, neck, arms, and chest is the superior vena cava, and the venous trunk for the legs and the abdominal organs is the inferior vena cava (see Fig. 10-2).

There are three important subdivisions of the general, or systemic, circulation. These subdivisions are the pulmonary circulation, the portal circulation, and the renal circulation.

The Pulmonary Circulation. The beat of the heart which forces arterial blood from the left ventricle into the aorta for its grand tour of the body also forces venous blood out of the right ventricle into the pulmonary artery for a side trip through the lungs. The venous blood in the right chamber is blood that has given up in the tissues the oxygen with which arterial blood is loaded. Also venous blood is heavily charged with carbon dioxide (CO_2). This gas is one of the end products of energy metabolism. The other end product is heat, the mechanical equivalent of which is energy. The carbon dioxide is a waste product and hence must be removed from the body. The heat is a vital product which keeps the fires of life burning and supplies the energy for all the work of the body.

Venous, or deoxygenated, blood is pumped from the right ventricle of the heart through the capillary networks in the lungs. There the carbon dioxide is exchanged for oxygen, and the aerated, or oxygenated, blood flows on through the pulmonary veins into the left auricle of the heart.

It takes less than half a minute for blood to make its round trip through the systemic and pulmonary circulations—from the right side of the heart through the lungs to the left side, and from the left side through the body and back to the right side.

The Portal Circulation. The portal circulation is an arrangement for sending blood to the liver from the stomach, small intestine, pancreas, and spleen. It is formed by veins which collect blood from the capillaries in these organs. These veins finally merge into one big vein, called the portal vein. After entering the liver the portal vein branches out into innumerable capillaries. This arrangement allows ample opportunity for the filtering out from the blood of various food substances and their absorption by the liver cells. Poisons or bacteria which the blood may have picked up also are filtered out and excreted by the liver in bile. After the blood has been acted on by the liver, it is carried by the capillaries into a new set of veins which return it to the inferior vena cava emptying into the heart.

The Renal Circulation. The renal circulation is the arrangement for sending blood to the kidneys for the filtering out of metabolic wastes produced by the breakdown of protein in foods. Blood is carried to the kidneys through branches of the renal arteries and is returned to the heart

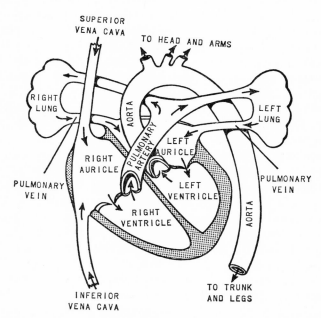

FIG. 10-2. The circulation through the heart and lungs. Blood flows into the right side of the heart from the two grand trunks of the tree of veins. From there it is pumped to the lungs, through the pulmonary artery and its branches. It returns to the left side of the heart through the pulmonary veins and is pumped into the aorta (the grand trunk of the arterial tree) for distribution to all parts of the body.

through the renal veins which empty into the inferior vena cava. (See The Kidneys and Their Work, in Chap. 13.)

The Pulse. Arteries have relatively thick elastic walls which are provided with a layer of circular muscle. Hence they can stretch and rebound to drive the blood along after the initial push given it by the heartbeat. Each time the heart forces a load of blood into the already full arterial tree, it starts a distending wave that can be felt as a "pulse" in any branch that lies comparatively close to the surface of the body. The principal places are in the wrist at the base of the thumb, at the temple in front of the ear, and at the back of the ankle on the inner side of the foot. The pulse rate is best taken by placing three fingers on the inner side of the wrist below the base of the thumb.

The pulse rate is regulated by the autonomic nervous system according to the needs of the body for oxygen and fuel food and for conserving or getting rid of heat. Vigorous physical activity, fever, and emotional excitement all make the heart beat faster than usual. The resting rate is normally more rapid in childhood than in adult life.

Blood Pressure. Any fluid that fills to capacity any closed system of tubes will exert pressure on the walls of the tubes. Blood actually overfills the closed system of tubes consisting of the blood vessels through which it circulates. Arterial blood pressure (which is the pressure measured when a physician takes a person's blood pressure by means of an instrument called a sphygmomanometer) varies rhythmically with the beating of the heart. It rises during contraction, when a fresh load of blood is driven into the arterial system (the systolic pressure), and falls during relaxation (the diastolic pressure), when the heart pauses to fill up between beats.

Except for the tempo and force of the heartbeat, the factor that has the greatest influence on arterial blood pressure is the resistance offered by the arterioles and capillaries (particularly the former) to the passage of blood from the tree of arteries to the tree of veins. The slightly elastic walls of the arterioles are composed mostly of rings of muscle. Nerves running from the autonomic nervous system to the muscles carry the impulses that make them contract or relax. Thus the bores of the arterioles may be made narrower or wider by nervous influences, as the occasion requires, to regulate the quantity of blood passing from the arteries to the veins by way of the capillaries.

The narrowing of the arterioles acts like a dam to back up the blood in the arteries. Naturally, the pressure in the arteries then goes up. The widening of the arterioles lowers the level of the dam and the pressure then goes down.

Temporary rises of blood pressure accompany muscular exertion and digestion (which increase the rate and force of the heartbeat) and periods of worry, joy, fear, anger, or other emotions (which give rise to nervous impulses that cause the arterioles to tighten up).

Hypertension. Hypertension is the medical name for persistently high blood pressure. It occurs when the arterioles throughout the body are kept in a more or less constantly constricted, or tightened-up, state. Hypertension increases the resistance that the heart must overcome in pumping blood into the arteries and thus greatly increases its work. This extra work tends to make the heart grow larger and weaker. Many cases of hypertension are associated with other diseases, especially diseases of the kidneys. Most cases of hypertension, however, are labeled "cause unknown." High blood pressure without discernible cause seems to run in families and is most common among people who are overweight. A veritable army of pressure-lowering drugs (including the major tranquilizers mentioned in Chap. 9) have been put at the doctor's command for the treatment of hypertension without detectable cause. Hypertension is most often encountered in middle age. It is rare in children.

The Traffic between the Blood and the Tissues

The most important thing to remember about the circulation is the fact that the whole elaborate system of pump and tubes exists solely for the purpose of getting blood into the capillaries where the exchanges between the body cells and the blood take place. The walls of all the blood vessels, except those of the capillaries, are too thick to permit the passage of materials from the blood into the tissue fluid surrounding the cells or from the tissue fluid into the bloodstream. The walls of the capillaries, on the other hand, are exceedingly thin. They are composed of a single layer of flat cells fitted together like paving stones. Digested food and oxygen and other dissolved substances can readily pass into the bloodstream through the capillary walls in the loading stations of the digestive tract and lungs and out again into the tissues. And wastes from the tissues can readily pass into the bloodstream and out again in the unloading stations of the lungs and kidneys.

SIGNS AND SYMPTOMS ASSOCIATED WITH CIRCULATORY DISTURBANCES

Serious circulatory disorders in children are for the most part due to congenital defects of the heart or large blood vessels leading into or out of it, or to rheumatic fever (see Young Hearts in Trouble, further on) or other infections that damage the heart. The lay observer has no means of checking up on the condition of the heart and blood vessels. Only the physician can do this in the course of a thorough cardiac examination. However, information about various signs and symptoms commonly associated with circulatory disturbances may be helpful to teachers in their observation and guidance of children.

Heart Murmurs

Heart murmurs are sounds produced as blood flows past the heart valves. By using his stethoscope, which amplifies chest sounds, the physician is able to detect heart murmurs or other sounds that indicate deviations from normal in the heart's action.

The presence of a murmur does not necessarily mean that the heart is diseased, damaged, or defective. A large percentage of healthy children have innocent murmurs. When the murmur is caused by some defect or deformity, it is called an organic murmur. Organic murmurs may be congenital or acquired. That is, a child may be born with a valvular deformity or he may acquire one as a result of a disease that attacks the heart. Rheumatic fever is the commonest cause of acquired heart disease.

Shortness of Breath

The medical name for difficult breathing is *dyspnea* (from two Greek words meaning "ill" and "breath"). It may be caused by anything that interferes with the oxygenation of the blood in the lungs or with the transport of the respiratory gases (oxygen and carbon dioxide). In children its most common cause is asthma.

Breathlessness during or after moderate exertion that has not previously caused breathlessness may be an early symptom of a weakened heart muscle. It most commonly occurs when the left side of the heart fails to pump on all the blood it receives from the right side by way of the lungs. As a result the lungs become congested with blood and their ability to distend during breathing is diminished.

Children who consistently "lose their breath" or get tired more quickly than their playmates do, or who consistently have trouble breathing during physical activities that give most children no respiratory distress, should be referred for a medical checkup.

Cardiac Misbehavior

The heart may act queerly without having anything organically wrong with it. Sometimes children, like their elders, experience common but annoying sensations such as skipped beats, palpitation, and very rapid beating of the heart. A child who complains of noticeable misbehavior of the heartbeat, pain or discomfort in the chest region, or any other annoying symptoms should always be referred for medical attention. If the physician after a careful examination can find nothing wrong with the heart, every effort should be made to reassure the child. Young people with sound hearts can be made very miserable and even develop emotional disturbances if they are allowed to grow up with the mistaken notion that something is wrong with their hearts.

Blueness

The normal color of the skin is determined partly by its natural pigmentation and partly by the red color of the blood in the blood-vessel network of the dermis. If the blood flowing through the superficial blood vessels contains less than its normal quota of oxygen, as may happen if any defect or disease of the heart or blood vessels sidetracks or obstructs the circulation of the blood through the lungs, the skin will look bluish. The medical name for this condition is cyanosis (from the Greek word *cyanos*, meaning blue). Most people are familiar with the term "blue babies," applied to infants who are born with a heart or blood-vessel defect that interferes with the oxygenation of the blood. (See Congenital Cardiac Defects further on in this chapter.)

Cyanosis is more clearly evident in regions where the skin is thin and unpigmented, such as the lips and under the fingernails, and also in regions where the skin blood vessels are normally well filled with blood, such as the face, ear lobes, and hands.

YOUNG HEARTS IN TROUBLE

Rheumatic heart disease and congenital malformation of the heart and great blood vessels are the chief causes of "heart trouble" in children and youth. Physicians and surgeons are becoming increasingly successful in dealing with both these types of cardiovascular (heart–blood-vessel) diseases.

Rheumatic Fever and Rheumatic Heart Disease

Rheumatic fever is the cause of rheumatic heart disease. Rheumatic fever manifests itself as polyarthritis (migration of pain and swelling from joint to joint with fever); as chorea or St. Vitus' dance (involuntary uncontrollable twitching or jerking movements of the limbs); or as carditis (acute inflammation of the heart muscle or lining). In some cases, however, it manifests itself merely as a low-grade, nonspecific illness (complaints of not feeling well or feeling tired all the time or vague pains in arms, legs, and joints).

The first attack of rheumatic fever is most likely to occur between the ages of six and ten, but it may occur at any age. The heart is nearly always involved in the acute phase. With subsidence of the acute illness, about one in three children is left with some scarring of the valves or other heart damage. The risk of heart disease increases with each subsequent attack. This is why it is important to recognize acute rheumatic fever and to treat all streptococcal infections properly.

Hemolytic streptococcal infections (notably scarlet fever and streptococcal sore throat) are responsible for triggering an attack of rheumatic fever in children or young adults who are susceptible to it. There is more in the picture than infection, however. Rheumatic fever occurs particularly in certain families, and it appears certain that a hereditary factor is involved. However, it has been impossible so far to find any mechanism by which the streptococcus exerts its effects. Lacking this knowledge, it is impossible to determine whether the hereditary factor is a familial allergy to one or more products of the streptococcus or some other kind of inherited sensitivity. All that can be said with certainty is that children of some families are more susceptible to rheumatic fever than are children of other families.

One of the worst features of rheumatic fever is its tendency to recur. A child doesn't "catch" rheumatic fever and set up an immunity as he does when attacked by measles, chicken pox, and other childhood diseases. Rather, a first attack makes him more vulnerable to a second; a second, to a third; and so on. Each attack provides a fresh opportunity for damaging the heart. Recurrent attacks occur most often during the first five years after an initial attack, become less frequent during adolescence, and are rare in adult life.

Attacks of rheumatic fever have become much less frequent since penicillin has come into use both for the treatment of streptococcal infections and for the prevention of streptococcal infections in children known to have had rheumatic fever. According to the American Heart Association and the American Academy of Pediatrics, every child who has had rheumatic fever should take penicillin by mouth twice a day or receive an injection of penicillin every month. This prophylactic treatment should be continued well into adult life.

Progress in the field of heart surgery also provides hope for those whose heart valves have been scarred or narrowed as a result of rheumatic fever. In many cases it is now possible to repair damage that formerly condemned the victim of rheumatic heart disease to a lifetime of restricted activity (see under Progress in Heart Surgery further on).

Signs and Symptoms of Rheumatic Fever. The fact that a first attack of rheumatic fever usually occurs during the school years suggests that teachers should be familiar with its signs and symptoms. In addition to what teachers observe, individual health histories may contribute significant information, especially if they contain records of frequent colds and sore throats, tonsil and adenoid operations (because they may indicate previous sore throats), scarlet fever or any other known streptococcal infection, or a history of previous rheumatic fever.

Rheumatic fever does not have a monopoly on many of the signs with which its early development is associated. Among the signs that may herald rheumatic fever as well as other slowly developing childhood diseases are failure to gain weight, pallor, poor appetite, and chronic fatigue. None the less, vague conditions of this kind may, if properly investigated by a physician, disclose early cases of acute rheumatic fever.

Even if rheumatic fever is not found, it is all to the good to have secured medical attention for school children with signs and symptoms of substandard health.

More definite signs of rheumatic fever are pain in joints and muscles; unusual restlessness, irritability, and twitching or jerking of the face, arms, or legs (chorea); repeated unexplained nosebleeds and unexplained fever. A period of medical observation and special tests are usually necessary to determine whether rheumatic fever is or is not the cause of these manifestations.

If the diagnosis is rheumatic fever, the child will be kept in bed to protect his heart until the doctor says it is safe for him to get up. After that he may lead a normal or near-normal life unless his heart has been severely damaged.

Follow-up Care. The attitude of parents and teachers toward children who have had rheumatic fever is very important to the mental health of these youngsters. Partly because of the close, regular medical supervision required to prevent streptococcal infections by chemotherapy and partly because of the fear that heart disease may develop, parents tend to worry excessively about their children who have had rheumatic fever, with or without heart damage. Yet parents who overprotect their children and constantly remind them to "be careful" may have a rebellious child or a cardiac cripple on their hands even if there is little or no heart damage.

The overanxious supervision of teachers also may engender fears in young children and resentment in adolescents, who cannot bear to be singled out for treatment different from that of their peers. The teacher must, of course, be guided by the physician's decision regarding physical activity. Fortunately, the tendency is to place fewer restrictions than formerly on children with rheumatic heart disease (see The Cardiac Child in School further on). These children need regular medical supervision, prophylactic treatment, and the common-sense health guidance teachers are in an excellent position to give. It is especially important for the rheumatic child to learn and practice good health habits so that he can help to build up his resistance and to protect himself from respiratory infections. By her unobtrusive supervision the teacher can make sure that he practices what he has learned from his doctor, his parents, and herself. And she can be on the alert for signs suggestive of the onset of a respiratory infection or of a recurrence of rheumatic fever, and see that he gets prompt medical attention.

Congenital Cardiac Defects

Some babies come into the world with abnormalities of the heart or of the great blood vessels that lead into or out of it. Such congenital abnormalities vary widely in severity. Some are so slight that they hardly affect a child's life or activities at all. Others are so severe that they cause death in the first few months or years of life. Still others show their effects only as the child grows older.

Most congenital defects in one way or another impose an added work load on the heart or interfere with the passage of blood through the lungs, or both. One of the most common defects is a narrowing of the opening between the right ventricle of the heart and the pulmonary artery through which blood from the right ventricle is pumped to the lungs to be oxygenated. The result is the distribution throughout the body of blood deficient in oxygen. This is one of the conditions that produces a bluish tint (cyanosis) of the lips, skin, and fingernails.

Two other common congenital defects have to do with the fact that in the unborn baby there is no air in the lungs and so blood is shunted from the right side of the heart to the left without passing through the lungs. The two shunts consist of an opening (foramen ovale) in the wall between the left auricle and the right auricle and a blood vessel known as the ductus arteriosus that runs from the pulmonary artery to the aorta. At birth the lungs expand, and normally the foramen ovale closes and the ductus arteriosus gradually shrinks up. It sometimes happens, however, that after birth the opening between the two auricles fails to close (patent, or open, foramen ovale). In that case blood leaks from the left auricle into the right because the pressure on the left side of the heart is greater than on the right. If the ductus arteriosus fails to close (patent ductus arteriosus), a passage is afforded for the transference of blood from the aorta to the pulmonary artery. In both cases blood that has already been pumped through the lungs is pumped through again, thus increasing the work of the heart. A number of others things can go wrong with the heart or great blood vessels. There may be a hole in the wall between the two ventricles or a hole permitting all four heart chambers to communicate. A narrowing of the aorta may greatly impede the flow of blood to the lower parts of the body. A valve may close improperly or perhaps fail to open wide enough to allow the free passage of blood or be scarred and narrowed as the result of rheumatic fever. The great blood vessels attached to the heart may not be hooked to the proper chambers.

Progress in Heart Surgery. Not long ago there was no solution to such problems. Today, because of spectacular progress in the field of heart surgery, an impressive number of congenital defects can be completely corrected or the function of the heart can be improved sufficiently to permit reasonably normal living. At present, however, not *all* hearts with defects in structure can be mended.

The invention of the heart-lung machine was perhaps the most important achievement in heart surgery because it permits repairs inside the heart itself. This elaborate and intricate machine is connected with the blood-vessel system in such a way that the patient's blood is pumped from his body into an artificial lung and is then pumped back into his body again without passing through the heart.

The heart-lung machine can assume for several hours the functions of the heart and lungs when the heart must be stopped for surgery. Other great steps toward the relief of congenital heart defects include the perfection of plastic blood vessels, synthetic patches for holes in the heart, and artificial valves to replace defective ones.

Getting Medical Attention for Children with Possible Heart Disease. Certain congenital defects, as we have seen, may not show appreciable effects until the child enters school. The actions and appearance of such a child may lead a teacher to suspect cardiac trouble or at least the need for a thorough medical examination. A child who restricts his own activity, who gets out of breath after slight exertion, or who becomes pale or looks tired after mild exercise is suspect. More definite signs are bluish lips, flushed cheeks, and chronic breathlessness. The teacher cannot, of course, diagnose heart trouble, but her alertness may lead her to refer the child to the school health service for medical investigation.

The physician serving the school who uncovers a case of suspected heart disease either as the result of his periodic health examination of the child or of referral by the teacher or school nurse, acts as a middle man, or go-between, for the school, the family, and the physician responsible for the child's treatment. He informs and persuades the family to seek medical attention for the child (avoiding a positive statement that the child has heart disease); interprets the findings of his own examination and other school information to the private physician or the clinic; interprets the reports from private physician or clinic to the nurse and to the teacher; and recommends adjustments in the school program on the basis of the medical findings.

The advantage of having a heart specialist study cases of probable heart disease is obvious. Public health units in many cities and communities maintain cardiac clinics to which private physicians can refer patients for accurate diagnosis. Also, in an increasing number of communities with well-organized school health programs, cardiac consultation service is being developed. Included in the functions of this service are: (1) accurate diagnosis of cardiac status, (2) education of school health personnel, including the administrator and teacher, in the modern concepts of heart disease and in the follow-up care of children who have had rheumatic fever, (3) recommendations as to suitable physical activity both in and out of school and advice on future occupation, and (4) consultation service for the private or clinic physician.

The Cardiac Child in School

Children or young people with either rheumatic or congenital heart disease can attend regular school unless their hearts have been damaged so severely that they should be at complete rest or have their physical activities markedly restricted. A number of cardiac school children have hearts that function normally and need no restriction of their activities. Others need no restriction of ordinary physical activities but are advised against severe or competitive physical exertion. Still others should have their ordinary physical activities moderately restricted and their more strenuous efforts discontinued. In most instances heart disease is not static, and the degree of activity considered advisable for any individual may change from less to more or from more to less as the heart condition gets better or worse with the passage of time. The medical recommendation regarding physical activity should be noted on the student's cumulative health record after each checkup of the heart so that the classroom teacher, physical education teacher, and the school nurse can plan an activity program adjusted to the student's needs.

Vocational Guidance. Children with heart disease or a history of rheumatic fever are in great need of vocational guidance if they are to make satisfactory progress in life. In the light of the findings of a pilot study conducted by the Vocational Advisory Service of New York City and sponsored by the American Heart Association and the New York Heart Association,[1] the following recommendations pertaining to the school's responsibility were made:

1. The schools should become more aware that if children with a history of rheumatic fever or with heart damage are to be prepared adequately for competition in the world of work, it is even more necessary for them than for physically normal children to have maximum education and training (in relation to ability). Because gaps occur in their education, very positive steps must be taken to hold these children in school. The educational, counseling, and personal adjustment services of the schools should be expanded at all levels and in all kinds of instructional situations, in order to provide more individual service. Where these children are eligible for official rehabilitation or community vocational counseling services, they should be referred to such services at an early age.

2. The schools and clinics should make increasing use, not only of the personal adjustment and social services provided within their framework, but also of family and youth casework services, child guidance services, and mental hygiene clinics in the community, to prevent, if possible, many of the social and emotional problems which develop in these children and to assist in the many adjustments they face in their childhood and adolescent years.

[1] American Heart Association: *Vocational Counseling for Children with Heart Disease or a History of Rheumatic Fever: A Pilot Study*, 1961, Chap. 6, Recommendations.

DEALING WITH CIRCULATORY EMERGENCIES

The circulatory system is involved in several conditions with which the teacher may have to deal while the school nurse or physician or someone trained in first aid is being summoned. Among such conditions are fainting, bleeding from an external wound, shock, and nosebleed.

Fainting

In fainting the person loses consciousness because of a lessening of the blood supply to the brain. Besides strong emotions such as fright or joy, other common causes of fainting are want of food, fatigue, pain, prolonged standing, and exposure to an overheated room. Some children may faint at the sight of blood or as a consequence of even a trivial injury. The face of a person about to faint gets very pale because of the constriction of the surface blood vessels, and perspiration usually breaks out on his forehead. He may say that he feels dizzy and weak, or that "everything looks black." In fainting he slumps into a chair or falls to the floor unconscious. His breathing is shallow, and his pulse weak and slow.

If you notice that a child is about to faint, have him sit down and thrust his head forward between his knees. This has the effect of improving the circulation of blood to the brain. If the child does not improve, or actually faints, lay him flat on his back and lower his head by elevating the lower part of his body. This may be done by placing a folded coat under his hips. If a nurse is available, ask someone to notify her. While waiting for her, or if no professional help is available, loosen tight clothing about the child's neck and waist. Cover him warmly, and see that he gets plenty of fresh, moving air. Open a window or fan him. Also it may help to sprinkle cold water on his face.

Usually a victim of fainting revives in a very short time. After he regains consciousness he should lie still for a while in a quiet place. If aromatic spirits of ammonia is on hand, he may be given half a teaspoonful in water.

If a fainting attack lasts for more than a few minutes, keep the child covered warmly and summon a physician at once. Any child who is subject to fainting spells should be referred for medical attention.

Bleeding from an External Wound

In most cases you can check bleeding from an external wound by placing a cloth pad directly over the wound and applying pressure with your hand. If the bleeding is from an arm or a leg, raising the limb will help. When a large blood vessel has been cut the injured person may bleed to death in a minute or so. Do not hesitate to apply direct pressure with your hand until a cloth pad can be obtained. The cleaner and more sterile the cloth the better, but don't be fussy in a real emergency. Use pieces of cloth torn from clothing or any other cloth immediately available.

If expert help has not arrived after the bleeding is stopped, apply additional layers of cloth to form a bulky dressing and bandage it snugly in place. This is called a pressure dressing. If blood seeps through the dressing *do not remove it* to apply a fresh one. Simply add more layers of cloth and tighten the bandage if that is necessary to stop the bleeding.

Nosebleed

Bleeding from the nose is a common occurrence among school children. It may happen spontaneously without apparent cause, or it may result from a blow on the nose. "Bloody noses" and "black eyes" are popularly interpreted as almost sure indications that a child has been in a fight. Recurrent nosebleeds without apparent cause should always be reported to the physician serving the school, as they may accompany some underlying disease such as rheumatic fever.

There are many things to try in stopping a nosebleed. First of all the child should be comfortably seated with his head thrown back. Then pinch the nostrils firmly together for four or five minutes. This may stop the bleeding by giving an opportunity for a clot to form. It may be necessary to plug the bleeding nostril with a bit of cotton or gauze and then pinch. Another measure to try is placing a little pad of soft paper or cloth under the upper lip and pressing with the fingers laid across the lip. It also may help to apply towels wrung out of cold water over the nose. After the bleeding stops have the child keep quiet for a while. Walking about, talking, laughing, or blowing the nose may cause resumption of bleeding.

Traumatic Shock

This form of shock is associated with serious injury to the tissues from wounds, burns, or fractures. It should not be confused with simple fainting which may occur as a result of minor injuries.

In shock, blood tends to collect in the capillary networks of the abdomen. As a result the blood supply to the brain and the surface of the body is lowered. The skin of a person in shock feels cold and clammy and looks pale. His tissues become starved for oxygen because there is less blood in circulation; hence he breathes faster than he usually does and occasionally gasps for breath. His pulse is rapid but may be very weak and impossible to detect. Shock is dangerous. To prevent it or lessen its severity, the following measures should be taken when the child (or older person) is severely injured even when few or no characteristic signs of shock are present.

1. Keep the child lying down, as this favors the flow of a greater amount of blood to the head and chest where it is needed most.

2. Place a blanket or newspapers under the child if he is lying on the

ground, but cover him lightly. The object is to prevent a loss of body heat without causing overheating. If the accident occurred out of doors in cold weather and not enough blankets are available to prevent chilling, a hot water bottle or some other heating device may be used. The heating device should be only slightly warmer than body temperature (98.6°F).

3. If the child is fully conscious and there is no abdominal wound or feeling of nausea, give him warm water, a little at a time, to quench thirst. If there is delay in getting medical care you may give drinks, about every fifteen minutes, of a salt and soda solution (one-half teaspoonful of salt and one-half teaspoonful of baking soda in a quart of water).

4. Give first aid for apparent injuries; for example, control external bleeding and splint fractures. Reassure the child as much as possible. If he must be moved, be very careful and gentle.

BLOOD AND ITS COMPOSITION

Until William Harvey announced his discovery of the circulation in 1628, nothing actually was known about blood except that it is essential to life. Now a great deal is known about this extraordinary fluid.

Blood Plasma

More than half the total volume of the whole blood is made up of a thickish liquid called plasma (see Fig. 10-3). Plasma is mostly water. The solid substances dissolved in it are proteins (which make up about 7 per cent of plasma) and a smattering of fats, sugar, and mineral salts. In recent years the proteins of plasma have been broken down into many different fractions, which are proving to be of the highest value in medical and surgical practice. One of these fractions is gamma globulin, which carries the antibodies developed in the body to fight germ invaders.

Other protein elements in blood plasma are the substances responsible for the highly complicated process of blood clotting (see further on in this chapter). If blood did not have the ability to clot over a break in the skin or mucous membrane and plug it, we might bleed to death from a very small wound. This actually has been known to happen in hemophiliacs, that is, boys or men suffering from a hereditary disease in which the blood fails to clot normally.

Serum Albumin. About 50 per cent of blood plasma is made up of a watery solution of albumin (white of egg is practically pure albumin). Serum albumin was the last protein to be separated from blood plasma in the famous blood fractionation program that was started in World War II under the direction of Dr. Edwin J. Cohn of the Harvard Medical School. It is often used now as a substitute for whole blood plasma in transfusions given to prevent or treat traumatic shock.

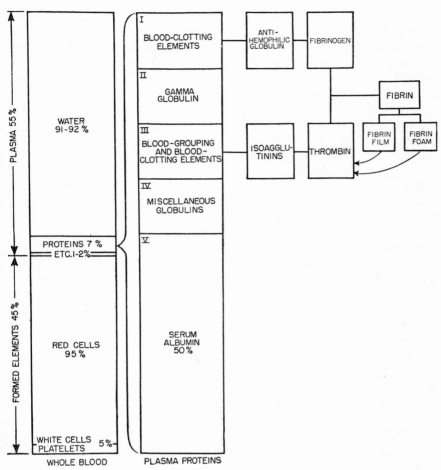

FIG. 10-3. Principal medical uses of blood and its derivatives. The size of the blocks indicating Fractions I, II, III, IV, and their subgroups is arbitrary.

Whole blood. To replace blood lost through hemorrhage.

Red cells. To treat anemias except those due to blood loss or infection.

Plasma. To prevent or treat (1) shock and (3) hypoproteinemia (a decrease in the normal amount of protein in the blood).

Fibrinogen and thrombin (blood-clotting elements). To make *fibrin foam* and *fibrin film* for the control of bleeding and for tissue repair in surgery.

Antihemophilic globulin. To shorten temporarily the blood-clotting time in hemophilia (a hereditary disease in which the blood fails to clot normally).

Gamma globulin (immune serum globulin). To prevent temporarily, or modify, measles and infectious hepatitis.

Isoagglutinins. To obtain anti-A, anti-B, and anti-Rh typing serums.

Serum albumin. To prevent or treat shock and hypoproteinemia.

Formed Elements

The Red Cells. A little less than half the total volume of whole blood is made up of formed elements. Of these, by far the most numerous are the red cells. There are about five million red cells in 1 cubic millimeter of blood (a small drop). Yet small as they are, one now and then has to squeeze to get through a capillary which is fifty times smaller than one of the hairs of your head.

The red cells are the oxygen carriers of the blood. Technically they are called erythrocytes (*erythro-*, meaning "red," plus *-cyte*, meaning "cell"). Erythrocytes are born in red bone marrow, where they go through several stages of development from infancy to maturity. When they are mature, capillaries in the red bone marrow open up and release them in batches into the bloodstream (see Fig. 10-4).

The mature red cell is an extremely small disk without a nucleus. Its groundwork is a spongelike jelly in which hemoglobin is enmeshed. Hemoglobin consists of an iron-containing red pigment (heme) combined with a protein substance (globin). The iron in hemoglobin gives it its red color and its property of combining with oxygen in the lungs and releasing it in the tissues.

In health the population of the red cells is kept within normal range by a nice balance between their birth rate and their death rate. The total number of red blood cells in the blood of the average man is about thirty trillion (30,000,000,000,000). This is about 200,000 times the population of the United States. The average length of life of each red cell is about 80 days, but some old-timers survive for 120 days or more. The average length of life of United States citizens at present is about seventy years. In health about ten million red cells are destroyed every second, or an average of 864 trillion every twenty-four hours. This is a daily death rate of about 28 per 1,000. The annual crude death rate per 1,000 of the United States population at the present time is less than 10.

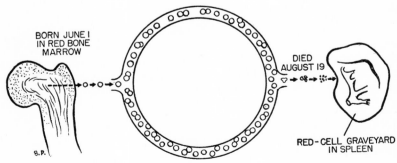

Fig. 10-4. Red cells born in red bone marrow circulate on the average for eighty days and then break up and are removed from the blood in the spleen.

The White Cells. The white cells of the blood are called leukocytes (*leuko-*, meaning "white," plus "cyte"). They belong to a class of cells widely distributed throughout the body which act as phagocytes (literally, "celleaters"). To the army of phagocytes all substances foreign to the body, including bacteria, are legitimate prey. Hence, phagocytosis (the eating up of bacteria by phagocytes) is one of the most powerful of all bodily defenses against infection.

There are two main types of leukocytes: granulocytes and lymphocytes. The granulocytes, as well as all red blood cells, are produced in the red bone marrow. The lymphocytes are produced in the lymph nodes and in tissue of similar structure (lymphatic tissue) in the spleen, tonsils, and other organs (see under The Lymph Nodes, further on).

In one small drop of blood (1 cubic millimeter) the number of white cells normally ranges from 5,000 to 10,000. Hence, for each white cell there are from 500 to 1,000 red cells. Unlike the red cells, to which the bloodstream is home, the white cells are transients in this stream. They use it as a highway in getting to places where they are needed to fight infection.

Normally the proportion of white cells to red cells is fairly constant. However, the white blood cells usually increase in number under the stimulus of an infection. This is an orderly mobilization set in motion by the body's need for new recruits to fight invading bacteria. When there is a wild disorderly overgrowth of white cells, leukemia (see Blood Disorders, further on) is the result.

The Blood Platelets. The blood platelets are infinitesimally small colorless bodies with no nuclei which are generally believed to be fragments of protoplasm broken off from giant cells in the red bone marrow. They get their technical name, thrombocytes, from the fact that they play a vital role in the clottting of the blood (*thrombo-* means "clot").

Blood Clotting

The changes in blood which make it clot begin as soon as blood escapes from a wound. Blood platelets break up at the site of the wound and an activating substance in the tissues called thromboplastin is set free. The thromboplastin then combines with a protein in blood plasma called prothrombin. Vitamin K (the coagulation vitamin) helps the body manufacture prothrombin. With the aid of calcium in the bloodstream, thromboplastin changes prothrombin into an enzyme called thrombin. In the next stage of blood clotting the thrombin changes fibrinogen, another protein in blood plasma, into fibrin. The fibrin is deposited in the form of very fine fibrous needles that make a network, in the meshes of which the red blood cells are caught. Thus a clot is formed.

Blood Grouping

The successful performance of whole-blood transfusions became possible when the discovery that every person belongs to one of four well-defined blood groups was announced by Dr. Karl Landsteiner in 1901. Each individual inherits the blood group to which he belongs. The four major blood groups (see Fig. 10-5) are characterized by different combinations of two factors capable of being agglutinated (agglutinogens A and B) in the red blood cells and two agglutinins (anti-A and anti-B) in the serum.

Compatibles and Incompatibles. In a whole-blood transfusion, the blood of donor and recipient must be compatible (match) to avoid the agglutination, or clumping together, of the red cells in the donated blood with serious and often fatal results. By referring to Fig. 10-5 it is easy to see that blood groups A and B are incompatible. If group A blood is transfused into a group B recipient, its red cells, which contain agglutinogen A, will be agglutinated by the anti-A agglutinin in the recipient's blood serum. A similar reaction will take place if the donated blood belongs to group B and the recipient to group A. The blood of a donor belonging to group O, however, can as a rule be given safely to a recipient in any of the other three groups because its red cells contain no agglutinogen to react with an anti-A or anti-B agglutinin. On this account, persons belonging to group O have been called "universal donors." As a person belonging to group AB has no agglutinin in his blood serum, he can as a rule receive blood safely from persons belonging to any of the other three groups. Persons belonging to this group, therefore, have been called "universal recipients."

It has been pointed out, however, that the terms "universal donor" and

GROUP	AGGLUTINOGEN IN RED CELLS	AGGLUTININ IN SERUM
A B	A AND B	NONE
A	A	ANTI - B
B	B	ANTI - A
O	NONE	ANTI - A AND ANTI - B

Fig. 10-5. The four major blood groups.

"universal recipient" may be dangerously misleading. To be on the safe side, blood of the same group to which the recipient belongs is employed in whole-blood transfusions unless it is unobtainable and the emergency does not brook delay.

The Rh Factor. In 1940, shortly before his death, Dr. Landsteiner and his coworker, Dr. Alexander S. Wiener, reported the discovery of another blood factor, which they named the Rh factor because they first identified it in the blood of rhesus monkeys. This hereditary factor is attached to the red cells of approximately 85 per cent of white persons regardless of blood group. These persons are called "Rh-positive." the 15 per cent who do not possess it are said to be "Rh-negative." The Rh factor is important clinically because of its antigenic activity. That is, it has the power to stimulate the development of anti-Rh antibodies (agglutinins) in the serum of Rh-negative blood.

At least eleven separate antigenic members of the Rh family have been identified since its discovery, and a great deal of detailed information regarding the inheritance of the Rh antigens has become available. The commonly used terms Rh-positive and Rh-negative, however, refer to the presence or absence of one antigen only (the D antigen) because it is clinically the most important factor.

Rh-negative individuals may become sensitized to Rh-positive blood in two different ways. The first way is by whole-blood transfusion. If the blood of an Rh-positive donor is transfused into an Rh-negative recipient, the development of Rh antibodies may be stimulated in the blood serum of the recipient. If an Rh-negative individual who has been sensitized in this way should be transfused later on with Rh-positive blood, the Rh antibodies in his serum will agglutinate and dissolve the red cells in the donated blood. It has been made an invariable rule, therefore, never to give Rh-negative persons Rh-positive blood by transfusion.

The second method of sensitization may take place during pregnancy, when the unborn child of an Rh-negative mother has inherited the Rh-positive factor from his father. In that case, the Rh factor in the child's blood may stimulate the development of Rh antibodies in the mother's blood. If that happens, the Rh antibodies in the mother's blood may clump the Rh-positive red cells in the child's blood. As a result the child may be born dead (stillborn) or born with erythroblastosis, a blood disease of the newborn in which the red cells are damaged. This "accident" seldom happens, as only about one in fifty Rh-negative mothers will become sensitized even if the unborn baby is Rh-positive.

It is now possible to be prepared for trouble by testing pregnant women and their husbands for the Rh factor. If it is found that the husband is Rh-positive and the wife Rh-negative, and the wife shows evidence of sensitization during pregnancy, the physician will be ready to exchange part of the newborn baby's blood for blood from an Rh-negative donor.

As exchange transfusions will temporarily make the child Rh-negative, the Rh antibodies in his blood serum can no longer hurt him. Later the baby makes his own fresh Rh-positive blood and becomes an Rh-positive individual.

BLOOD DISORDERS

Blood does so many things for us, as it courses through the body on its rapid rounds from the heart and back to it, that any change in its own composition or in the freight or passengers it normally transports has significance from a health point of view. Information regarding such changes can be gained only by submitting a blood specimen to various types of laboratory examination, depending upon what the physician wishes to find out.

Teachers, parents, and other lay observers have no means of checking up on the condition of the blood, but they may be of service in getting medical attention for children who show persistent changes in skin color (see Observing Changes in Skin Color, in Chap. 15) or easy fatigability or some other possible indication of a deviation from normal in the composition of the blood. The more common disorders in which such changes occur are described here.

The Anemias

It sometimes happens that the balance between the death rate and the birth rate in the red-cell population is tipped one way or another. The number of red cells turned out by the red-cell factories in red bone marrow may be below normal; or the number of red cells destroyed or lost from the circulation (as in hemorrhage) may be above normal; or the quality of the red cells may be below standard—for example, too large or too small or deficient in hemoglobin. When any of these things happens the capacity for transporting oxygen to the tissues is inadequate.

Anemia means literally "bloodless" (Greek *an*, meaning "not," plus *haima*, "blood"). Any disease in which the red-cell population, or the quality of its individual members, is adversely affected may be characterized by anemia.

Types of Anemia. The many different types of anemia fall roughly into two broad classifications: (1) anemias in which the red cells are abnormally large and contain an abnormally large amount of hemoglobin; and (2) anemias in which the red cells are abnormally small or normal in size but deficient in hemoglobin. Anemias in the first class include pernicious anemia and other anemias which are caused by anything that interferes with the normal manufacture of red cells in the red-cell factories. These anemias are very rarely found in school children. Anemias in the second class include those caused by a deficiency of iron and other blood-building substances (the so-called "nutritional anemias"). Iron-deficiency anemia is fairly common in infancy, early childhood, and about the age of puberty.

Laboratory examination of a blood specimen is the only sure way of telling whether a child is anemic and, if so, which one of the manifold forms of anemia is present.

Pallor. In the popular mind pallor[2] is so often associated with anemia that it is tempting to think or say of any persistently pale child that he is "anemic." As a matter of fact, the color of the blood may be normal, reduced, or heightened, according to the type of anemia from which an individual is suffering.

It is chiefly in the nutritional anemias, especially those caused by iron deficiency, that the blood is paler than usual. The low color index of the blood is due partly to the smaller size of the red cells and partly to the fact that each red cell has received less than its normal quota of pigment. The iron deficiency responsible may result from not getting enough iron in the diet or from defective absorption of iron from the food.

One form of nutritional anemia, once very common in girls and young women, is called chlorosis ("green sickness") because of the peculiar greenish pallor of the skin which characterizes it. A favorite explanation of green sickness, before its true nature was discovered a few decades ago, was "love sickness" (mal d'amour or febris amatoria). No less than fifteen paintings by seventeenth-century Dutch painters were on this theme. Garrison[3] points out that in these canvases "the representation of the pallor and feverish discomfort of the greensick lovelorn maidens is very life-like." Chlorosis is now very rare, not, one surmises, because the course of young love runs smoother, but rather because the diets of young maidens are now much better than they were one or two generations ago.

While pallor is frequently misleading as an indication that anemia is present or, if so, in what degree it exists, its presence is a valuable diagnostic aid to the physician. The history of its onset as obtained from parents is occasionally vague and unsatisfactory, especially in the chronic forms of anemia. Physiological adjustments in chronic anemia may be so efficient that physical activity can be carried out for long periods of time with a decidedly lowered hemoglobin level. Hence, a teacher who observes that a child is beginning to look paler than usual and seems tired or generally not up to par will be doing that child a great service by referring him for a medical examination.

---

[2] Pallor is also associated with constriction of the surface blood vessels. Withdrawal of blood from the surface blood vessels takes place under all circumstances in which the body must conserve blood to carry on the vital activities of its internal organs. This explains the pallor in extensive hemorrhage, in shock, and in fainting. See also Normal Temporary Changes in Skin Color, in Chap. 15.

[3] Fielding H. Garrison: *An Introduction to the History of Medicine* 3d ed., W. B. Saunders Company, Philadelphia, 1924, pp. 304–305.

The Leukemias

The name leukemia means literally "white blood." It was invented about a century ago by Rudolph Virchow, a famous German pathologist who found some cases in which the blood had turned white as a result of the replacement of the red cells by white ones.

Actually, cases of leukemia in which this phenomenon occurs are extremely rare. In many cases, however, the blood is paler than normal, because the wild uncontrolled overgrowth of the white blood cells crowds out the red cells and eventually destroys their manufacturing centers and those of the blood platelets as well.

There are several different types of leukemia, but they are all characterized by runaway growth of the white cells. For this reason leukemia is sometimes referred to as cancer of the blood. Largely because of the decrease in deaths from the communicable diseases of childhood, leukemia (classified under malignancies) has advanced to first place in the ranks of the leading causes of death by disease in the school ages (five to nineteen). The cause of leukemia in human beings is unknown, but viruses are known to be responsible for the development of leukemia in certain animals. There is now suggestive evidence to indicate that leukemia in man, and especially in children, also may somehow be caused by viruses.

Certain chemicals, hormones, and other forms of treatment are being used to prolong the lives of children suffering from acute leukemia. Anything that delays death in these cases is all to the good because some day some group of workers is going to "hit the jackpot" in their efforts to find a way to control this disease.

DISEASES SPREAD BY BLOOD-SUCKING INSECTS

The parasites responsible for several infectious diseases depend upon blood-sucking insects for their passage from host to host, and in some species for the completion of their life cycles. The most important insect-borne disease problems in our country up to the middle of this century were malaria, endemic typhus, and Rocky Mountain spotted fever. Today malaria is on the run; only a relatively few cases of endemic typhus are reported annually; but Rocky Mountain spotted fever is still a problem. Information on these three diseases in addition to that given below may be found in Sec. 4, Appendix B.

Malaria

Although malaria has practically disappeared from the United States and Canada, it is the single most serious widespread communicable disease in the world today. For centuries it has been found in all regions of the earth wherever *Anopheles* mosquitoes breed freely. It still continues to weaken some thirty-five million people each year.

A problem as big as this is of concern to everyone engaged in health education and in the work of protecting public health. No country today can be an island like the England extolled by Shakespeare as a "fortress built by nature for herself against infection and the hand of war." The ease and rapidity of transportation and the constantly rising tide of global travel impose the need for taking all steps required to prevent the importation of infected *Anopheles* mosquitoes from malarious regions into an area or country from which malaria has been eradicated. In the meantime the World Health Organization (WHO) is carrying on a worldwide campaign designed to wipe out *Anopheles* mosquitoes in malarious lands.

Malaria is caused by any one of four different species of *Sporozoa* of the genus *Plasmodium*. *Sporozoa* belong to a class of parasites which reproduce by forming spores. The *Sporozoa* of malaria spend part of their life cycle in *Anopheles* mosquitoes and part in the bloodstream of human hosts.

About a week after entering the human bloodstream, the parasites invade the red blood cells. The destruction of the invaded red cells as a result of the growth and development within them of the parasites is responsible for the periodic attacks of "chills and fever" characteristic of malaria. As large numbers of blood cells cannot be destroyed time and again without causing anemia (see The Anemias in this chapter), repeated attacks of malaria leave a person pale, tired, and often too weak to work. Children particularly suffer badly from malaria. They often become thin and pale and do not grow as they should.

Methods of Control. The most important modern weapon used in fighting malaria is the insecticide known as DDT. In 1945 the U.S. Public Health Service in cooperation with the health departments of the Southern states launched a great campaign to eradicate malaria. The workers sprayed DDT at appropriate intervals on the inside walls of dwellings and on other surfaces upon which *Anopheles* mosquitoes habitually rest. By doing this they killed the mosquitoes before the insects could pass on malarial parasites from infected people to well people. The people helped by screening their living and sleeping quarters and by staying inside their dwellings after dark as much as possible because *Anopheles* mosquitoes usually bite only after dark. This teamwork has been responsible for the virtual eradication of malaria from the United States.

DDT also is the insecticide usually employed by WHO workers in countries where intensive campaigns for wiping out malaria are under way. Speedly eradication of *Anopheles* mosquitoes is considered essential because of the tendency of insects to develop immunity from DDT. The original time limit placed on the WHO global campaign against malaria was fifteen years. In highly malarious areas the use of suppressive drugs has special value. Such drugs keep malaria from developing in persons after they have been bitten by infected mosquitoes. Very effective drugs for treating chronic and acute cases of malaria are also available. There is good reason to hope that this disease—one of the oldest enemies of mankind—will be wiped off the face of the earth.

Typhus Fever

There are two kinds of typhus, one endemic, the other epidemic. An endemic disease is a disease that has a low incidence but is constantly present in a given locality. An epidemic disease, on the other hand, attacks many people at the same time but is only occasionally present in a given locality. Both epidemic and endemic typhus are caused by a species of rickettsia (see Rickettsia, in Chap. 7).

Epidemic Louse-borne Typhus. The rickettsia that cause epidemic typhus are spread by lice, mainly body lice, which have fed upon infected persons. Prior to modern methods of control, epidemics were frequent among military and refugee populations and in areas suffering famine or war. Epidemic typhus is a thing of the past in our country but it still exists in many areas of the world, and vaccination is recommended for travelers to those areas.[4]

Endemic Flea-borne Typhus. Endemic typhus is a much milder disease than its close relative, epidemic typhus. The great majority of persons who contract it recover completely. Primarily it is a disease of rats. For that reason it is sometimes called murine typhus, from *mus*, the Latin word for "rat." The rickettsia causing it are carried from rat to rat and from rat to man by rat fleas that have become infected by biting a rat suffering from the disease. It cannot be transferred directly from person to person.

Formerly several thousand cases of endemic typhus occurred each year in the United States. Currently only about 100 cases are reported annually, mainly in the Gulf and South Atlantic seaboard states during the summer months when fleas are abundant. Endemic typhus was once most common in seaboard cities and centered around feed and grain stores where rats could find plenty of food. An increase in the rat population of farms now makes the disease primarily rural.

Methods of Control. For rapid control when cases occur, insecticide powders (10 per cent DDT or other compounds) are applied to rat runs, burrows, and harborages. A murine typhus vaccine was made available some time ago but its development and testing has been abandoned because of the effectiveness of insecticides in controlling outbreaks and also because endemic typhus can be treated successfully with antibiotics.

Eradication of murine typhus from endemic areas depends upon reducing the rat population. Rats are such destructive animals, besides being involved in the spread of endemic typhus and several other diseases, that public health authorities sometimes launch rat-control pro-

[4] A booklet, "Immunization Information for International Travelers" is available from local or state health departments or any office of the U.S. Public Health Service.

grams including the extermination of living rats, a cleanup of rat-infested premises, and the ratproofing of dwellings. Such a program may involve an entire town or large section of a town or city. Teachers and their students have often helped in this important work.

Spotted Fever

This serious rickettsial disease is transmitted by ticks. Although it is now known to occur widely throughout the United States, it was first recognized in the Mountain states, particularly in Montana and Idaho. For that reason it is usually called Rocky Mountain spotted fever.

The disease is passed from generation to generation in ticks. The ticks probably become infected in the larval stage of development by feeding upon infected wild rodents. Adult female ticks hibernate during the winter months and do not become active until the first warm days of spring. The lay their eggs in the late spring and early summer after a meal of blood and then die. That accounts for the fact that spotted fever is limited to the spring and summer months.

Once attached to an animal or human host, a tick may feed for several days. A blood meal seems to make the spotted fever organisms increasingly active and virulent.

Methods of Control. A vaccine is available for lessening the chances of infection from tick bites, but with the advent of antibiotics in treatment vaccination is generally limited to persons whose work takes them into tick-infested areas during the spotted fever season. For the general population the avoidance of tick bites is the only practicable means of prevention. The simplest way to avoid tick bites is to stay out of underbrush and tall grass in tick-infested localities during the tick season. Some insect repellents are of value against ticks.

The dog tick is by far the most common carrier of spotted fever in the East. Familes that keep dogs in Eastern tick-infested areas should take special precautions to avoid infection. The dogs should be examined periodically for ticks and the ticks carefully removed as described below.

Since spotted fever is usually not transmitted until an infected tick has been feeding for several hours, careful search for attached ticks and their prompt removal reduces the risk of infection. In tick-infested localities parents should be urged to look their children over carefully for ticks at the end of the day. It is especially important to examine the nape of the neck and the scalp. The tick has a small-toothed probe on its head. In attaching itself it sinks its probe into the skin of the victim and hangs on. Great care should be taken in removing ticks to avoid crushing them with the bare fingers and to make sure that the probe does not break off and remain embedded in the flesh. Contamination of the skin with the crushed tissues or feces of infected ticks may lead to infection.

To make a tick withdraw its probe cover it with salad, mineral, or machine oil to close its breathing pores. It may remove its probe right away. If not, leave the oil in place for half an hour. Then remove the tick carefully with tweezers or with a bit of cotton or paper tissue held between the fingers. After removing the tick, scrub the tick-bite area with soap and water. Burn the tick or flush it down a drain.

THE CIRCULATION OF LYMPH

The cells that form the tissues of the body are water dwellers. They must be surrounded by fluid or they would surely dry up and die. Even the living tissues that must of necessity be in contact with the air are all kept moist. You see the lines you are now reading, for example, through a film of salty water covering the living "windows" of your eyes. The fluid that occupies all the cracks and crannies between the closely packed cells is tissue fluid. It drifts slowly in thin streams like sea water in wet sand until it enters the lymph vessels which empty it into the bloodstream. It is customary to speak of tissue fluid after it has entered the lymph vessels as lymph. Tissue fluid and lymph, however, are identical.

Fluid Interchanges between the Blood and the Tissues

Tissue fluid and all other special body fluids come from blood plasma. The hydraulic (water) pressure of the blood within the capillaries tends to squeeze fluid out of the capillaries. Too steady a seepage, however, would not only deplete the water content of the blood but also would swell and waterlog the tissues. The counterforce that keeps this from happening ordinarily is osmotic pressure.

Osmotic pressure may be simply defined as the drawing force that salt, sugar, and many other substances dissolved in water exert upon the water molecules when water and a solution of any of these substances are separated by a semipermeable membrane. In Fig. 10-6 you see water separated from a solution of sugar by such a membrane.

The water molecules (represented by small dots) can pass through this membrane into the sugar solution, but the sugar molecules (represented by large dots) cannot pass into the water. However, the sugar molecules exert a force which attacts, or draws, the water molecules across the semipermeable membrane into the sugar solution. As a result, the volume of the sugar solution increases and its pressure rises. This pressure is called osmotic pressure.

The blood plasma inside the capillaries contains in solution more protein particles than are contained in the tissue fluid outside the capillaries. As a result, the protein particles exert a drawing force which tends to draw water into the bloodstream through the semipermeable capillary walls. Thus a nice balance is achieved between the hydraulic pressure tending to force water out of the capillaries and the osmotic pressure tending to draw it in.

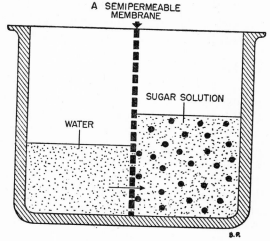

A SEMIPERMEABLE
MEMBRANE

SUGAR SOLUTION

WATER

FIG. 10-6. Osmotic pressure. Water passes through the semipermeable membrane and into the sugar solution, in the direction of the arrow, causing the pressure in the sugar solution to rise.

Edema. Edema, which literally means "swelling," is the term applied to an excessive accumulation of fluid in the tissue spaces. The old-fashioned name for it is dropsy, which literally means "water." Edema occurs when the balance between the inward and outward flow of fluid through the capillary walls is upset. Among the possible causes of edema are (1) an abnormally low concentraton of protein particles in the plasma as a result of kidney disease (see The Kidneys and Their Work, in Chap. 13); (2) a rise in the pressure of blood in the capillaries which takes place when the blood flow is abnormally slow because of a weakened heart muscle; (3) increased permeability of the capillary walls as a result of bacterial toxins or other injurious agents; and (4) obstruction of the lymph channels.

It is important to remember that shifts in tissue fluid take place constantly in health. Just standing up for a long time, for example, may make the legs or ankles swell, because of an increase in the amount of fluid outside the blood vessels. However, any persistent swelling of the legs and ankles or of any other part of the body open to observation indicates the need for medical attention.

The Lymphatics

Fluid does not normally collect in stagnant lakes in the tissues. It is kept moving slowly in thin streams by the rhythmical pressure of working muscles and also by the currents set up by the constant shifting of tissue fluid out of and into the bloodstream through the capillary walls. These sluggish streams eventually enter channels of their own which drain directly into the bloodstream. The lymph channels are called the lymphatics, or lymph-vessel system. The lymph capillaries originate as tiny blind tubes in the tissues in the close neighborhood of the blood capillaries. They converge to ever-larger vessels with ever-thicker walls. Through these vessels the tissue fluid drifts eventually into two large ducts that drain into two large veins in the upper chest.

The Lymph Nodes

Glandlike structures called lymph nodes are situated at strategic points in the course of the lymph vessels. All the tissue fluid on its way back from the tissue spaces to the bloodstream must pass through these nodes, which act as filters to remove any bacteria or other injurious agents that might otherwise be carried into the blood. On passing into a lymph node from an incoming lymph vessel, lymph spreads out in a relatively large umbrella-shaped lake where the rate of flow at once becomes exceedingly slow. Thus there is every opportunity for the settling of bacteria or other small particles. In this water trap, so to speak, bacteria are attacked by phagocytes within the lymph nodes. Hence the lymph nodes must be looked upon as an important line of defense against the invasion of the bloodstream by bacteria traveling by way of the lymphatics from beachheads of infection in the tissues (see Fig. 10-7).

Solving the Mystery of the Thymus

The lymph nodes and lymphatic tissue in the spleen and other organs produce the white blood cells known as lymphocytes. The lymphocyte populations in the lymph nodes and blood contain certain cells that are responsible for the formation of antibodies by which the body builds immunity from communicable disease (see Antigen-antibody Reactions

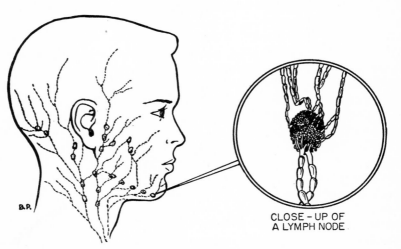

CLOSE - UP OF
A LYMPH NODE

Fig. 10-7. Lymph vessels and nodes in the face and neck.

in Chap. 7). In 1962 the announcement was made that lymphocytes get their start in life in the thymus gland.

At the beginning of 1961 the function of the thymus gland was unknown. This gland, as we have learned, is relatively large at birth. At about age twelve it begins to grow smaller and after puberty a definite shrinkage in size commences. In the adult there is hardly any thymus left. Why this should be remained a mystery until it occurred to Jacques F. A. P. Miller (an Australian scientist carrying on cancer research in England) that the thymus shrinks after childhood because its work is done. Using mice as his experimental animals, Miller was able to demonstrate that the work of the thymus is to raise lymphocytes for the job of forming antibodies. These lymphocytes are seeded in the lymph nodes and spleen where they multiply and become fully competent to perform their antibody-producing function. As time goes on the lymph nodes and other lymphoid tissue can continue to carry on the production of lymphocytes on their own, and, therefore, the thymus is no longer needed. As a result of this research, the thymus is now looked upon as the body's "immunity organizer."

Challenges for Thymus Research. Further research on the thymus is expected to throw light on several puzzling medical and surgical problems. One such problem arises because the body forms antibodies that react to foreign proteins, that is, to proteins different from those that the body itself produces. As a result it is practically impossible to graft skin, bone, or other tissue from one person to another unless donor and recipient are identical twins. There are a few exceptions. The cornea of the eye, for example, does not arouse such antibody response, and so corneal transplants can be made. Also one person can receive another person's blood so long as their blood groups match (see Blood Grouping in this chapter).

There is now strong experimental evidence to support the belief that the thymus gives rise to lymphocytes tuned to produce the antibodies that react to alien proteins. One experiment, for example, disclosed that grafts took on mice whose thymuses had been removed soon after birth. When enough is known about the thymus and how it works, it may be possible to control a person's immunity system so that even whole organs can be transplanted from one person to another. The day may come, for example, when an entire heart may be taken from a person killed in an accident and grafted into another whose heart is diseased. Fantastic? "Merely a matter of time," says one surgeon.

Infected Lymph Glands

Adenitis (Swollen Glands). Swollen or infected glands and adenitis are terms applied to infected lymph nodes, especially those in the neck. The cervical lymph nodes in children frequently become involved in respiratory infections, especially colds, streptococcal sore throat, and scarlet fever. The lymph nodes in back of the ears and at the back of the neck nearly always become enlarged in German measles.

Infected cervical lymph nodes may steadily feed bacteria into the slowly moving lymph stream. From being a filter the node becomes a cesspool, draining eventually into the blood. A child with "swollen glands" should be under the care of a physician (see Plate 5). In some cases the condition may clear up with rest and medication. In others it may be necessary to set up surgical drainage.

Infectious Mononucleosis. An acute infection involving the lymph glands, known as infectious mononucleosis, has become increasingly common. Its incidence is greatest among children and young adults. Epidemics are most frequently recognized in schools and institutions for children. Probably it is spread by direct contact with, or droplets from the nose and throat of, infected persons.

The cause of infectious mononucleosis is unknown. One form, commonly called "glandular fever," is characterized by fever and enlargement of the lymph glands (especially those at the back of the neck) and the spleen. Glandular fever is common in children. Another form in which the physical signs are fever and sore throat, with or without lymphatic gland involvement, is common in older children and adults.

A great variety of unusual manifestations occur often enough in infectious mononucleosis to make doctors keep it in mind when confronted with any fever of unknown origin. A diagnosis can be made only by the laboratory examination of blood samples. Although there is no specific remedy for the disease, most cases end with complete recovery. Serious complications may arise, however, particularly if the central nervous system becomes involved in the infection.

Tonsils and Adenoids

Tonsils are composed of masses of spongy lymphoid tissue covered with mucous membrane. One pair of olive-shaped tonsils, the palatines, stands guard between the pillars (folds of mucous membrane) on each side of the passage leading from the mouth to the pharynx (Fig. 11-2). Another pair of tonsils, the linguals, is located, one on each side of the tongue near its base. A third set of tonsils, the pharyngeals, is located on the back wall of the pharynx near the place where the nose opens into the pharynx and between the openings of the eustachian tubes that lead to the ears. The pharyngeal tonsils are popularly called adenoids (adenoid means "resembling a gland").

The tonsils, as part of the lymphatic system, contain the same kind of phagocytic cells that attack bacteria in the lymph nodes. They are honeycombed with crypts in which the bacteria are trapped and devoured. The tonsils, located as they are at the portals of entry from the mouth and nose to the throat, are exposed to frequent mass attack by bacteria from the air, and on the objects that children seem to enjoy putting into their mouths. The tonsils do all they can to destroy as many bacteria as possible. But in the process they may themselves become infected and abnormally enlarged. Infected and swollen tonsils may interfere with normal breathing, swallowing, and speech. Enlarged adenoids also may interfere with hearing by blocking the throat openings of the eustachian tubes. In addition bacteria, and the toxins (poisons) produced by them, can spill over and spread to other tissues resulting in infections of the ears, nasal sinuses, or digestive system.

In the past, before the development of chemotherapy, it was practically routine procedure to remove children's tonsils and adenoids as a means of solving the problem of frequent or chronic respiratory ailments in childhood. At the end of World War II, the operation known as T and A (short for tonsils and adenoids) was described in the *Journal of the American Medical Association* as the most frequent surgical procedure in the United States, with nearly two million operations performed annually. Even in recent years one of the important findings of the U.S. National Health Survey[5] is the large number of tonsillectomies reported for school-age children. In one year, for example, 61 per cent of all operations performed on girls in the five to fourteen age group were tonsillectomies. A more critical attitude is developing, however, with the result that physicians nowadays usually recommend surgery only after other methods of treatment have failed.

Selection of Children in Need of Operations. The recorded observations of teachers and nurses are of great help to physicians in making decisions about the advisability of removing tonsils and adenoids. A history of recurrent colds, earache or discharge from the ears, frequent sore throats or swollen glands has direct bearing on the problem. The child's manner and appearance also are significant. Persistent mouth breathing (almost the sign manual of the adenoidal child), mannerisms suggesting hearing loss (see Loss of Hearing and Its Detection, in Chap. 17), easy fatigability, slowness in gaining weight, and listlessness are among the signs that the physician will wish to consider in interpreting his physical findings.

FOR REVIEW AND DISCUSSION

1. If you were give the task of labeling a "road map" of the circulation, where would you find and how would you label

[5] *Illness among Children*, Children's Bureau Publication No. 405, U.S. Department of Health, Education, and Welfare, 1963, p. 7.

    a. The points of arrival and departure for the round trip of blood through the body? *Ventricle* *Heart*

    b. The points of arrival and departure for the round trip of blood through the lungs? *Ventricle*

    c. The highroads leading away from the heart?

    d. The highroads leading toward the heart?

    e. The loading stations where supplies for the tissues are delivered to the blood?

    f. The unloading stations where wastes from the tissues are removed from the blood?

    g. The stations en route where supplies are delivered to, and wastes removed from, the tissues?

2. If you were on a hunting trip through the body, in which of the places named after each quarry should you expect to find it?

    a. Hemoglobin: phagocytes, erythrocytes, blood platelets

    b. Gamma globulin: blood plasma, spleen, red bone marrow

    c. Carbon dioxide: arterial blood, venous blood, serum albumin

    d. Trapped bacteria: lymph vessels, tissue fluid, lymph nodes

    e. Heart murmurs: auricles, heart valves, ventricles

3. Match each disease or condition listed in the box with the word or phrase below the box which you associate with it

Nutritional anemia	7 Adenitis
Malaria	8 Cyanosis
Hypertension	9 Congenital cardiac defect
Rheumatic fever	10 Leukemia
Traumatic shock	11 Endemic typhus
Spotted fever	12 Edema

6 Ticks

Swollen lymph glands

4 Streptococcal infections

11 Rat fleas

3 Persistently high blood pressure

9 Patent ductus arteriosus

5 A severe injury

10 Runaway growth of white blood cells

1 Iron deficiency

2 Anopheline mosquitoes

Accumulation of fluid in tissue spaces

8 "Blue babies"

4. Have pairs of students demonstrate interviews between teacher and nurse in which sets of signs and symptoms suggestive of rheumatic fever, nutritional anemia, infectious mononucleosis, and chronically

infected tonsils and adenoids are discussed with reference to particular children. Have the rest of the class guess which condition is indicated in each case.

5. Have demonstrations in class of the first aid procedures to be followed to prevent shock following an injury; to stop bleeding by applying pressure over the wound; to stop a nosebleed; and to revive a child who has fainted.

SELECTED REFERENCES

American Medical Association: *The Facts about Leukemia,* The Association, Chicago.

American Medical Association: *The Heart,* Part 4 of *The Wonderful Human Machine* series (the workings of the human body in words and pictures).

American National Red Cross: *The Story of Blood,* The Association, Washington, D.C. (A pamphlet describing the composition, functions, and medical uses of blood and its derivatives.)

American Public Health Association: *Control of Communicable Diseases in Man* (first given as reference in Chap. 7).

Best, C. H., and N. B. Taylor: *The Human Body* (first given as reference in Chap. 1). Part III, *The Fluids of the Body,* Chaps. 6–10; Part IV, *The Circulation of the Blood,* Chaps. 12–18.

Blakeslee, Howard: *Blood—Your Gift of Life,* Public Affairs Pamphlet No. 145, Public Affairs Committee, Inc., New York. (A comprehensive pamphlet on human blood and its medical uses.)

Blakeslee, Howard: *Know Your Heart,* Public Affairs Pamphlet No. 137, Public Affairs Committee, Inc., New York.

Engel, Leonard: *The Operation,* McGraw-Hill Book Company, New York, 1958. (The fascinating account of a 4½ hour "miracle" heart operation. Gives a good idea of progress in heart surgery.)

Marvin, H. M., and others: *Your Heart; A Handbook for Laymen,* Doubleday & Company, Inc., New York, 1960.

Richardson, Robert G.: *The Surgeon's Tale: The Story of Modern Surgery,* Charles Scribner's Sons, New York, 1959. (The absorbing story of the development of major surgery from the discovery of anesthesia to the almost magical heart operations of today.)

Riedman, Sarah R.: *Your Blood and You,* Abelard-Schuman, Limited, New York, 1952. (An interesting, simply written story of human blood.)

Schneider, Leo: *Lifeline: The Story of Your Circulatory System,* Harcourt, Brace and Company, Inc., New York, 1958. (A clear and simply written description of this system.)

Zinsser, Hans: *Rats, Lice and History,* Little, Brown & Company, Boston,

1935. (A classic "biography" of typhus by a distinguished bacteriologist.)

Organizations

American Heart Association
American Cancer Society

Chapter 11   ON THE AIR ROUTE

The Respiratory System
Respiratory Infections
The School and Respiratory Disease Control
Respiratory Allergies
What to Do in Respiratory Emergencies

The respiratory system is the arrangement evolved for meeting the body's need for oxygen from the surrounding atmosphere and for removing from the body the waste gas (carbon dioxide) produced by the body's use of oxygen.

Of all the natural portals of entry into the body, the respiratory tract is the one most open to infection. Reference has already been made to the fact that colds and other infections of the breathing passages are the most common causes of illness among school children. A brief sketch of the plan and defensive arrangements of the air route into the body is given here to help teachers visualize the terrain, so to speak, of this most important beachhead.

THE RESPIRATORY SYSTEM

The plan of the respiratory system is quite simple. Air containing oxygen passes through an air-conditioning system (the nose) and enters what may be visualized as a hollow upside-down tree (the respiratory tree, Fig. 11-1). The trunk of this tree is the windpipe (trachea). After passing through the windpipe, the air spreads out through its hollow branches (the bronchial tubes) and comes to a stop in the tiny blind air sacs (alveoli) at the ends of the hollow twigs (bronchioles).

A fine network of capillaries surrounds the alveoli, or air sacs. It is through the double partition represented by the exceedingly thin alveolar and capillary walls that the continuous, rhythmic exchange of oxygen and carbon dioxide between the air in the lungs and the blood in the capillaries takes place.

The Mechanics of Respiration

The mechanics of respiration is also quite simple. It is based primarily upon the increase and decrease in the size of the chest cavity brought about by the action of the great muscle (the diaphragm), which forms the floor of the chest and the ceiling of the abdomen, and of the muscles in the chest walls. When the chest is expanded during inspiration, air rushes into the elastic lungs, which stretch out fanwise to occupy the extra space made available. When the capacity of the chest is made smaller during expiration, the air is literally squeezed out of the lungs by the pressure of the rising floor and inward-moving walls of the chest. The elastic alveolar walls, by recoiling during expiration, also help to drive out the air.

Nervous Control of Respiration

Breathing is essentially an involuntary act. We can hold the breath for only so long and then we are forced to resume breathing.

The respiratory center that controls the breathing muscles is a group of nerve cells located in the lowest portion of the brain (the medulla oblongata). Breathing stops automatically when the respiratory center is put out of commission as in electric shock, for example, or in bulbar poliomyelitis.

The rate of breathing is also controlled by the respiratory center. One "respiration" consists of one inbreath, or inspiration, and one outbreath, or expiration.

The respiration rate, like the pulse rate, is subject to many different influences. Among those which speed it up are vigorous exercise, emotional excitement, and fever. An ingenious automatic arrangement makes

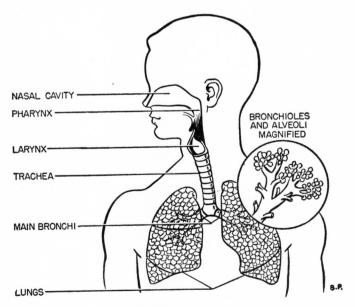

NASAL CAVITY
PHARYNX
BRONCHIOLES AND ALVEOLI MAGNIFIED
LARYNX
TRACHEA
MAIN BRONCHI
LUNGS

FIG. 11-1. The respiratory tree.

possible faster, deeper breathing when this is called for as a result of an increased need for oxygen. When a person is not breathing fast enough and deep enough to ventilate the lungs thoroughly, the blood flows through and out of the lungs without unloading its normal quota of carbon dioxide. Arterial blood with this extra heavy load of carbon dioxide reaches the respiratory center in the course of its regular rounds. The nerve cells of this center are very sensitive to an increase in the carbon dioxide content of the blood. Instantly stronger impulses from the center go to the breathing muscles to stimulate these muscles to more vigorous action.

Topography of the Nose

"It's as plain as the nose on your face" is a saying that emphasizes the obviousness of the nose. Yet we are not so much interested in noses from the outside as in what goes on inside. The primary function of the nose is to act as an air-conditioning system. It is especially designed to warm, moisten, and filter the air in the first stage of its journey to the lungs.

The nose is designed to permit inhaled air to spread out over as large an area as possible in flowing through it. Structural features that help to increase the nasal area exposed to inhaled air include (1) the division of the nose lengthwise into two nostrils by a wall, or septum, of bone and cartilage; (2) the extension from the side walls of the nose into the nasal cavity of three shelves, or ledges, of bone called the turbinates; and (3) cavities called sinuses in the bone of the skull and face which lead into the nasal cavity through very small openings.

Mouth Breathing. Since the nose is especially designed to act as an air conditioner, children should be encouraged to breathe through it. Those who are consistent mouth breathers should be referred to the nurse or the physician serving the school. The habit of mouth breathing nearly always indicates that some sort of obstacle is interfering with nasal breathing. In children, as we have seen, the chief cause usually is overgrowth of the adenoids (see Tonsils and Adenoids, under the Circulation of Lymph, in Chap. 10). Blocking of the nasal passages may also be caused by any one of several different anatomical abnormalities—for example, a deviated nasal septum or enlarged turbinates. Malocclusion, too, may favor mouth breathing, if it is difficult or uncomfortable to keep the lips closed over protruding teeth.

Mouth breathing has many disadvantages. An open mouth with droopy lower jaw gives the face a dull, vacuous expression, and many a bright child looks stupid if he is obliged to breathe through his mouth. The passage of air over the tongue has a drying effect, and the sense of taste may be blunted. Also, interference with the aeration of the nose and sinuses may favor the development of infection.

A Busy Traffic Circle

The pharynx, or throat, is something like a traffic circle into which several different routes open. The posterior, or back, portion of the nostrils leads into the upper part of the pharynx. This meeting place of nose and throat is called the nasopharynx. The throat openings of the eustachian tubes, which lead to the middle chambers of the ears, are located near the throat openings of the nostrils. The lower portion of the pharynx communicates with the mouth above and with the esophagus, or food pipe, and the larynx below.

The Larynx

The larynx is an oblong hollow organ composed of cartilage, muscles, and ligaments which connects the lower part of the pharynx with the trachea, or windpipe (see Fig. 11-2). Hence it forms an integral part of the passage through which air is carried to and from the lungs. One of the cartilages of the larynx projects forward and in boys and men may be quite prominent. It is called the Adam's apple.

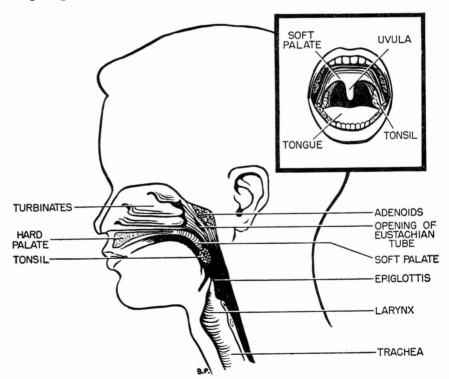

Fig. 11-2. Important points along the air route through the nose and pharynx, with an inset showing the location of the tonsils (the palatines).

During the act of swallowing, a muscle raises the larynx so that its opening is brought under the shelter of the epiglottis and the root of the tongue. This keeps food from "going down the wrong way" into the larynx and on into the trachea instead of into the food pipe (esophagus). It was once believed that the epiglottis snapped down to make a sloping lid for the larynx when food and drink were being swallowed. However, this structure stands erect, like a screen, and the food slides over its back surface into the food pipe. If the larynx is not lifted quickly enough during swallowing to bring its opening under the shelter of the epiglottis, food may get into the larynx. When this happens, the sensitive larynx contracts and at the same time the person begins to cough in an effort to expel the food.

Choking. If a piece of food or a foreign object slips into the larynx and lodges in the windpipe before it can be coughed out, it may cause asphyxia (see Asphyxia, further on in this chapter). Slapping the back sharply between the shoulder blades may succeed in dislodging the object. The victim can help by bending forward or by lying crosswise on a table or desk on his abdomen with his head and shoulders hanging over the side. A child small enough to be picked up in the arms may be held upside down by the heels while his back is being slapped. If the object is not dislodged immediately after these measures are started, send for a doctor at once or rush the child to a doctor's office or hospital. It may be necessary to give artificial respiration if the child is in great respiratory distress and starts to become blue in the face before or after the object is removed (see Artificial Respiration further on in this chapter).

The Respiratory Mucous Membranes

The air-conditioning activities of the upper respiratory tract are carried on by the mucous membranes that cover the inner surface of the nose and throat and extend into the passages leading from the throat to the lungs. The mucous membrane lining the nose contains many tiny blood vessels. These vessels are dilated by several different conditions, for example, by infections, local irritants, and a rise in temperature of inspired air. As a result, the mucous membrane swells and the air passages are narrowed. Cool air and certain drugs (Adrenalin and ephedrine) contract the blood vessels.

Normally the respiratory mucous membranes are covered with a blanket of mucus—a sticky, slightly antiseptic fluid secreted by mucous glands—which warms, moistens, and cleans air entering the nose. Tiny whiplike extensions of special cells in the membranes, called cilia, keep this "mucous blanket" on the move from the back of the nose downward to the throat and from the windpipe and bronchial tubes in the lungs upward to the throat.

The Cilial Escalator. The moving mucous blanket with its propulsive force supplied by the cilia has often been called the "cilial escalator." Always riding on the escalator down to the throat from the nose and up to the throat from the lungs are the stray germs, dirt, and other foreign particles inhaled at every breath and normally caught and held in the sticky mucous blanket. Those which fall off in the throat are disposed of by being swallowed or coughed out.

The respiratory mucous membranes play a most important part in both the background and the foreground of the respiratory infection picture. In the transfer of airborne infections they act as the reservoirs from which the causative agents are expelled into the air. And they provide a formidable barrier against the invasion of the tissues by virulent bacteria and viruses. The mucous membrane of the nasopharynx is never sterile. Whatever visitors from outside come to rest in the nose, the windpipe, or the bronchial tubes are eventually passed by the cilial escalator to the nasopharynx.

Resistance to Respiratory Infection

The strong local resistance of the respiratory mucous membranes and good general physiological resistance constitute our best defense against many germ invaders of the nose and throat. Other things being equal, children in good health stand a better chance of resisting colds and other respiratory infections than do children whose natural defense forces have been weakened by substandard health. There are several ways in which the local resistance of the mucous membranes may be upset.

Fatigue. Various experimenters have shown that physical exhaustion may render an experimental animal susceptible to disease-causing (pathogenic) germs to which it is ordinarily highly resistant. Similarly, studies on human beings have shown that fatigue may make a person temporarily susceptible to colds. Exactly what combination of causative factors makes it possible for fatigue to lower resistance to infection is not known.

Malnutrition. It is not yet known just how malnutrition in general lowers resistance, although there is no doubt that it does. Many studies have been made on the role of specific nutrients in maintaining good resistance. It has been demonstrated that vitamin A, for example, is required for upholding the integrity of the mucous membranes of the body, which are our first line of defense against bacterial invasion. Recently it has been shown that adequate protein is essential in maintaining the mechanism of resistance because this nutritional element is necessary for building up the protein substance (gamma globulin) in the blood plasma which carries the antibodies developed to fight disease-causing germs.

Chilling. The local cellular resistance of the respiratory mucous membranes may be temporarily upset by the adjustments associated with abrupt changes in temperature and perhaps with other atmospheric changes, such as those of humidity or air pressure. The fact that these adjustments are most frequently made necessary in the colder seasons and coincide with the congregation of large groups of people indoors (thus increasing chances of exposure to airborne germs) accounts for the marked seasonal fluctuation in the prevalence of respiratory infections.

A "cold" (in England, called a "chill") gets its name from the fact that chilling of the body has long been associated with catching cold. Chilling may be brought on by sitting around with wet feet, exposure to drafts, cooling off too quickly when overheated, or wearing unsuitable clothing in cold or wet weather.

Chilling of itself, however, cannot cause a cold. This has been amply demonstrated in numerous experiments. Volunteers taking part in such experiments allowed themselves to be doused in cold water after taking hot baths and stood in drafts until their teeth chattered. Others wore wet socks all day. No volunteers caught cold unless cold virus was dropped in their noses. It appears, however, that chilling may contribute to the development of a cold after getting a large dose of cold virus because it causes reactions that change the consistency of the nasal mucous membranes.

Chilling makes the surface blood vessels shrink, thus reducing the blood supply to these membranes. And cold also slows down or stops the action of the cilia responsible for keeping the mucous blanket with its freight of germs on the move toward its dumping ground in the nasopharynx. Normally, the healthy nose has a new mucous blanket about once every ten minutes over its posterior, or back, portion and once every hour or two over its anterior, or front, portion. Halting the cilial escalator makes it more difficult to dispose of stray bacteria and viruses. Hence, they may accumulate and be given an opportunity to multiply and mobilize. Since the resistance of the mucous membranes depends upon their ability to prevent the massing and combining of hostile invaders, it is easy to see that any chance for team play on the part of these invaders tends to interfere with the resistance of the mucous membranes and to break it down.

Virus Activity. Another way in which the resistance of the mucous membranes may be lowered is by the activity of viruses. The nature of this activity is not known with certainty. However, it is logical to suppose that theft of essential vital materials from the cells of the mucous membranes by the robber viruses may impair, if not actually destroy, the cells. The depletion of the cells may make them a better culture medium for pathogenic bacteria. Whether this is the true explanation or not, it is an established fact that an initial virus invasion sets up a beachhead for a secondary bacterial invasion of the respiratory tract.

RESPIRATORY INFECTIONS

Many different kinds of bacteria find the moist, warm, dark nasopharynx a congenial place in which to settle down. They make up the normal but constantly changing flora of the nasopharynx. Ordinarily, they do not cause trouble. But into this innocuous bacterial garden—or culture medium—come the virulent transient visitors—the pneumococci, streptococci, bacilli, and viruses. Their fate depends upon their numbers and the conditions they find. They may be disposed of before they penetrate the mucous membrane barrier by being swallowed or by being sent forth in coughing, sneezing, talking, and laughing on aerial expeditions to other throats. Or they may be able to stage a successful invasion, that is, to produce the disease of which they are the causative agents.

The extreme sensitivity of the respiratory mucous membranes to the activity of viruses and bacteria readily accounts for the early signs and symptoms characteristic of the most common respiratory infections. In an acute cold, for example, the blood vessels of the nose swell to accommodate extra blood. As a result, the air passages are obstructed, the normal drainage openings are swollen shut, and the nose feels stuffed up. Also the irritated membranes of the nose and throat feel sore and scratchy. To get rid of the virus both the flushing action of mucus and the mechanical action of coughing and sneezing are employed. It is the greatly increased secretion of mucus that makes the nose (and sometimes the eyes) water. The irritation of the sensitive nose lining is responsible for the sneezing. And the tickling of the throat and windpipe linings by the activities of the virus and by the postnasal drippings of excess mucus causes the coughing.

The bare facts about common respiratory diseases and other diseases spread by discharges from the respiratory tract are given in Secs. 1 and 2, Appendix B. In addition, teachers may find it helpful to have fuller information about several of the more important current respiratory disease problems and the progress now being made in solving them.

The Common Cold and Its Hangers-on

There is no longer any doubt that the cause of a plain cold in the head is a virus, of which there are several different strains and probably more than one type. Cold viruses have been recovered from the nasal washings of persons sick with colds by passing the washings through filters which hold back bacteria. The filtered washings produce colds in many, but not all, human volunteers when dropped or sprayed into their noses.

As one British virologist[1] put it, "We strongly suspect that catching a cold depends on receiving quite a small dose of virus at a time when one's defenses are off guard."

In a long-term study of colds begun in 1946 by the British Common Cold Research Unit in Salisbury, England, scientists have established that the cold virus is of extremely small size (only 1/300 the size of the average bacterium). They have succeeded in growing the virus in test tubes in a special culture medium. Fluid from the test tubes produced colds in human volunteers after several passages from tube to tube.

The next step in fighting colds is the development of a vaccine. The main obstacles to be overcome before this step can be taken is the complexity of the cold virus. Several strains of this virus have been identified. Each strain produces antibodies that work against it alone. Much more must be learned about the varieties of the virus strains that cause colds before a safe and effective vaccine can be prepared.

The common cold is not in itself a serious disease. Doctors define it as a mild, self-limiting infection, usually without fever, in which most of the symptoms are caused by inflammation of the upper respiratory tract (nose and throat). Its importance lies in the fact that it is a major cause of disability, resulting in about half of all absences from school or work, and also in the fact that it predisposes to more serious respiratory tract infections.

As we have seen, the activity of viruses weakens the defense mechanisms of healthy mucous membrane, thereby setting up favorable conditions for the moving in and multiplication of a wide variety of bacteria. Many of these bacterial invaders are responsible for the secondary infections that so often follow in the wake of neglected colds. Among these frequent complications are catarrh (a chronic cold), sinusitis, bronchitis, and infections of the middle ear.

There is no drug of any kind that attacks the cold virus itself. Chemotherapeutic drugs (the sulfonamides and antibiotics) are, however, effective in treating the bacterial complications of colds.

The most effective "cold cure" is rest. In one study of 2,500 colds treated with rest alone, about half began to clear up after one day and the remainder in about a week. Parents should be urged to keep children home from school for at least the first day or two of a cold and see that they get plenty of rest and sleep. Not only will this measure help a child to get over a cold more quickly but also it will help to limit the spread of the virus to others.

Chronic Colds (Catarrh). A common secondary infection is the cold

[1] Sir Christopher Andrewes, quoted in an article entitled "Closing in on the Common Cold" by J. D. Ratcliff, *Today's Health*, October, 1961.

that "hangs on." An ordinary viral cold clears up in a few days. Long-continued colds are characterized by the secretion of a thick yellowish mixture of mucus from the mucous glands and pus produced in the fight with bacteria that are ordinarily present in too small numbers to cause trouble. They are often accompanied by a persistent cough, which is caused by the continual or frequent dripping of mucus from the back of the nose into the throat.

Sinusitis. A sinus infection in acute or chronic form is usually characterized by pain or soreness in the cheeks or over the eyes. Sometimes the teeth may ache. The severe pain of acute sinusitis is caused by the pressure of pus which accumulates in one or more of the sinuses, when these air-containing spaces are invaded by pus-producing germs from the nasal cavity. The sinuses most often affected are the frontals above the eyes and the maxillaries on each side of the nose in the upper jawbone (Fig. 11-3).

As the openings leading from the sinuses into the nose are very narrow, they frequently swell shut when the mucous membranes lining the sinuses are inflamed. The pain and soreness persist until drainage is re-established either by natural subsidence of the infection or by medical treatment.

A child who complains of headache, pain or soreness in the cheeks or above or behind the eyes, or of aching teeth when he has a cold should always be referred to the physician or nurse, as neglect of acute sinusitis may lead to chronic sinusitis. A head cold that hangs on, or repeated attacks of head colds, particularly when they are accompanied by a dull headache or pain or soreness over the affected sinus, are signs that chronic sinus disease may be present.

Bronchitis. Acute bronchitis is an inflammation of the bronchial tubes. It may develop independently, but usually it extends from an upper-respiratory-tract infection, such as a head cold or influenza. Acute bronchitis most commonly starts with laryngitis, that is, inflammation of the larynx, which is located near the top of the windpipe. The chief character-

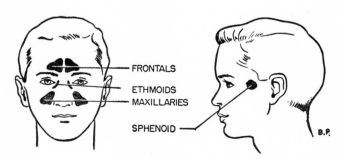

Fig. 11-3. The nasal sinuses.

istic of laryngitis is hoarseness. As the infection progresses downward into the bronchial tubes there is usually a feeling of tightness and heaviness in the chest, accompanied by wheezing and a dry cough which later becomes loose.

Acute bronchitis is commonly referred to as a "chest cold" or a "cold in the chest." In the beginning it may or may not be accompanied by fever. If the temperature is normal, the child may not feel ill. Yet it is extremely important to see that a child gets medical attention at the first signs of a chest cold, as the bronchial infection may prepare the way for pneumonia.

Chronic bronchitis may follow repeated attacks of acute bronchitis. However, this form of bronchitis affects old people chiefly, and is often associated with other diseases and conditions common in middle and old age.

Middle-ear Infections. Otitis media, or inflammation of the middle ear, is a common complication of colds and of many other respiratory infections. This condition is discussed in connection with the ear (in Chap. 17).

Adenovirus Infections

A whole new family of respiratory viruses known as the adenoviruses has been discovered in recent years. The first members of the adenovirus family to be recognized were described in 1953. These viruses were isolated by scientists of the U.S. Public Health Service from the cells of human adenoid tissue. The adenoviruses are readily grown in tissue cultures; so far more than twenty-three separate and distinct types have been described.

As a group the adenoviruses have certain characteristics in common. But one or more individual members of the group are associated with specific infections of the throat or eyes or of both. To find out which type is responsible for a particular infection it is necessary to grow virus obtained from the patient in a tissue culture and show that antibodies against it have developed in the patient after recovery.

The three main categories of adenovirus infections are briefly described below.

Pharyngitis. This infection is most frequently associated with type 3 adenovirus. It begins with fever, headache, sore throat, and sometimes with conjunctivitis (inflammation of the conjunctiva, that is, the delicate membrane that lines the eyelids and covers the eyeball in front) and lasts for from three to five days. It occurs most commonly in epidemics during the summer months among children in close association with one another as in institutions, summer camps, and densely populated urban areas. A vaccine against type 3 adenovirus is available and may be useful in institutions and summer camps when high attack rates are anticipated.

Adenovirus vaccines are not recommended for general or widespread use in the population as a whole.

Acute Respiratory Disease. Adenovirus types 4 and 7 are responsible for an acute respiratory infection which almost exclusively attacks large numbers of military recruits shortly after their arrival in basic-training camp. This infection is called ARD (short for acute respiratory disease). Its principal signs are fever, cough, and hoarseness. The attack rate is high; from 20 to 40 per cent of recruits may require hospitalization and an equal number may be infected in a less severe or less apparent manner. To combat ARD a highly effective vaccine against adenovirus types 4 and 7 has been developed; it was first used for immunizing recruits during the latter part of 1958.

Conjunctivitis and Keratoconjunctivitis. Since the discovery of adenoviruses more than twelve types of these viruses have been isolated from the eye washings of persons with conjunctivitis. Keratoconjunctivitis, a more serious eye infection than conjunctivitis, occurs in epidemic form particularly among workers in industrial plants and shipyards where the eyes are subject to injury from dust and dirt. Type 8 adenovirus has been established as a major cause of keratoconjunctivitis in the United States. (See Infectious Conjunctivitis, and Epidemic Keratoconjunctivitis, in Chap. 16.)

Influenza

In any line graph showing the death rates from pneumonia and influenza during the first half of the twentieth century, the observer is struck by a sharp peak which abruptly rises and as abruptly drops within the short period of three years (from 1917 to 1919). This is the indelible imprint of the influenza pandemic of that period. A pandemic is a worldwide epidemic. Influenza is an interesting disease historically, because it made such a deep and lasting impression upon the generations of mankind whom it visited that we have records of pandemics as far back as 1580.

Since the 1918–1919 pandemic, the long-term trend of the death rate from influenza has been sharply downward (see Fig. 11-4.) Although fluctuations in mortality have continued to occur, the peaks have definitely become lower. However, this virus disease continues to be an important medical and public health problem. It still causes widespread illness and heavy loss of time from school and work, particularly in years when epidemics occur.

Description. Influenza (flu for short) is an acute, highly contagious disease marked by sudden onset with fever, chilliness or a chill, aching especially in the back and limbs, malaise (feeling ill), and prostration (extreme weakness). The disease may be accompanied by signs of a

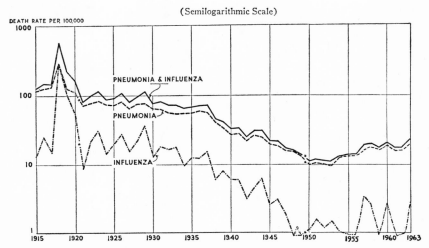

(Semilogarithmic Scale)

Fɪɢ. 11-4. Mortality from pneumonia and influenza, 1915 to 1962, ages one to seventy-four. (*From Metropolitan Life Insurance Company, Industrial Department.*)

cold, sore throat, and cough. If there are no complications, flu usually runs its course in two or three days (forty-eight to seventy-two hours), but the acute stage may be followed by a period of exhaustion. Susceptibility to flu is greatest in childhood, with the disease most common at about ten years of age. When deaths occur, they usually result from complications, especially pneumonia. To lessen the severity of flu and to prevent secondary infections, a person who comes down with it should go to bed immediately and stay away from school or work until the doctor says it is safe to return.

The Cause. Influenza is caused by a virus, of which three types have been identified. Type C, more recently recognized, has appeared only in localized outbreaks. Types A and B include numerous distinct strains.

When invaded by the virus of one strain, the body produces antibodies to fight it. These antibodies remain in the blood for varying lengths of time. While they are in the blood they give protection from the virus of that particular strain but they cannot prevent infections caused by the virus of other strains. The picture is complicated by the fact that the strains currently prevailing tend to be replaced by other strains within periods as short as from ten to fifteen years.

Flu Vaccine. Effective influenza vaccines have been developed that give protection from prevailing strains of type A and type B virus. Routine immunization is not feasible for the whole general population but is recommended for those for whom influenza poses the greatest risk of death or severe illness. Those who run the greatest risk are persons of all ages who suffer from chronic debilitating cardiac, respiratory, metabolic, renal, or neurological diseases. These individuals should be given flu vaccine routinely at yearly intervals well before the expected seasonal occurrence (late fall and winter). Consideration also should be given to the immunization of groups employed in essential community services (medical and health services, education, public safety, public utilities, transportation, and communication).

Anticipating Epidemics. The World Health Organization (WHO) operates a worldwide influenza alerter system around the clock without most people even knowing about it. The World Influenza Center is located in London, England.

An outbreak of influenza in any part of the world is promptly reported to the World Influenza Center. In the United States the news of an epidemic travels by telephone or telegraph in an unbroken chain from the local physician to the local health department to the state health department to the Influenza Information Center in Washington, directed by an officer of the U.S. Public Health Service, to the World Influenza Center.

The exchange of information through official health agencies makes it possible for the World Influenza Center to chart the movements of epidemics. In April, 1957, for example, an outbreak of flu was reported in Hong Kong, China. Then hundreds of thousands of people throughout Asia were stricken. The United States and other countries were alerted by the World Influenza Center so that they would be ready to fight "Asian flu" when it arrived.

An important item included in the report of a flu epidemic is the type and strain of the virus responsible. This information is obtained by sending the necessary blood samples or throat washings to one of the official influenza detection centers, which now number close to sixty and are widely distributed in many countries. Once the virus is identified, physicians are notified so that they will know what flu vaccine to use. If a new strain of virus is found, work is started at once to produce a new vaccine to combat it.

This is what happened in the Asian flu epidemic. The strain of type A virus which was found to be responsible was so different from previously isolated strains that the vaccines available were useless against it. So United States drug manufacturing companies immediately set to work to produce the vaccine which proved to be helpful in controlling the Asian flu epidemic.

Pneumonia

The most important complication of a neglected head or chest cold or of epidemic influenza is pneumonia. This serious inflammation of the lungs may be caused by any one of a large number of different types **of**

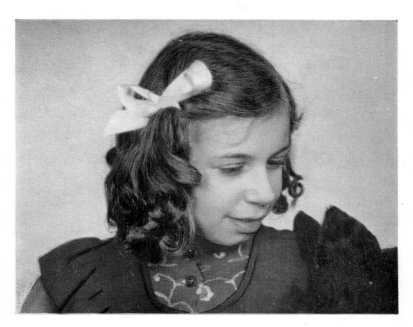

PLATE 1. This is a picture of Jane as her teacher sees her when she is healthy and happy.

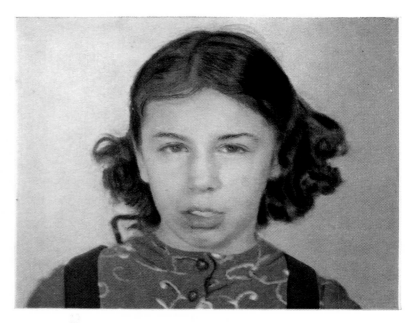

PLATE 2. This is a picture of Jane as her teacher saw her when she returned to school after an illness.

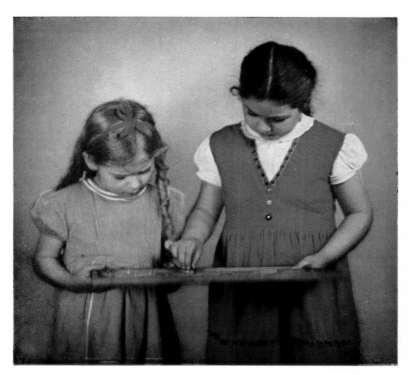

PLATE 3. Both Jean and Frances are six years old. This is a good illustration of the fact that each healthy child develops along his or her own pathway.

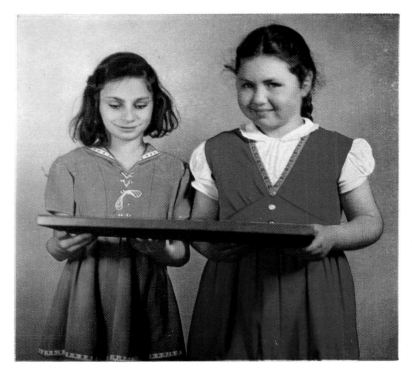

PLATE 4. In this picture ten-year-old Rosalie is compared with six-year-old Jean. Rosalie is definitely undersized for her age and shows other signs that made her teacher suspect malnutrition.

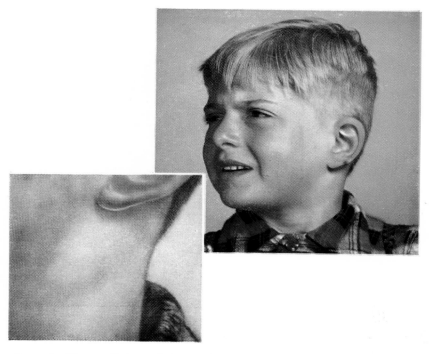

PLATE 5. The small lump below the lobe of Tommy's left ear indicates a swollen gland. The swelling is barely noticeable because Tommy is almost well now, and his physician has given him permission to return to school.

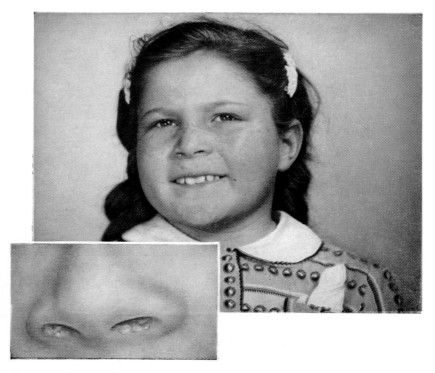

PLATE 6. If you will look closely, as her teacher did, you will notice that Lois has a slightly running nose.

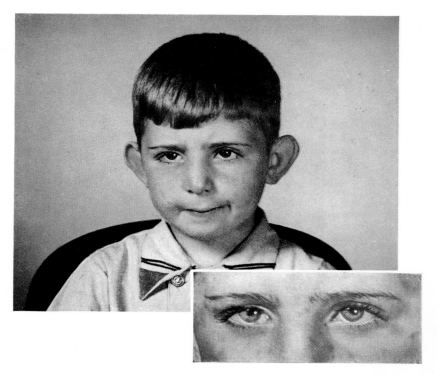

PLATE 7. Johnny is not very happy today. His eyes are red and watery, with puffiness of the lower lids. He is just coming down with the measles.

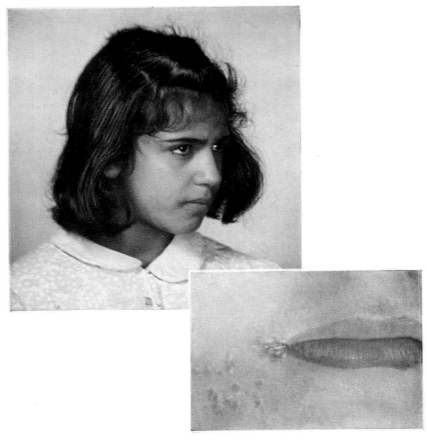

PLATE 8. Anne was referred by her teacher for a medical examination because her general appearance and posture indicated fatigue. Also, the teacher had noticed a persistent cracking and slight redness at the corner of Anne's mouth. The physician discovered that Anne was suffering from inadequate nutrition, and more particularly from a B-vitamin deficiency.

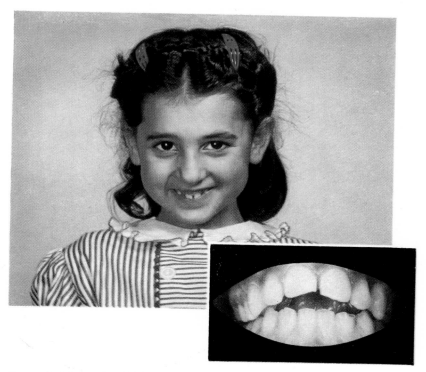

PLATE 9. The only thing that keeps Evelyn from being a pretty little girl is the possession of teeth that do not come together properly. Malocclusion may spoil a child's looks and interfere with happy adjustment to life.

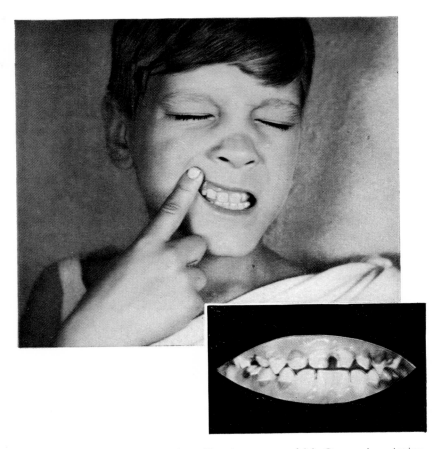

PLATE 10. A slight dental defect, like the one to which George is pointing, may not be visible to his teacher. On the other hand, no one can miss obviously decayed teeth like those shown at the right.

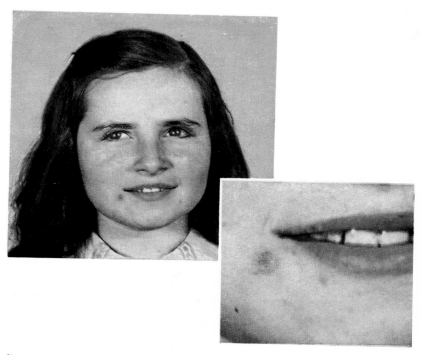

PLATE 11. The small red spot near the right corner of Peggy's mouth is impetigo. This very contagious skin infection is marked by groups of little blisters, which later turn to crusty sores.

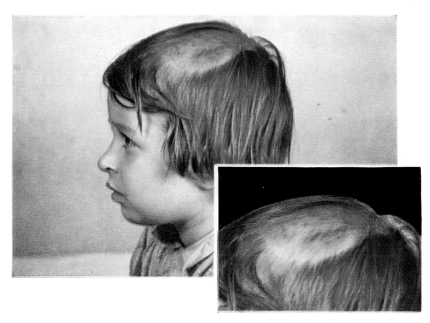

PLATE 12. Dorothy has an advanced case of ringworm of the scalp. The affected hairs become dull and brittle and snap off near the root, leaving bald spots on which raised gray scaly patches appear.

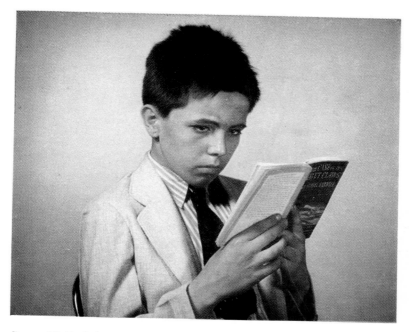

PLATE 13. Both in appearance and in behavior, Kenneth shows the signs that signal "nearsightedness" to a keen observer. In this picture he is holding his book too close to his eyes.

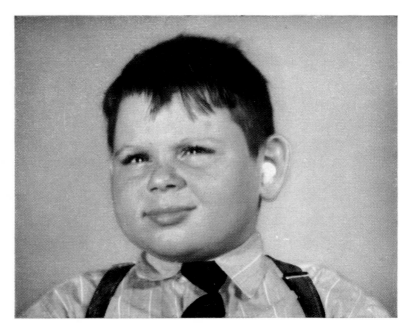

PLATE 14. Teddy is a big boy for his eight years. He is robust and has good color, but the piece of cotton in his ear indicates that his ear is draining. Teddy's look of watchful waiting is typical of children who do not hear well.

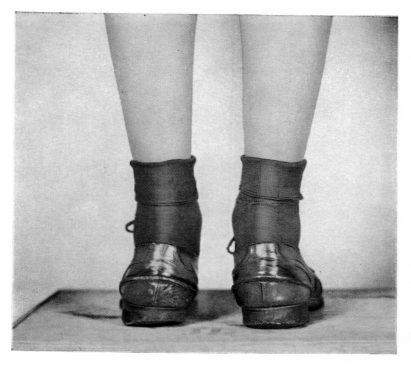

PLATE 15. Nina's teacher has observed that Nina wears down the heels of her shoes toward the inside in a short time. Besides indicating something wrong that needs correction, run-down heels are hard on the feet and are frequently the cause of bad falls and "turned" ankles.

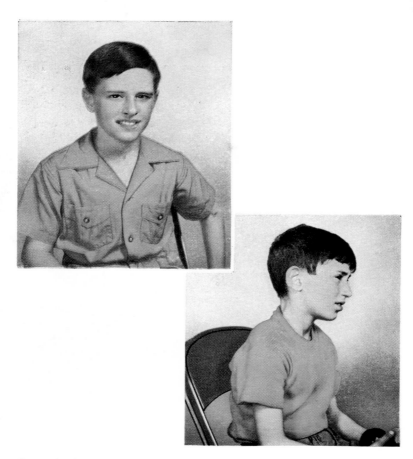

PLATE 16. By comparing postures and expressions it is easy to tell which of these two boys is suffering from chronic fatigue. Charlie, at the left, is a healthy alert youngster, whereas poor Freddie cannot enter whole-heartedly into any activity. Freddie's teacher referred him for a special medical check-up, and a physician found that he had large adenoids, which were interfering with his breathing and lowering his vitality.

pneumococci (in which case it is called pneumococcal pneumonia), or by some other species of bacteria, or by a virus of one kind or another.

Pneumonia is the extension of a respiratory infection into the air sacs (alveoli) of the lungs. It is in these tiny, pouchlike blind endings of the smallest branches of the bronchial tree that the exchange of oxygen and carbon dioxide between the air and blood takes place. The extension of infection into the pulmonary air sacs is very much like the extension of an infection of the nose into the sinuses or through the eustachian tube into the middle ear. What happens is that the causative agents, or germs, get into places that cannot be kept clean by the moving mucous blanket of the respiratory passages. Pneumonia is invited and encouraged by anything that interferes with the normal escalatorlike operation of this blanket which, as we have seen, keeps virulent visiting pathogens from accumulating and mobilizing for invasion. That is why the development of pneumonia is so often associated with chilling of the body following exposure to cold and wet, with exhaustion from any cause, or, more especially, with a forerunning attack by the virus of the common cold or influenza virus.

Attack by a virus may prepare the way for bacterial invasion of the lungs, the most common being that staged by the pneumococci. Or the virus itself may extend to the alveoli of the lungs and set up an inflammation in its own right, that is, a lung infection known as virus pneumonia.

Pneumococcal Pneumonia. The classic signs and symptoms of pneumococcal pneumonia are a shaking chill, followed by high fever; sharp pain in the side, chest, or shoulder; cough; difficult breathing; and the raising of sticky, rust-colored sputum.

The use of penicillin and other antibiotics in treatment have greatly reduced the death rate from pneumococcal pneumonia (see Fig. 11-4), and also from pneumonia caused by bacteria other than the pneumococci.

Virus Pneumonia. Also called primary atypical pneumonia, this is generally a mild disease, but it can be severe. It develops slowly, beginning with headache, fever, chilliness, fatigue, malaise, and respiratory symptoms of cough and expectoration. The average duration of the illness is about a week, and complications are uncommon. Recognized virus pneumonia is most frequent among adolescents and young adults. Certain antibiotics have been used in treatment with beneficial results in individual cases.

Recurrences of Colds, Influenza, and Pneumonia

One of the conspicuous features of colds, influenza, and pneumonia is their tendency to recur in the same individual. Unlike many other diseases caused by bacteria or viruses, one attack does not confer long-lasting immunity from further attacks.

Any child who has more colds than most children do (the average number of colds per person per year is three) should be brought especially to the attention of the physician who examines the child periodically. Also, a child who is subject to repeated colds or who has once had pneumonia or rheumatic fever should be given the benefit of whatever measures we now possess for controlling respiratory infections. Such measures include education regarding the things the child can do to build up good general health and to keep the respiratory mucous membranes in good condition. In some cases the doctor may prescribe one of the drugs that act to suppress secondary bacterial invaders when the child has a cold.

Chronic Diseases Associated with Cigarette Smoking

Lung cancer, chronic bronchitis, emphysema, and coronary heart disease are rarely, if ever, encountered in school-age children. Formation of the habit of cigarette smoking in youth may, however, give these disorders a head start. The findings of the Advisory Committee on Smoking and Health of the Surgeon General of the Public Health Service[2] leave no doubt that there are very serious risks to health attached to the habit of cigarette smoking. The major risks are briefly summarized below:

In comparison with non-smokers, average male cigarette smokers have about a 9- to 10-fold risk of developing lung cancer and heavy smokers at least a 20-fold risk. The risk of developing lung cancer increases with the duration of smoking and the number of cigarettes smoked per day. The risk is diminished by discontinuing smoking.

Cigarette smoking is the most important of the causes of chronic bronchitis and increases the risk of dying from it. It has not been established that cigarette smoking is causally related to the development of emphysema (another chronic disorder of the lungs), but it is definitely associated with the risk of dying from emphysema.

It has not been proved that cigarette smoking is causally linked to coronary artery disease, but smokers have a higher death rate from this disease than have non-smoking men. Higher mortality also is associated with many other cardiovascular diseases in smokers.

The combined results of seven long-term studies comparing the mortality experience of smokers with that of non-smokers show that the death rate for all causes of death taken together is 70 per cent higher among smokers than among non-smokers.

Polonium 210 and Lung Cancer. Shortly after the Committee's report was published, two Harvard School of Public Health investigators announced that one natural contaminant of tobacco may prove to be the

---

[2] *Smoking and Health,* Report of the Advisory Committee to the Surgeon General of the Public Health Service, Public Health Service Publication No. 1103, 1964.

link between cigarette smoking and lung cancer.[3] This contaminant is the radioactive element known as polonium 210. It occurs naturally in all green plants. Its danger to smokers lies in the fact that it vaporizes at the burning temperature of the cigarette and is carried into the lungs by attaching itself to smoke particles. For a man smoking two packs of cigarettes a day, the radiation dose to the bronchial linings from polonium 210 inhaled in cigarette smoke is at least seven times that of the normal radiation dose from background sources. It has long been known that radiation can produce cancer in man. Radiation from inhaled cigarette smoke may, therefore, act as an important initiator of bronchial cancer in smokers. Much further research will be necessary to determine whether polonium 210 is indeed the long-sought link between cigarette smoking and lung cancer.

Schools with comprehensive health education programs have for many years included whatever information was available on the harmful effects of smoking. Now that the cup of scientific and statistical evidence is full to overflowing, the opportunities for developing realistic educational programs that will appeal to the intelligence of thoughtful junior and senior high school students have been substantially increased.

Cystic Fibrosis

The disease commonly called cystic fibrosis is due to an abnormality in many of the glands of the body that secrete their products directly onto the surface of the skin or mucous membrane. The disease, which is not uncommon, is both congenital and hereditary. The mucous glands of the respiratory tree, the glandular tissue of the pancreas which secretes pancreatic juice, the minute biliary canals of the liver, the salivary glands, and the sweat glands of the skin may be involved in cystic fibrosis. A child may be born with a mild, a moderate, or a severe case. A minimal case may go unrecognized for years only to erupt into a very serious case at or near puberty.

The most serious effects of cystic fibrosis are produced by a disturbance in the functioning of the mucous glands of the trachea and bronchial tubes. These glands instead of secreting a thin clear mucus secrete a thick sticky fluid that is difficult to clear away. Its retention predisposes to infection and airway obstruction. Often a doctor suspects cystic fibrosis when a child fails to recover promptly from a "chest cold," the flu, or whooping cough. Certain children with bronchitis, "chronic pneumonia," or "whooping cough pneumonia" are now correctly diagnosed as having cystic fibrosis.

The laboratory diagnosis of cystic fibrosis is based primarily upon the "sweat test." The sweat of children with this disease contains much more

[3] Edward P. Radford, Jr., and Vilma R. Hunt, "Polonium-210: A Volatile Radioactive element in Cigarettes," *Science,* Jan. 17, 1964.

salt than is found in the sweat of normal children. Parents of these children may observe that their children "taste salty" when kissed.

There is at present no cure for cystic fibrosis, but doctors can do a great deal to relieve its distressing symptoms. Antibiotics are most useful in preventing or combating lung infection. A solution to the cystic fibrosis problem is now being sought in several research centers throughout the country.

Scarlet Fever and Streptococcal Sore Throat

Group A hemolytic streptococci, of which there are at least forty distinct types, are the infectious agents of scarlet fever and streptococcal sore throat. These streptococci are capable of producing erythrogenic toxin which causes a diffuse red skin rash. A susceptible person infected with Group A streptococci will come down either with scarlet fever or with streptococcal sore throat, depending upon whether he is or is not immune from the erythrogenic toxin they produce. To put it in its simplest terms, scarlet fever is streptococcal sore throat *with a rash;* streptococcal sore throat is scarlet fever *without a rash.*

Immunity from erythrogenic toxin develops within one week of the onset of scarlet fever. However, many persons acquire immunity from this toxin without having scarlet fever. Many strains of streptococci are such poor toxin producers that they do not cause a skin rash. A person infected with one of these strains has streptococcal sore throat but may —and often does—acquire immunity from the erythrogenic toxin responsible for the rash of scarlet fever. Immunity from the infecting type of streptococcus develops and lasts several years. Many persons also develop immunity from the erythrogenic toxin or from the infecting type of streptococcus or both, as a result of inapparent infections (that is, infection without recognizable symptoms). In untreated cases streptococci may be present in the nose and throat discharges for months after recovery. Nasal carriers are particularly likely to contaminate their environment.

Cases of scarlet fever and cases of streptococcal sore throat frequently occur in the same epidemic. If a group of children is exposed to a person with scarlet fever, or a carrier, some may not be affected, some will develop scarlet fever, and others will develop no more than an acute pharyngitis and yet be able to transmit scarlet fever to other susceptible children. Susceptibility to scarlet fever is greater among children (particularly in the five- to nine-year-old age group) and young adults.

During epidemics of scarlet fever and streptococcal sore throat, penicillin may be used to protect intimate contacts and household contacts of a case and those known to have been exposed to contaminated milk or other food. It is especially important to protect persons in whom recurrent streptococcal infections provide a special risk, such as individuals who have had rheumatic fever or chorea. When a streptococcal infection occurs in a household which includes someone who has rheumatic fever or who has had rheumatic fever, all members of the family should receive a course of penicillin treatment.

Even in mild cases, scarlet fever and streptococcal sore throat may have serious complications, of which cervical adenitis, otitis media, rheumatic fever, and acute glomerular nephritis are the most common. Various forms of penicillin are used in the treatment of persons sick with scarlet fever or streptococcal sore throat. This treatment serves to lighten the illness, reduce the frequency of complications, and prevent the development of rheumatic fever or acute glomerular nephritis. Adequate treatment with penicillin also eliminates within twenty-four hours the probability of transmission of the disease from patients or carriers.

Septic Sore Throat. This term is used to describe epidemics of streptococcal sore throat of explosive onset. Generally, such epidemics are caused by the consumption of unpasteurized milk or milk products which have been contaminated with hemolytic streptococci either from the infected udder of a cow or from an infected milk handler. The signs and symptoms resemble those of acute streptococcal sore throat except that the disease is often more virulent and is accompanied by various manifestations of a systemic infection such as high fever and prostration.

Measles

Measles has long stood as the classic example of a contagious disease that we must learn to live with rather than hope to eradicate. It now appears that it can be effectively controlled by active immunization.

Although the usual case of measles is a self-limiting illness of short duration, moderate severity, and low fatality (see Sec. 1, Appendix B), it can pave the way for serious bacterial infections, notably pneumonia. Occasionally it is complicated by encephalitis, a dangerous inflammation of the brain. According to the most conservative estimate, measles causes a minimum of eight million days of illness a year in one million individuals—mostly children—in the United States.

Passive Immunization. For some time immune serum globulin (gamma globulin) has been used successfully to prevent the development of measles after exposure in very young or chronically ill children. This protection, however, lasts only for that particular exposure. Gamma globulin in a smaller dose also is used after exposure to make measles milder in susceptible older children and adults. This mild measles confers active immunity but is as communicable as regular measles. Furthermore, it is not always possible to tell whether or when a child has been exposed or to be sure that an exposed child will receive medical care.

Active Immunization. Two types of measles vaccine that promise to end the misery of measles became available for general use in the early

1960s: (1) attenuated live-virus vaccine and (2) inactivated, or killed, virus vaccine. The first type was developed by Dr. John F. Enders, whose pioneering work in demonstrating that polio viruses can be grown on nonnervous tissue led directly to the production of polio vaccines (see Poliomyelitis, in Chap. 8). Starting with measles virus from the blood of a boy in the early stages of measles (the Edmonston virus), Enders succeeded in attenuating (weakening) the virus by passing it through more than fifty generations of human tissue cells. He then weakened it still further by growing it in chick embryos and chick-cell cultures.

After extensive tests of the safety and effectiveness of the vaccine prepared from this attenuated live virus, thirteen susceptible children were inoculated with it in September, 1958. Since then thousands of children have received the vaccine. The results show that the vaccine causes a mild reaction lasting about five days, during which many of the children develop a rash and fever and in some cases other typical signs of measles infection. "Modified measles," as this response to the vaccine is called, is not communicable. The rash and fever can be significantly reduced by administering the live-virus vaccine in conjunction with an injection of gamma globulin. The data obtained so far indicate that live-virus measles vaccine combined with gamma globulin gives solid lasting protection against naturally occurring measles.

Killed-virus measles vaccine consists of attenuated live-virus measles vaccine inactivated with formaldehyde. Studies show that three injections of this vaccine at monthly intervals produce a good antibody response in children who receive it. The protection rate tends to fall off in the first year, but the effect of a booster dose is excellent. Two doses of killed-virus vaccine followed from one to three months later by the administration of live-virus vaccine dramatically reduce the undesirable side effects that are usual with the live-virus vaccine. It has been demonstrated that the protective effect of this vaccine combination lasts for at least six months; further study is needed to determine how much longer it will persist.[4]

Tuberculosis

Tuberculosis is a chronic infectious disease caused by the tubercle bacillus. Tubercle bacilli may set up infection in many parts of the body, but tuberculosis of the lungs, or pulmonary tuberculosis, is by far the most common form of the disease in our country.

Where we now stand with regard to tuberculosis has been described in Chap. 2 (under Stories of High Achievement). The most important

[4] Report of the Committee on the Control of Infectious Diseases, American Academy of Pediatrics, Evanston, Ill., 1964.

fact to keep in mind about it is that it is a preventable disease. Whether TB is to be or not to be in the years ahead is up to the people living today.

In general there are two fundamental types of pulmonary tuberculosis, (1) the primary, or first-infection type, and (2) the reinfection type.

First-infection Tuberculosis. First-infection, or primary, tuberculosis takes place when tubercle bacilli invade the body of a person who has never before been infected. The bacilli bring about destruction of tissue at points where they lodge in the lungs, resulting in the typical lesions of pulmonary tuberculosis. Phagocyte cells are quickly mobilized to fight the invaders, however, and if all goes well from the body's point of view there is complete healing of the lesions of first-infection tuberculosis in from one to two years. In healed lesions the destroyed areas are walled off from the surrounding healthy tissue by fibrous capsules or by nodules called tubercles, which in time may become calcified. Living bacilli may be imprisoned within the capsules or tubercles, but they can do no harm unless the walls break down and let them out.

Primary tuberculosis is most dangerous for babies and young children up to five years of age because of the possibility of serious complications, especially miliary tuberculosis and tuberculous meningitis. In miliary tuberculosis large numbers of the bacilli get into the bloodstream and are carried throughout the body. Wherever they lodge, tiny lesions (like millet seeds, hence the designation "miliary") develop. In tuberculous meningitis, the coverings of the brain (cerebral meninges) become involved.

In children of elementary school age, first-infection tuberculosis is usually a benign disease. Many children with first-infection tuberculosis show no outward signs and symptoms whatever. Others who were formerly alert and active may act tired and listless until the infection is arrested. Tubercle bacilli are extremely difficult to find in simple primary tuberculosis. On this account, children with uncomplicated primary tuberculosis are usually noninfectious.

Allergy and Immunity. The great majority of children with healed primary lesions will live out the rest of their lives without any further trouble from tuberculosis. One reason for this is that the first struggle between the body and the bacilli gives some protection from subsequent infections. During a first infection the body becomes highly sensitive—"allergic"—to tubercle bacilli. If tubercle bacilli should again enter the body or should escape alive from healed primary lesions, the defense forces of the body sensitized by their former encounter are mobilized much more quickly and effectively. As a result, the same sort of defense reactions take place as in a first, or primary, infection, but they happen much more quickly and vigorously.

With the development of allergy, therefore, some measure of immunity is acquired. This protection is far from absolute, however. In some cases the sensitized tissues are destroyed faster than the defense forces of the body can deal with the invaders. When this happens, the destructive, progressive form of tuberculosis, known as reinfection tuberculosis, develops.

Reinfection Tuberculosis. The infecting bacilli in reinfection tuberculosis may enter the body from the outside or escape from healed primary lesions. The development of reinfection tuberculosis appears to be favored by (1) a breakdown of the body's defense forces as a result of poor nutrition or fatigue or an illness or some other debilitating condition, and (2) an overwhelming of the relative resistance or immunity acquired during a first infection by frequently repeated or massive reinfecting doses of bacilli such as might occur in day-by-day contact with an active case of tuberculosis or in the breaking loose of large numbers of bacilli from previously healed primary lesions.

When tuberculosis was much more common than it is today, the rate of primary infection steadily mounted during the childhood years. Then came the onset of puberty and with it a lowering of the body's ability to resist attack by reinfecting doses of tubercle bacilli. With greater opportunities for tuberculosis infection than now exist, many young people who had had primary tuberculosis in childhood without even knowing it developed reinfection tuberculosis in their late teens and twenties. Consequently, tuberculosis in our country was once a disease of youth. Even as recently as 1924 half of those who died of tuberculosis were thirty-three years old or younger.

The picture has changed greatly in recent years. Now more than half of those who die of tuberculosis are persons more than fifty years of age. It is believed that many of the new active cases in late life are flare-ups of infections which took place years ago in childhood and youth. Although first infections usually cause only a trivial illness, there is always the danger that the disease may become active later on. That is why it is so important to keep from becoming infected in the first place. But no one can be safe from infection so long as people who do not even know they have active tuberculosis are in a position to spread it.

For every 150 persons in our country who know they have tuberculosis, it is estimated that there are 100 persons who do not know they have it. The lesions of reinfection tuberculosis may begin to form without producing any signs and symptoms whatever. Among the earliest noticeable danger signals that the observant teacher or parent may detect are persistent fatigue, loss of weight, chronic cough with or without expectoration, flushed face in the afternoon indicating fever, night sweats, poor appetite, and digestive upsets. The sooner such signs and symptoms are brought to a physician's attention, a diagnosis made, and, if the verdict is active tuberculosis, proper treatment begun, the better are the chances of a satisfactory recovery.

Case Finding. Fortunately there are ways of finding active tuberculosis without waiting for its victims to develop obvious signs and symptoms. Case-finding programs are one of the most important activities of the local public health units (city or county) and local tuberculosis associations affiliated with the National Tuberculosis Association. The tuberculin test and photofluorography (X-ray photography) are the main tools used in case-finding programs. The tuberculin test is used mostly in case-finding programs in the schools.

The Tuberculin Test. This test is based on the fact that the body becomes allergic to the products of the tubercle bacilli while fighting a first infection. Tuberculin is the filtered, sterilized fluid medium in which tubercle bacilli have grown, or the proteins of the tubercle bacilli extracted from it. In giving the test, a very small amount of tuberculin is injected between the layers of the skin (the *Mantoux test*), or tuberculin is injected into the skin through multiple punctures (the *Heaf test*), or a piece of gauze moistened with tuberculin is fastened to the skin with adhesive tape (the *patch test*). If the test is positive, redness and swelling develop in forty-eight hours at the spot on the skin where the test was made.

A reaction to the tuberculin test indicates only that the person is allergic to the products of tubercle bacilli. To have become allergic, tubercle bacilli must at some time have entered his body. At the time of the test he may have (1) an active primary infection; (2) a healed primary infection; (3) active reinfection; (4) healed reinfection.

Chest X Rays. Everyone who reacts to the tuberculin test must be given a thorough medical examination, including an X-ray picture of the chest to determine whether the infection is active or inactive. A child with X-ray evidence of a healed tuberculous lesion may engage in the normal activities of children of his age without danger. He should have a chest X ray periodically, however, so that any signs of fresh trouble can be detected in their very earliest stages when tuberculosis is most quickly and easily arrested.

In case-finding programs among groups of adults, chest X-ray examinations are usually made without preliminary tuberculin testing. For more than half a century, mass X-ray surveys have resulted in the finding of thousands of unknown cases of tuberculosis.

Routine chest X-ray examinations are recommended for groups having a higher prevalence of tuberculosis than the general population, such as nurses, medical students, patients and outpatients in general and mental hospitals, and selected groups of industrial workers. In communities where the frequency of tuberculosis is known to be excessive, X-ray screening of the entire adult population may be considered advisable.

Routine chest X rays for individuals who constitute a special hazard to others if they have active tuberculosis is of great importance. Teachers and other school personnel, including school bus drivers, belong in this category. The measures recommended are the requirements of a negative X ray of the chest as a condition for the employment of any school employee who comes in direct contact with the students and of subsequent periodic chest X rays to find cases in employees who may later develop tuberculosis. These measures are now in effect, wholly or in part, in many cities and towns and in some states. Not only do they protect school children from infection through day-by-day close contact with unsuspected active cases of tuberculosis, but also they are proving instrumental in the saving of useful productive lives with a minimum of time lost from work.

Progress in Treatment. The chances of recovery from tuberculosis are now excellent and are continually getting better. They are especially good when the disease is discovered early. Rest in bed and a good diet were about the only aids to recovery in the early days of tuberculosis treatment. They are still very important, but today's treatment also includes the use of drugs and various surgical procedures.

Streptomycin was the first drug that was found to be effective in stopping the growth of tubercle bacilli. But any tubercle bacilli which are not quickly stopped by streptomycin develop resistance to it. These resistant bacilli keep on growing and multiplying. Another drug known as para-aminosalicylic acid (PAS, for short) delays the development of streptomycin-resistant bacilli. A third most valuable drug in tuberculosis treatment is Isoniazid. This drug made its dramatic entrance in March, 1952. Isoniazid and streptomycin are most effective when used together. When either Isoniazid or streptomycin is used alone, it is combined with PAS to prevent the development of drug-resistant bacilli. Other new drugs also are being investigated. But no drugs have yet been found that destroy all bacilli so promptly that no resistance develops or that do not produce bad side effects in some patients. And so the search goes on with increasing hope that a drug will be found which will combat this ancient disease with complete success.

Great advances also have been made in the use of surgery as an aid in the treatment of tuberculosis. In an increasing number of operations the diseased portion of a lung, or even an entire lung, is removed. In others, all or part of a diseased lung is collapsed permanently.

Recovery and Rehabilitation. The use of the new drugs in treatment not only speeds up recovery from tuberculosis, but also makes the patients noninfectious within a few months. In spite of these new aids to recovery, however, a child found to have active tuberculosis will usually need to spend some time in a hospital where he is sure of getting rest and the proper food and of receiving the prescribed drugs regularly.

During the recovery period it is important to provide opportunities for continuing the child's education as soon as the physician permits. This is being done through educational programs in tuberculosis hospitals and through visiting teachers and other specialized workers if the child is being cared for at home.

When the child is permitted to return to regular school his teachers may be called upon to help with the plans for his scholastic and recreational activities. Over a period determined by the physician it may be necessary to adjust his curriculum to a shorter school day and to provide recreational occupations that do not require strenuous physical effort.

In helping the student to make the transition from invalidism to a normal school life, it is an advantage to know that exaggerated personality traits, such as overaggressiveness or withdrawal, are not uncommon after a long illness. As a rule, such manifestations will be temporary if they are understood and accepted by his teacher and other adults as a natural reaction to the prolonged thwarting of his normal desires for fun and companionship. Interest in the student as a person will do much to enable him to make satisfactory adjustment to everyday school routine.

Progress in Prevention. Ever since Robert Koch discovered the cause of tuberculosis in 1882, research workers have been trying to develop a vaccine to immunize people from tuberculosis. So far no vaccine that gives complete protection has been found. However, encouraging results have been obtianed in the use of BCG vaccination.

BCG vaccination is based upon the quickened response of a body sensitized to tubercle bacilli as a result of a first infection. BCG is the abbreviation for "bacillus Calmette-Guerin." This strain of tubercle bacillus was developed by two French scientists, Calmette and Guerin, and their fellow workers. It is so weak that it cannot cause active tuberculosis. However, it is strong enough to make the body allergic to tubercle bacilli and hence heightens resistance against those bacteria. The protection given is only partial, not complete. Resistance can be broken down by large or frequently repeated doses of tubercle bacilli at a time when the body's natural defenses have been weakened.

BCG is given only to tuberculin-negative individuals. As it makes these individuals tuberculin-positive, its widespread use would cancel out the effectiveness of the tuberculin test in finding infected persons. Medical and public health authorities in our country recommend that the use of BCG be restricted to individuals who are exposed to high risk of infection. In this category are household contacts of active cases, and persons who are exposed to infection by reason of occupation, such as medical and nursing students. BCG is advised also for tuberculin-negative children who have a high probability of exposure to tuberculosis either at home or in an area with a high infection rate. The American

Academy of Pediatrics recommends that daily administration of Isoniazid alone be considered for tuberculin-negative children obliged to live in close contact with adults suffering from infectious tuberculosis.[5] BCG should not be given during Isoniazid administration.

THE SCHOOL AND RESPIRATORY-DISEASE CONTROL

Most of the communicable diseases with which a school may have to contend are spread by discharges from the respiratory tract. Many cases of such diseases are discovered in school, where the threshold of suspicion is lower than in the home. Cooperation with other community agencies in the education of parents and other adults in the measures required to protect children from respiratory and other infections is an important part of the school's responsibility in communicable-disease control. These measures include (1) the immunization of children from diseases for which immunization procedures are available (see Immunization Timetable, Appendix A); (2) seeing that children do not come to school when they show early signs and symptoms of illness; (3) sending children home with an escort when they become ill in school; (4) protecting children as far as possible from exposure to infection while in school; and (5) notifying parents when a serious communicable disease breaks out in school, so that children who show early signs and symptoms of the disease may be kept at home.

Observing Children for Signs of Infection

Every teacher should know how to detect early indications of communicable disease, and, when any of the danger signals appear, she should refer the child to the physician or nurse serving the school. If professional assistance is not available, she should isolate the child from the other pupils and arrange to have him taken home. Information about the common respiratory diseases of childhood is given in Secs. 1 and 2, Appendix B. In addition to information about specific diseases, the teacher should have a general picture of the symptom complex—set of symptoms—that indicates the possible onset of one of the contagions most commonly suffered in childhood. The following signs and symptoms, whether occurring singly or in combination, should be looked on with suspicion:

A chill or chilliness
Fever (flushed face, lassitude, malaise)
Sore or scratchy throat
Red, watery eyes
Watery nasal discharge

Tight, dry cough
Sneezing
Headache, earache, or aching in back or legs
Nausea or vomiting

[5] *Ibid.*

It will be noted that several of the signs and symptoms resemble those of the common cold. The characteristic signs of a particular communicable disease rarely appear at onset. For example, the eruption of vesicles characteristic of chicken pox, the typical rashes of measles and scarlet fever, the swelling of the salivary glands in mumps, and the spasmodic cough of whooping cough usually do not appear for one or more days after onset (Secs. 1 and 2, Appendix B).

Procedures during Epidemics

Dealing with epidemics of communicable disease in a community is the responsibility of the local public health unit. School officials should follow the recommendations of public health officials regarding special precautions, such as regular daily inspection and continuing observation of school children, when a communicable disease is especially prevalent.

It is not considered advisable, in communities that have well-organized public health facilities, to close schools during epidemics (of scarlet fever, for example, or of influenza). Unless the medical and nursing staffs are inadequate to exercise proper supervision, children are usually better off in school, where they are under constant, experienced observation. The alert teacher can play an invaluable part in limiting the spread of infection by reporting immediately any children who show signs and symptoms of illness.

Protecting School Children from Airborne Infections

The avoidance of exposure to respiratory infections is at the present time impossible. With regard to the common cold, for example, many of us have good reason to know that careful observance of all the classic hygienic rules, such as washing our hands before eating and giving careless coughers and sneezers a wide berth, does not keep us from catching cold two or three times a year. Also, the extreme contagiousness of influenza, measles, and chicken pox has made it practically impossible to control these and other easily transmitted airborne diseases by erecting the barrier of isolation.

A better understanding of what we have to contend with in attempts to control airborne infection has been reached by the discovery that droplets sprayed from the mouth and nose evaporate faster than they fall, leaving small residues called droplet nuclei. These tiny germ-laden particles may float about for long periods of time in the air of enclosed spaces in much the same manner as particles of tobacco smoke. It doesn't take much imagination to think of indoor atmosphere during late fall, winter, and early spring as being pervaded by a sort of invisible miasma, or fog, arising from the mucous membranes of those present. This picture gives us some idea of the way in which we are almost continually exposed to the respiratory flora of other people by the simple act of breathing air that contains their exhalations.

Although there are as yet no specific practical measures available for protecting school children completely from airborne infection, the following general preventive measures may have some value.

Correct Use of Handkerchiefs. The proper technique of coughing and sneezing is a form of good manners as well as a means of avoiding the broadcasting of infection. Children should be trained in this technique until it becomes habitual. The first requirement is the possession of a handkerchief (preferably a supply of disposable paper handkerchiefs). In blowing the nose children should learn to blow gently, leaving both nostrils open so as to avoid the risk of driving the infection into the sinuses or middle ear.

In coughing, the handkerchief should be held so that it completely covers both mouth and nose. In sneezing, it is best to sneeze naturally through the mouth, with the handkerchief held as in coughing, rather than politely through the nose. Also, children should learn not to pull out used handkerchiefs with a flourish or to shake them. Experiments have shown that the shaking of dry used handkerchiefs releases thousands of germs into the surrounding air.

Proper Seating. Children should be seated as far apart as possible. During epidemics advantage should be taken of empty seats to increase the spacing. To prevent the exposure of large numbers of children to the early or missed case of an airborne disease or to a carrier, it is considered best to preserve the same relative position of children to one another in class and to avoid the mingling of classes so far as possible. If this cannot be done ordinarily, children should be "frozen" at once if a case of infectious disease occurs.

Good Ventilation. Whatever the heating and ventilating arrangements of the school are, provision should be made to keep the air of occupied classrooms constantly in motion. Moving air helps to break up concentrations of airborne germs. Also, fresh outdoor air, or air properly cleaned, moistened, and warmed (as in an air-conditioning system) helps to keep the mucous membranes of the nose and throat in a healthy condition. The classroom should be neither too hot nor too cold. For moderately active children wearing ordinary indoor clothing, a room temperature of about 70°F, with 50 per cent relative humidity, is considered to be about right in cold weather.

Hand-washing Facilities. Although hand washing may not materially affect the spread of airborne infection, it is a good hygenic habit for children to form. Always washing the hands with soap and water before eating or handling food and after every visit to the toilet is an important factor in the control of diseases that are spread sometimes or usually by indirect contact, that is, by handling, eating, or drinking anything soiled with the body discharges of a sick person or carrier. The facilities required to make hand washing effective are warm water (preferably running water from a tap), soap, and individual cloth or paper towels.

Dry Clothing. There will be fewer colds caught in school if provision is made for the children to dry wet clothing and to change into dry footwear on rainy or snowy days. Children should learn to remove rubbers or overshoes and outdoor wraps when they come indoors. The moisture from perspiring bodies is as effective in making clothing and footwear damp as are rain and snow!

School Cleaning. Airborne germs in droplet nuclei or on dust particles eventually settle on the floor and on furniture. They are given a second chance to find victims if they are stirred into the atmosphere during cleaning. The floor and furniture finishes and the methods of cleaning in modern schools reduce the raising of dust to a minimum. In schools without these improvements, the use of damp sweeping and damp dusting is recommended as a means of reducing the contamination of air by germs.

Staying Home from School. In some schools so much emphasis is placed on good attendance records that many children come to school who ought to stay at home. Certainly children should be encouraged to stay home when they have early signs of respiratory infection, such as the sniffles or a sore throat. Talks with parents by nurses or physicians serving the school, or by teachers, will help to emphasize the need for keeping children home and consulting a physician when the children do not seem to be in their usual good health.

RESPIRATORY ALLERGIES

Children who show signs of a respiratory allergy usually come from allergic families (see Types of Allergy in Chap. 7). Specialists both in allergy and in child care emphasize the importance of early recognition of such conditions in children. Prompt diagnosis and early treatment will not only make a big difference in the child's day-by-day comfort and happiness but also will help to prevent complications which are difficult to cure and which may seriously interfere with the child's health, growth, and personality development. For example, an untreated nasal allergy, such as hay fever, may result in deformities of the face or teeth, or the development of nasal polyps or a chronic nasal infection, or chronic bronchial asthma.

Nasal Allergy

Nasal allergy may be either seasonal or nonseasonal. The seasonal type occurs in persons who are sensitive to the pollen of various trees, grasses, and weeds when the offending pollen (or pollens) is in the air. This type of nasal allergy is called hay fever. The allergens most commonly responsible for the nonseasonal type are various inhalants such as dust, orris root, and animal danders. A less common cause is sensitivity to other substances such as certain foods or drugs.

Hay Fever. The symptoms of pollen allergy are similar to those of a cold in the head, that is, obstruction of nasal breathing, sneezing, watering of the eyes, and itching of the roof of the mouth, the eyes, and the nose. When the lungs become involved, a form of bronchial asthma (see below) called pollen asthma is set up.

Tree pollens are the allergens responsible for hay fever in the spring, and the pollens of grasses and weeds, in the summer and fall. The worst offender in most places in the late summer and fall is ragweed pollen. For this reason an effort is being made in some communities to stamp out ragweed either by spraying the weeds with a chemical plant killer or by cutting them down and burning them before they mature.

Helping Children with Nasal Allergies. It is now easy for doctors to diagnose hay fever. The appearance of the nasal mucous membranes is typically allergic, and the exact pollens responsible can be detected by sensitization tests of the skin (intradermal or patch tests) or of the mucous membrane (nasal sniff test and eye test).

However, a child suffering from a nasal allergy sometimes fails to get medical attention because he is considered merely to be subject to frequent head or chest colds. Or a child may be kept home from school for a cold when the condition is allergic. This is one more important reason for referring for medical checkup any child who seems to have one cold after another. Also certain mannerisms that may pass simply as bad habits are characteristic of children suffering from hay fever or allergic rhinitis. Among them are rubbing or wrinkling the nose and frequent sniffing. Using the fingers to push the tip of the nose upward and inward, both to relieve itching and to spread the walls apart in an effort to improve ventilation, is such a common mannerism that it has been called "the allergic salute."

There is as yet no cure for hay fever. Specific treatment only relieves the symptoms. The most generally used treatment consists in eliminating pollen sensitivity by injecting increasing doses of an extract of the pollen or pollens to which the patient is allergic. This treatment is begun early so that the patient reaches the maximum dose at the beginning of the hay-fever season. The maximum dose is then injected at intervals through the season. A single massive dose of pollen extract in mineral oil may in certain cases be substituted for the multiple-shot treatment. The mineral oil acts as a repository so that the pollen extract can be absorbed gradually during the pollen season.

Several antihistamine drugs also are proving very helpful for lessening the discomforts of the hay-fever victim. The physician also may prescribe drops or sprays for the eyes or nose.

Bronchial Asthma

This allergic disorder is marked by recurrent attacks of paroxysmal difficulty in breathing, wheezing, and a cough. These attacks frequently occur in the early morning hours. In children the only warning may be a persistent unexplained cough, coming on in paroxysms with little or no wheezing and without difficulty in breathing. There may be other causes of asthmatic symptoms besides allergy. Only after careful medical study of the individual is it possible to arrive at the correct diagnosis.

The manifestations of bronchial asthma are caused by swelling of the mucous membrane that lines the bronchial tubes and by spasms of the muscles in their walls. The allergens responsible may be pollens and other inhalants, foods, drugs, substances handled in the course of one's work, and so on. The common cold and other acute infections of the respiratory tract often precipitate asthmatic attacks or increase their severity. For this reason the asthmatic patient is usually worse in the fall and winter, when respiratory infections are common. Emotional disturbances, exertion, and sudden temperature changes likewise play an important part in precipitating or contributing to the severity of an asthmatic attack. In children, particularly, untreated hay fever may lead to development of asthmatic symptoms toward the end of the pollen season.

WHAT TO DO IN RESPIRATORY EMERGENCIES

A respiratory emergency is any condition that interferes with breathing. The body has in storage enough food to last, in a pinch, for weeks and enough water to last for several days, but no provision has been made for the storage of oxygen. In the hemoglobin of the red blood corpuscles, there is available at any one time only enough oxygen to keep us alive for two or three minutes. When suddenly it becomes impossible for the body to get oxygen from the outside world, survival is a matter of moments only. In the ordinary course of events this is not likely to happen. We are surrounded by an ocean of air which contains about 21 per cent oxygen. It is necessary only to be able to breathe to get all we need. Under certain circumstances, however, that is just what it is impossible to do. Any accident that results in interference with the delivery of oxygen to the body cells causes asphyxia.

Asphyxia

The following are the most common causes of asphyxia:

1. Obstruction of the air passages to the lungs, either from without, as in smothering and strangulation, or from within, as in choking and submersion.

2. Paralysis of the respiratory center of the brain, as in electric shock, so that the breathing muscles cannot work.

3. Interference with the oxygen-carrying function of the red blood cells, as in the inhalation of carbon monoxide, which combines more rapidly, easily, and firmly with hemoglobin than oxygen can.

4. Lack of oxygen in the air breathed in, as in old wells, storage bins, or airtight vaults, where oxygen has been replaced by carbon dioxide through the process of oxidation.

An asphyxiated person is not breathing or breathes only with great difficulty. Even after breathing ceases, the heart usually continues to beat for a few minutes, and in this time the person's life may be saved by prompt action. To restore natural breathing, artificial respiration must be administered immediately after rescue.

Artificial Respiration

Proficiency in administering artificial respiration is a very useful accomplishment both for teachers and for older boys and girls. Instruction in giving artificial respiration is often included in high school first aid classes.

The mouth-to-mouth (or mouth-to-nose) technique is now considered by the American National Red Cross, the American Medical Association, and other national organizations to be the most practical method for artificial respiration in the absence of equipment or of help from a second person regardless of the cause of the cessation of breathing. In rescue breathing, as the method is often called, the rescuer uses his own breath to revive a person who is unable to breathe for himself. How to administer rescue breathing, as described by the American Red Cross, is shown on the following pages.

HOW TO PERFORM RESCUE BREATHING

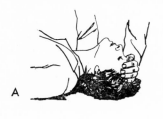

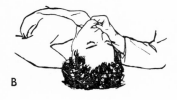

Step 1. Place the victim on his back and quickly remove any foreign material visible in his mouth by wiping it out with your fingers or with your fingers wrapped in cloth.

Step 2. Place one hand under the victim's neck and the other hand high on his forehead and tilt his head back with his chin pointing upward (see A). Then pull or push his jaw into a jutting-out position. The jaw can be *pulled* forward by hooking your thumb over the lower teeth (see B). Or it can be *pushed* forward by placing the fingers of both hands at the angle of the jaw

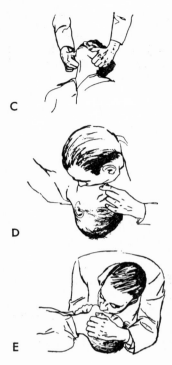

C

D

E

just beneath the victim's ears and gently and cautiously sliding the jaw forward (see C). These procedures should keep the base of the tongue from pressing against and blocking the upper air passage.

Step 3. Open your mouth, take a deep breath and tightly seal your lips over the victim's mouth. At the same time pinch his nostrils shut or close them with your cheek pressed against them to prevent air leakage (see D). OR close the victim's mouth and place your lips over his nose (see E). (For a young child cover both mouth *and* nose with your mouth.) Inflate the victim's lungs by blowing vigorously into his mouth or nose until you see his chest rise. (Air may be blown through the victim's teeth even if the teeth are clenched.) The first blowing effort should determine whether any obstruction exists. (See step 6.)

Step 4. Remove your mouth, turn your head to one side, and listen for the sound of air rushing from the lungs.

Step 5. Repeat blowing vigorously at the rate of about twelve breaths per minute for an adult. For a child take relatively shallow breaths and blow at the rate of about twenty breaths per minute.

Step 6. If you do not hear the sound of exhalation after the first blowing effort, recheck the head and jaw position (see A to C) and blow again. If you still do not get air exchange, turn the victim on his side and administer a sharp blow between the shoulder blades in the hope of dislodging foreign matter that may be obstructing the throat. Then again sweep your fingers through the victim's mouth to remove any obstruction. If the victim is a small child, hold him up by the ankles or invert him over one arm and give him two or three sharp pats between the shoulder blades to help in dislodging the obstructing material.

FOR REVIEW AND DISCUSSION

1. In the following mix-up, words and terms have become separated from their definitions; bring them together again: alveoli; the great muscle responsible for changes in the size of the chest cavity during respiration; respiratory center; air passages in the lungs; sinuses; shelves of bone extending from the side walls of the nose into the nasal cavity; larynx; the air sacs in the lungs where the exchange of respiratory gases takes place; nasopharynx; the group of nerve cells

that controls the rate of breathing; diaphragm; the meeting place of nose and throat; bronchial tubes; cavities in the bone of the skull and face; epiglottis; the hollow organ connecting the lower part of the pharynx with the windpipe; turbinates; the structure that keeps food out of the air passages during swallowing.

2. Tell the difference between

   a. First-infection tuberculosis and reinfection tuberculosis
   b. Tuberculin test and BCG vaccination
   c. Scarlet fever and streptococcal sore throat
   d. Asphyxia and emphysema
   e. Epidemic and pandemic
   f. ARD and BCG

3. What specific contribution to the present or future well-being of children as individuals or in groups may be made by the teacher who

   a. Refers for medical attention a child who is subject to frequent head or chest colds? a child who complains of a sore throat? a child who persistently breathes through the mouth?
   b. Encourages parents to keep children at home when they show early signs and symptoms of illness?
   c. Is familiar with the early signs and symptoms of the common respiratory infections of childhood?
   d. Trains children in the proper use of handkerchiefs?
   e. Can give artificial respiration?
   f. Has periodic chest X rays?

4. Discuss in class what the teacher can do to help

   a. A child who has returned to school after a long illness
   b. A child who is subject to frequent colds or sore throats
   c. During an epidemic of respiratory disease
   d. In preparing for the tuberculin testing of school children

SELECTED REFERENCES

Allergy Foundation of America: *A Story of Millions,* Public Affairs Pamphlet No. 275, Public Affairs Committee, Inc., New York.

American Academy of Pediatrics: *Report of the Committee on the Control of Infectious Diseases* (first given as reference in Chap. 7).

American Medical Association: *Allergies from the Air and What to Do about Them,* The Association, Chicago.

American Medical Association: *The Lungs,* Part 5 of *The Wonderful Human Machine* series, The Association, Chicago. (The workings of the human body in words and pictures.)

American Public Health Association: *Control of Communicable Diseases in Man* (first given as reference in Chap. 7).

Best, C. H., and N. B. Taylor: *The Human Body* (first given as reference in Chap. 1); Part V, *The Physiology of Breathing*, Chaps. 19–21.

Blakeslee, Alton L., and Maxwell S. Stewart: *TB—Can It Be Vanquished?*, Public Affairs Pamphlet No. 156, Public Affairs Committee, Inc., New York.

Dubos, Rene, and Jean Dubos: *The White Plague*, Little, Brown & Company, Boston, 1952. (A fascinating story of man's fight against tuberculosis.)

Grant, Madeleine Parker: *The Wonder World of Microbes*, McGraw-Hill Book Company, New York, 1956. (Answers such questions as: What are the different kinds of microbes and viruses? What do they do and how do they live?)

Holly, Hazel: *What's in the Air?*, Public Affairs Pamphlet No. 275, Public Affairs Committee, Inc., New York. (A booklet on respiratory allergies.)

Maurois, André: *The Life of Sir Alexander Fleming*, E. P. Dutton & Co., Inc., New York, 1959. (A fascinating story of how chance and a prepared mind joined hands in the discovery of penicillin.)

Waksman, Selman A.: *My Life with The Microbes*, Simon and Schuster, Inc., New York, 1958. (An interesting story by the discoverer of streptomycin about his experiences in search of new antibiotics.)

Organizations

National Tuberculosis Association
Allergy Foundation of America

Chapter 12   NUTRITION AND MALNUTRITION

How the Body Uses Food
Meeting the Nutritional Requirements of School-age
  Children
Observing the Nutritional Status of School Children
Overweight and Underweight
Nutrition Education

The word nutrition embraces all the processes by which the body makes use of the various raw materials in food and achieves that state which we all recognize as normal and healthy. Faulty diet or any condition that interferes with the digestion, absorption, or use of food by the body results in the state that we call malnutrition. In this chapter we are concerned with the food needs of the body, what materials in food meet these needs, and what happens when one or more needs are not met.

HOW THE BODY USES FOOD

Foods are complex substances made up of many different kinds of raw materials. We may think of any food—meat, potatoes, milk, or bread, for example—as if it were a complicated design built up of blocks of several different compositions and shapes. The blocks, then, would be the foodstuffs of which that particular food is synthesized or built. If we had a whole box of such blocks and could use them to synthesize a food, as actually we cannot do, we should first have to separate them into six groups, or classes, of foodstuffs: (1) carbohydrates, (2) fats, (3) proteins, (4) vitamins, (5) mineral salts, and (6) water. If we wished to go further into the matter, we should find that these raw materials are in turn built up of much simpler elements.

The body uses the raw materials in food (1) to produce heat and energy; (2) to grow and to replace worn-out tissues; (3) to manufacture entirely new substances of various sorts for use in specialized types of work essential to life and health; and (4) to assist various organs and tissues to function normally and keep in good condition.

Meeting the Need for Energy

The most urgent need of the body is for energy, that is, the ability to do work. Without a constant supply of energy the continuous activities of the body, such as the beating of the heart and the rhythmic movements of respiration, would quickly cease.

Energy Metabolism. The transformation by which energy is made available for the uses of the body is called energy metabolism. Essentially it consists in the juggling of oxygen from the air into new combinations with the carbon and hydrogen atoms in food. As a result carbon dioxide (CO_2) and water (H_2O) are formed and energy in the form of heat is set free. This process is called oxidation. When a person has had no food for several hours and is resting quietly oxidation goes on at a very slow rate. This minimum rate is called basal metabolism.

Energy in the form of heat can be transformed into other forms of energy. The form of energy required to do any kind of mechanical work is called mechanical energy. About 25 per cent of the heat produced by oxidation is converted into mechanical energy for all types of muscular activity and for the maintenance of vital functions. Another portion is used to maintain body temperature (see Reactions to Internal Temperature Changes, in Chap. 7). Excess heat is lost through the skin. The other by-products of oxidation (carbon dioxide and water) are removed by way of the lungs.

Calories. All forms of energy can be changed into heat. It is customary, therefore, to measure the energy supplied by food simply in terms of heat. The heat value of a food is expressed in terms of calories, which are units of heat just as inches or feet are units of length. One calorie is the amount of heat required to raise the temperature of 1 liter (about 1 quart) of water 1°C, or 1 pint of water 4°F.

Carbohydrates, fats, and proteins all supply calories because they all contain carbon. One gram of fat when oxidized in the body yields 9.3 calories; 1 gram of carbohydrate yields 4.1 calories; and 1 gram of protein yields 4.1 calories. Only a fraction of the proteins in food can be oxidized, however, as protein molecules are made up partly of nitrogen which will not burn. Besides, the body uses protein mainly as building and repair material.

Carbohydrates. Carbohydrates are the sugars and starches in food. They come mainly from the plant kingdom (see Table 12-1). The plant builds them up with the aid of energy absorbed from sunlight by combining carbon obtained from the carbon dioxide in the air with water drawn from the earth. Carbohydrates, therefore, are simply carbon and water, hence their name. The Latin word *carbo* means charcoal (carbon) and the Greek word *hydor* means water. During the process of digestion all sugars and all starches are converted into the simple sugar glucose. The glucose molecule is made up of six atoms of carbon and six molecules of water ($C_6H_{12}O_6$).

Glucose is the body's favorite source of heat and energy. If more glucose is made available than is needed at the moment, it is put into "live storage." The readily soluble sugar is changed for storage purposes into an insoluble starch called glycogen. Glycogen is stored in the liver and the muscles. When the glycogen is needed for muscular work, enzymes help to turn it back into glucose.

Fatty Acids. The most common fats contain three molecules of a fatty acid attached to one molecule of glycerin. Fatty acids are classified as saturated or unsaturated according to the amount of hydrogen the chain of carbon atoms in the fatty acid molecule can hold. In a saturated fatty acid, the carbon atoms are incapable of holding more hydrogen. In an unsaturated fatty acid the chain of carbon atoms lacks one or more pairs of hydrogen atoms. If only one pair of hydrogen atoms is lacking, the fatty acid is said to be monounsaturated; if two or more are lacking the fatty acid is said to be polyunsaturated.

Fats that contain a large amount of unsaturated fatty acids are liquid like soybean oil and cottonseed oil. Fats that are made up mostly of saturated fatty acids are solid like butter and the fat of meat. With few exceptions unsaturated fats are vegetable fats and oils, and saturated fats are animal fats.

Unsaturated fatty acids can be forced to pick up extra hydrogen by a process called hydrogenation. As they do so they become saturated and the liquid fat, or oil, changes to a solid. As a result of hydrogenation we have margarine and solid vegetable shortenings.

Fats in the Diet. Pure fats when oxidized furnish more than twice as much energy weight for weight as glucose, but when glucose is provided abundantly through a diet rich in carbohydrates it is preferably utilized and the oxidation of fats is almost completely stopped.

One advantage of fat in the diet is its "staying power." Its digestion and absorption are extended over a much longer period of time than those of carbohydrates. Hunger, emptiness, and fatigue are experienced more frequently upon a high-carbohydrate, low-fat diet than upon a diet containing an adequate amount of fat. Eskimoes, lumbermen, and others doing heavy work in cold climates eat large amounts of fat. Even in temperate zones most people seem to eat more fats in cold weather than in warm weather.

Besides furnishing energy, some fats contain polyunsaturated fatty acids that are absolutely essential in nutrition. The most important is linoleic acid that makes up from 40 per cent to 55 per cent of corn, soybean, and cottonseed oils. The essential fatty acids are compounds that the body cannot manufacture and hence must be included in the diet. Fats also are important because they are the carriers of fat-soluble vitamins (vitamins A, D, E, and K).

Production of Fatty Tissue. Fatty acids that are not oxidized right away and glucose that is not required for immediate use and for "live storage" are changed into fat droplets and stored in the fat depots of the body. The internal fat depots form soft elastic shock absorbers between

Table 12-1

CHIEF SOURCES OF BODY ENERGY

Food groups	Foods	What may happen if children do not get enough
Starches...............	Grain foods: breakfast cereals, rice, tapioca, and all foods made of flour or meal (breads, macaroni, spaghetti, noodles, crackers, pancakes, etc.)	Underweight Listlessness
	Vegetables: potatoes, root vegetables (carrots, turnips, beets, etc.), legumes (peas, beans)	Fatigue Hunger
Sugars.................	Sugar in practically pure form: table sugar, sirups, honey, molasses, jams, jellies, candy Fruits: most kinds, dried or fresh Sweet desserts	Burning of protein to get energy, leaving too little for growth and repair
Fats...................	Animal products: bacon, other fat meat, lard, cream, butter, cheese made from whole milk or cream, egg yolk	Underweight Fatigue Hunger Vitamin deficiencies
	Plant products: salad and cooking oils, mayonnaise, margarine, nuts, chocolate	Burning of protein for energy

various organs and help to hold them in place. The fat deposits just beneath the skin (subcutaneous fat) help to cushion blows and hold in heat.

Another important function of the fat depots is the storage of fat for nutritional purposes. The body does as Joseph advised Pharaoh to do—that is, it sets aside a store of food to be used in the time of famine, so that it will not perish through the famine.

The Cholesterol Question. The whole question of the kinds and amount of fat in the diet has become a matter of intense public concern because medical research and statistical studies appear to indicate that saturated (animal) fats are related to the development of coronary atherosclerosis. The coronary arteries supply the heart muscle itself with blood. In atherosclerosis solid deposits of a fatlike pearly substance called cholesterol thicken the walls of these arteries. As a result the arterial passageways become too narrow for blood to get through in large enough amounts to keep the heart muscle well nourished. Also, the roughening and scarring of the thickened arterial walls favor the formation of blood clots. Coronary heart disease is the general term applied to the most serious complication of coronary atherosclerosis. A heart attack occurs when a coronary artery or one of its branches closes (occludes) or is blocked by a blood clot (thrombus).

Cholesterol occurs in combination with the saturated fatty acids in animal fats. It belongs to a group of alcohols called sterols that are classified with the fats because, like fats, they are insoluble in water. There is a tendency to consider cholesterol as "bad for us" because of the publicity given to it as a prime suspect in the development of coronary heart disease. Nothing could be further from the truth. Cholesterol is essential to life. It is an important component of all cells and is used in the manufacture of the steroid hormones. Most of the cholesterol the body needs is synthesized in the liver. Even if it were completely absent from the diet, the body would draw on stored fat to continue its manufacture.

Some cholesterol in combined and free forms is normally present in the serum of the blood at all times. It is only when much more cholesterol than the body needs or can metabolize is supplied in food or released from the liver that the concentration of cholesterol in the blood serum may become abnormally high.

Medical interest in cholesterol is based on several pieces of evidence. The results of clinical studies indicate that abnormally high levels of blood-serum cholesterol are related to the development of coronary atherosclerosis and coronary heart disease. Many statistical studies indicate that in the United States and other countries where the living standard is high and the diet rich in calories and saturated fats (animal fats and hydrogenated vegetable oils) the death rate from coronary heart disease is much higher than in countries in which the caloric intake is not excessive and the fats in the diet are mostly unsaturated (nonhydrogenated vegetable fats and oils). Several dietary studies show that the substitution of polyunsaturated vegetable oils for saturated animal fats reduces the concentration of blood-serum cholesterol in almost every person. The mechanism by which polyunsaturated fatty acids lower cholesterol levels is poorly understood. One reason appears to be related to the fact that polyunsaturated fatty acids cause an increased secretion of bile acids, which are the end products of the breakdown of cholesterol in the liver.

In the light of all this knowledge, should we make specific changes in the fat content of our diets? Some medical authorities say yes. Others say no largely because no direct causal relationship between diet and atherosclerosis has yet been proved. A middle-of-the-road answer is the suggestion that a reasonable substitution of polyunsaturated fats (cooking oils and oils used in salad dressings) for saturated fats (animal fats and solid shortenings) may be a possible means of preventing atherosclerosis and lessening the risk of heart attacks and strokes. For individuals in certain groups, most medical authorities agree that changes in the fat content of the diet, made under a physician's direction, are advisable. These groups include (1) persons in whom the blood-serum level of cholesterol is abnormally high; (2) persons who have already had a heart attack or stroke; and (3) persons who have a family history of early death from heart disease.

Proteins for Building and Repair of Tissue

We have seen that the carbohydrates and fats are "burned" by the tissues to produce heat for warmth and energy for the accomplishment of work. But neither of these two food materials can take the place of protein. The reason for this is that protein contains large amounts of nitrogen—an element missing from the other two. All living things—plants, animals, and humans—must have nitrogen in order to build up the protoplasm of which their bodies are largely composed. Protoplasm, which has been called the "stuff of life," is a clear jelly-like substance composed of water (about 75 per cent), protein (about 25 per cent), and small amounts of various salts.

Proteins are broken down during digestion into long chains of organic compounds called amino acids. All amino acids contain a basic nitrogen group in addition to carbon, oxygen, and hydrogen groups.

The amino acids are split up by the body cells and regrouped in the most varied ways to build the protein molecules characteristic of human protoplasm. There are twenty-two known amino acids. Hence each tissue has a wide variety from which to choose the materials for building and repair which are adapted to its particular style of cell architecture. Various tissues also use amino acids in manufacturing hormones, enzymes, and other products that are used in regulating the body's work.

Amino acids play a fundamental role in maintaining both natural and acquired resistance to infection. Protein is required for the formation of phagocytes (see Blood and Its Composition, in Chap. 10); also, the production of the globulin in blood plasma (gamma globulin) which carries bacterial antibodies depends upon a sufficient intake of protein.

Surplus amino acids, unlike surplus glucose and fat, are not stored in specific depots. However, the body maintains in the blood plasma and in the cells a large pool of circulating amino acids that may be drawn upon by any body cell needing protein or capable of storing surplus protein. When more protein is taken in than the body needs at the time for building and repair, manufacturing operations, and the emergency pool, most of the excess amino acids are deaminized. That is, the amino group is converted by the liver to urea, which is then excreted by the kidneys in the urine (see The Kidneys and Their Work, in Chap. 13). The leftover nonprotein fraction is changed by the liver into carbohydrate and fat and, as such, is stored or oxidized to furnish heat and energy.

Proteins are present in both animal and plant products. All proteins, however, do not have the same value. The proteins of plants, such as grains and legumes, lack one or more essential amino acids and are therefore called incomplete. All animal proteins, such as meat, milk, and eggs, contain the essential amino acids and are therefore called complete proteins (see Table 12-2). When grains (cereals and foods made from

Table 12-2

CHIEF SOURCES OF PROTEIN

Proteins	What may happen if children do not get enough

Complete:
    Animal products: milk (all kinds), eggs,
    cheese, meat, fish, and poultry
Incomplete:
    Plant products: dried peas, beans, and
    lentils, bread and cereals, nuts, peanut
    butter
	Retarded growth
	Muscular weakness
	Decreased vitality
	Mental and physical fatigue
	Lowered resistance to infection

flours) and legumes (peas, beans, and similar foods) are combined with animal proteins such as milk or its products, or eggs, they can provide a balanced, adequate intake of amino acids at comparatively low cost.

Meeting the Need for Minerals

The minerals in the human body weigh about 6¼ pounds and commercially are worth about 97 cents. To the living organism, however, they are priceless because without them it could not exist. Minerals are present in a wide variety of foods in the form of water-soluble salts. They do not require digestion, as they are present in foods in molecules small enough to pass through the walls of the small intestine into the bloodstream.

Mineral salts are used by the body (1) as building materials (for example, calcium and phosphorus for the building of bones and teeth, and iron for the manufacture of red blood cells); (2) as essential ingredients of several body secretions (for example, iodine in the thyroid secretion, thyroxine); (3) as aids in making a favorable environment for the cells (for example, sodium chloride to keep the blood and tissue fluid slightly salty or brackish, and sodium bicarbonate to protect the blood and tissue fluids from any considerable change in the acid direction); and (4) as regulators for many different body processes (for example, the clotting of blood, the beating of the heart, and the functioning of nerves and glands).

Some of the minerals known to be required by the body are calcium, iron, phosphorus, iodine, copper, sodium, chlorine, fluorine, sulfur, magnesium, manganese, molybdenum, cobalt, potassium, chromium, selenium, and zinc. Many minerals are utilized better in the presence of other minerals, certain vitamins, and protein. Iron and calcium, for example, are used to greater advantage in the presence of a generous amount of ascorbic acid. Vitamin D is necessary for the absorption and deposition of calcium, especially important during growth periods. Adequate protein and fluorine also promote the utilization of calcium. Minerals are widely distributed in different foods, which is one of the reasons for encouraging the use of varieties of food (see Table 12-3).

Table 12-3

GOOD SOURCES OF CALCIUM, IRON, AND IODINE

Minerals	Foods	What may happen if children do not get enough
Calcium...............	Animal products: milk and cheese (except cream cheese) Plant products: all green leafy vegetables (except spinach, beet greens, and Swiss chard)	Abnormalities in bone growth (for example, bowlegs and chest malformations) Possibly poor teeth Stunted growth
Iron..................	Animal products: lean meat, liver, heart, kidneys, oysters, egg yolk Plant products: green leafy vegetables, whole-grain and enriched bread and cereals, dried beans and peas, potatoes, and dried fruits	Nutritional anemia (pallor, easy fatigability)
Iodine................	Sea food, iodized salt	Simple goiter (swelling in neck below Adam's apple)

Meeting the Need for Vitamins

Vitamins are organic compounds built up by plants and animals of carbon, oxygen, hydrogen, and in some cases of other elements. Each one has its own distinctive chemical pattern, which can now be duplicated in the laboratory. That is, the known vitamins can be synthesized outside the living plant or animal body. Some of them are dissolved in the fat (fat-soluble vitamins) and others in the water (water-soluble vitamins) of many different foods.

The vitamins all play essential roles in nutrition and bodily welfare. Those which are recognized as important in meal planning are A, B complex, C, and D. If one or more is lacking in the daily diet for any length of time, a characteristic disease or disorder appears. Table 12-4 contains a summary of the principal food sources of specific vitamins and the effects produced by a deficiency of each one.

Vitamin A. This vitamin exists in animal food sources in the form of fat-soluble crystals which are readily destroyed by oxidation at all temperatures. In plant food sources it exists in the form of carotene, which must be converted into active vitamin A in the body. When more vitamin A is consumed than is immediately required, the surplus is stored in the liver.

Vitamin A is needed by the bone-building and tooth-forming cells in childhood and youth and throughout life for keeping the skin, mucous

Table 12-4

CHIEF SOURCES OF VITAMINS

Vitamins	Foods	What may happen if children do not get enough
Vitamin A..............	Animal products (in form of active vitamin A): liver, fish-liver oils, egg yolk, butter, cream, whole milk, cheese made with cream or whole milk Plant products (in form of carotene): yellow and green vegetables and fruits, such as sweet potatoes, yellow corn, pumpkin, bananas, cantaloupe, apricots, yellow peaches, spinach, watercress, string beans, peas, and green peppers Margarine fortified with vitamin A	Rough scaly skin Papular eruption (like gooseflesh) on skin Dry, coarse, brittle, lusterless hair Inflammation of eyelid margins (blepharitis) Night blindness and glare blindness Retarded growth
Thiamine (B_1)............	Animal products: liver, heart, kidneys, lean meats (especially pork and ham), oysters, milk, eggs Plant products: whole-grain and enriched bread and cereals; wheat germ, peanuts, green or dried beans (especially soy beans), and peas	Nervous irritability Headaches Fatigue Limited ability to concentrate Listlessness Loss of appetite Faulty digestion Constipation due to poor intestinal muscle tone
Riboflavin (B_2)...........	Animal products: liver, heart, kidneys, fish, milk, cheese, egg yolk Plant products: whole-grain and enriched bread and cereals, green leafy vegetables, peanut butter	Redness at angles of lips with scaling and fissuring (cheilosis) Sore, beefy red or magenta tongue (glossitis) Tiny red lines (engorged capillarries) extending around or across cornea and inward toward pupil (keratitis) Inflammation of eyelid margins (blepharitis) Eye fatigue and sensitivity to light Lowered resistance and vitality

Table 12-4 (Continued)

Vitamins	Foods	What may happen if children do not get enough
Niacin...............	Animal products: heart, liver (especially pork liver), kidneys, lean meats, poultry, fish Plant products: whole-grain and enriched bread and cereals; beans (especially soy beans), peas, peanuts, almonds, bananas	Dermatitis (pellagra) Gastrointestinal disturbances (diarrhea, for example) Mental depression
Ascorbic acid (vitamin C)	Plant products: canned, frozen, or fresh citrus fruit (oranges, grapefruit, lemons, and limes), raw apples, strawberries, cantaloupe, papayas, tomatoes (canned or fresh), raw cabbage, raw green peppers and other raw vegetables, potatoes (baked or boiled in skins)	Tender, swollen, bleeding or spongy gums (subclinical scurvy) Easily bruised skin Sore joints
Vitamin D.............	Animal products: the oils of many different bony fishes (cod, halibut, etc.), irradiated (vitamin D) milk (Egg yolk, butter, and cream contain vitamin D in very small amounts. These amounts are increased when hens and cows are exposed to summer sunlight or are fed irradiated substances.)	Rickets (malformation of bones and teeth)

membranes, and eyes in a healthy condition. It protects these structures through its influence on the glands that secrete substances that moisten and lubricate them. In vitamin A deficiency the glands waste away and as a consequence the skin, hair, eyes, and mucous membrane linings of body openings and tracts become excessively dry.

The specific vitamin A deficiency disease is xerophthalmia (from two Greek words meaning "dry" and "eyes"). The tear glands dry up, and the eyes, having lost the protective and lubricating action of tears, become the prey of invading germs.

Vitamin A also is necessary for the prevention of "night blindness," that is, inability to see in dim light. A rose-red pigment called "visual purple" in the retina of the eye is essential for normal vision in dim light. It becomes exhausted when the eyes are exposed to bright light and vitamin A is required for its regeneration.

Vitamin B Complex. The vitamin B complex includes a whole family of vitamins, many of which are now known by their chemical names (for example, thiamine, riboflavin, niacin, and folic acid). The B vitamins have intimate functional relationships. They are of the highest importance for the growth and energy metabolism of all forms of life from the highest to the lowest—from microbes to mammals—presumably because they form an essential part of the enzyme systems that underlie living processes.

Thiamine in pure form consists of water-soluble white crystals which break down under prolonged heating and are destroyed in alkaline media, such as water to which bicarbonate of soda has been added. Surplus thiamine is not stored to any extent in the body and so it is needed regularly.

Thiamine is necessary for healthy nerves, for good muscle tone in the digestive tract, and for the oxidation of carbohydrates in the body. The classic thiamine deficiency disease is beriberi. Beriberi is an inflammation of the nerves (polyneuritis) resulting in progressive paralysis of the limbs. Because thiamine prevents its development, this member of the vitamin B complex is sometimes called the antineuritic vitamin.

Riboflavin in pure form consists of water-soluble yellow crystals which are stable to heat but are destroyed by alkalis and light. It increases vigor at all ages through its influence on the nerves, digestion, skin, and general body resistance. It also helps to prevent degenerative changes in the cornea of the eye (keratitis). Like thiamine, riboflavin is not stored in the body in appreciable amounts.

Riboflavin deficiency produces a set of symptoms which includes cheilosis (an inflammation and cracking of the lips and corners of the mouth) and glossitis (inflammation of the tongue).

Niacin in pure form consists of water-soluble white crystals. It helps to protect the health of the skin and nerves and aids digestion. There is little evidence that surplus amounts are stored in the body.

The classic niacin deficiency disease is pellagra (literally "rough skin"). Pellagra is the most common form of nutritional deficiency characterized by dermatitis. In addition, nervous and digestive disorders usually occur. Red, dry, scaly patches form upon skin surfaces exposed to the sun's rays, for example, the back of the hands, the neck, cheeks, and bridge of the nose. These patches usually appear as matched spots, as on both hands, or both cheeks. Because it prevents pellagra, niacin is frequently referred to as the pellagra-preventive (P-P) factor in the vitamin B complex.

Vitamin C (Ascorbic Acid). Pure ascorbic acid exists in the form of water-soluble white crystals which are readily destroyed by oxidation when exposed to the air in the presence of certain enzymes or traces of copper, iron, and alkalis. Surplus amounts consumed are not stored, and so regular supplies are needed.

Vitamin C is known as the antiscorbutic vitamin. It was a lack of this element in the diet of seafaring men that was responsible for the scurvy, which was once the curse of all those who went in for long-range navigation. In the eighteenth century it was discovered that eating fresh vegetables and fruits (especially citrus fruits) would prevent scurvy.

Ascorbic acid is required for the formation of the intercellular cement that binds together the cells forming the walls of the capillaries. A lack of it makes the walls of the capillaries so weak that blood can leak through. This accounts for the hemorrhages into the gums and other tissues which are characteristic of scurvy. A very small amount of vitamin C is needed to prevent this disease. Well-defined cases have practically disappeared in lands of plenty. However, much more vitamin C is needed for health than for the prevention of frank scurvy.

Vitamin D. Vitamin D is indispensable for the normal calcification of bones and teeth. Its absence from the diet causes the disease called rickets (see Rickets, in Chap. 18). This disease is characterized by defective ossification of the bones and the development of various bone deformities. Because it prevents rickets, vitamin D is called the antirachitic vitamin.

In the search for this vitamin, the discovery that sunlight possesses antirachitic properties came first (1919). Then it was found that cod-liver oil, halibut-liver oil, and the oils of other bony fishes are potent rickets preventives.

The antirachitic power of sunshine comes from the ultraviolet rays in sunlight, which activate a fatty substance in the skin. This activated substance (vitamin D_3) is the form of vitamin D present in fish-liver oils and in milk and other foods exposed to ultraviolet irradiation. In pure crystalline form vitamin D exists as calciferol. The fat-soluble crystals of calciferol (vitamin D_2) are stable to heat and oxidation.

Children need more vitamin D than grown-ups do. However, they get very little vitamin D from ordinary foods, and the antirachitic effects of sunshine are lessened during the winter months in temperate climates. Even in summer the haze hanging over most cities filters out the ultraviolet rays. Hence children's diets should be reinforced with a fish-liver oil, or vitamin-D milk should be used instead of ordinary milk.

Cellulose

Cellulose is the woody carbohydrate substance used by plants as structural material. It may contain small amounts of valuable minerals and vitamins that are released and absorbed into the blood stream during digestion, but mostly it consists of a mass of fibers that cannot be digested. This indigestible bulk, which is sometimes called "roughage," is pushed into the colon for removal from the body. As it helps to stimulate the movements of the colon and exerts a favorable effect on the intestinal flora, it is a valuable part of the diet. The parts of plant foods that are rich in cellulose are edible leaves, edible stems, the hulls of grains, and the edible skins and fibers of fruits and vegetables.

Water

Water is used in the body to maintain the water level of the vast inland sea in which the cells live, to keep the blood volume uniform, and to carry on most of the body's activities. It is essential to the processes of removing waste products and excess heat. Hence there is a necessarily large loss of water from the body every day via the kidneys (urine), the sweat glands (perspiration), the lungs (water-laden expired air), and the large intestines (defecation). To balance this daily loss of water, we take in already formed water in liquids and in solid foods and potential water in foodstuffs containing hydrogen that unites with oxygen to form water in the process of oxidation. The water content of food varies greatly. Green vegetables contain 90 to 95 per cent; fruits, 85 per cent; and meats, 50 to 75 per cent. An average day's meals contain about two quarts of potential and already formed water.

The amount of water we need to drink every day depends both upon the amount we get from other beverages and from soups and solid foods and upon the amount of water we lose in perspiration and other ways. Four glasses of drinking water a day is about the minimum amount recommended for young people.

MEETING THE NUTRITIONAL REQUIREMENTS OF SCHOOL-AGE CHILDREN

To meet all the nutritional needs of the body it is necessary to have a well-balanced daily diet. Such a diet supplies the body with enough of all the different materials it needs from food. But how much is enough?

The Nutrition Yardstick

To answer this question, the Food and Nutrition Board of the National Research Council developed what is often called a "yardstick of good nutrition." This yardstick consists of a table of recommended daily allowances of specific nutrients for men and women according to degree of activity and for boys and girls according to age. That part of the table which applies to boys and girls is reproduced as Table 12-5.

A Daily Food Guide

In using the nutrition yardstick to measure the adequacy of daily meals, it is necessary to have it translated in terms of food. We don't eat calories, for example; we eat bread and butter. We don't eat protein by the gram; we drink milk and eat meat. Most foods, moreover, contain more than one nutrient, but no single food contains all the nutrients in the amounts needed. It is possible, however, to group foods according to the food materials in which they are richest. In the National Food Guide developed in the 1940s by the U.S. Department of Agriculture, foods were classified according to their nutritional content. This guide was popularly known

Table 12-5

RECOMMENDED DAILY DIETARY ALLOWANCES FOR BOYS AND GIRLS*

	Calo-ries†	Pro-tein, gm	Cal-cium, gm	Iron, mg	Vita-min A‡ I.U.	Thi-amine, mg§	Ribo-flavin, mg§	Nia-cin, mg§	Ascor-bic acid, mg	Vita-min D, I.U.
Girls and boys¶										
3–6 yr (40 lb)	1,600	40	0.8	10	2,500	0.6	1.0	11	50	400
6–9 yr (53 lb)	2,100	52	0.8	12	3,500	0.8	1.3	14	60	400
Girls¶										
9–12 yr (72 lb)	2,200	55	1.1	15	4,500	0.9	1.3	15	80	400
12–15 yr (103 lb)	2,500	62	1.3	15	5,000	1.0	1.5	17	80	400
15–18 yr (117 lb)	2,300	58	1.3	15	5,000	0.9	1.3	15	70	400
Boys¶										
9–12 yr (72 lb)	2,400	60	1.1	15	4,500	1.0	1.4	16	70	400
12–15 yr (98 lb)	3,000	75	1.4	15	5,000	1.2	1.8	20	80	400
15–18 yr (134 lb)	3,400	85	1.4	15	5,000	1.4	2.0	22	80	400

* The allowance levels are intended to cover individual variations among most normal persons as they live in the United States under usual environmental stresses. The recommended allowances can be attained with a variety of common foods providing other nutrients for which human requirements have been less well defined.

Table of measures used: A gram (gm) equals approximately 1/30 part of an ounce. 1 milligram (mg) equals 1/1,000 part of a gram. 1 international unit (I.U.) of a vitamin is the activity of a certain specified very small amount of that vitamin. 1 milligram of thiamine equals 333 international units. 1 milligram of ascorbic acid equals 20 international units. There are no international units for riboflavin and niacin.

† Proper calorie allowance is that which maintains body weight or rate of growth at the level most conducive to well-being.

‡ Four-fifths of the vitamin A value of the average diet is contributed by the provitamin carotene (from vegetables and fruits) and one-fifth by preformed vitamin A (from animal products, such as liver and eggs).

§ Other members of the vitamin B complex also are required, though no value can be given. Foods supplying adequate thiamine, riboflavin, and niacin will tend to supply sufficient amounts of other B vitamins.

¶ Allowances are based on the needs for the middle years in each age group (4½, 7½, 10½, 13½, 16½) and are for moderate activity and for average weight at the middle year of the age group.

Source: "Recommended Dietary Allowances," Sixth Revised Edition, 1964, A Report of the Food and Nutrition Board, National Academy of Sciences, National Research Council, Publication 1146.

as the "Basic 7." In the late 1950s the Basic 7 plan was simplified so as to include only four groups of food. This dietary pattern is entitled "A Daily Food Guide" (see Table 12-6) and is now widely used in teaching nutrition in the schools. The students learn that their basic food needs will be met by including in each day's meals some foods from each of the four groups in the amounts recommended.

OBSERVING THE NUTRITIONAL STATUS OF SCHOOL CHILDREN

The observant teacher, because of her familiarity with optimum growth and healthy appearance in general and normal variations from them in

Table 12-6

A DAILY FOOD GUIDE

Milk group	Meat group
For calcium, protein, riboflavin, vitamin A, and many other nutrients	For protein, iron, and B vitamins
Foods included: Milk—whole fluid, evaporated, dried, buttermilk Cheese—cottage, cream, cheddar-type, natural, or processed	Foods included: Beef, veal, lamb, pork, variety meats such as liver, heart, kidneys Fish and shellfish Poultry and eggs As alternates—dried beans, peas, and lentils; nuts, peanut butter
Amounts of milk recommended: Children—3 to 4 cups Teen-agers—4 or more cups Adults—2 or more cups	Amounts recommended: 2 or more servings Count as 1 serving: 2 to 3 ounces lean meat, fish, poultry 2 eggs 1 cup cooked legumes 4 tablespoons peanut butter
Cheese and ice cream may replace part of the milk. Their equivalent in calcium is: 1-inch cube hard cheese $= \frac{2}{3}$ cup milk $\frac{1}{2}$ cup cottage cheese $= \frac{1}{3}$ cup milk $\frac{1}{2}$ cup ice cream $= \frac{1}{4}$ cup milk	

Vegetable-fruit group	Bread-cereal group
For vitamins and minerals	For protein, iron, B vitamins, and calories
Foods included: Citrus fruits, cabbage, peppers, salad greens, tomatoes, melons, berries, and other good sources of vitamin C Dark-green vegetables and deep-yellow vegetables and fruits as good sources of vitamin A All other fruits and vegetables, including potatoes	Foods included: All kinds of whole-grain or enriched breads and other baked goods All kinds of cooked or ready-to-eat whole-grain or enriched cereals Macaroni, spaghetti, noodles
Amounts recommended: 4 or more servings 1 serving of a good source of vitamin C every day 1 serving of a good source of vitamin A at least every other day The remaining servings of any vegetable or fruit	Amounts recommended: 4 or more servings Count as 1 serving: 1 slice bread 1 ounce ready-to-eat cereal $\frac{3}{4}$ cup cooked cereal, macaroni, noodles, or spaghetti

Other Foods. To round out meals and satisfy the appetite, everyone will naturally have some foods not specified in these four main groups. These foods include (1) butter, fortified margarine, mayonnaise, and salad oils added to foods at the table and used in cooking, and (2) sugar, syrups, honey, and preserves used for flavoring and in the preparation of sweetened baked goods and other desserts. These "other foods" make up the total daily calorie requirements and supply other nutrients depending upon the ingredients used in the preparation of made dishes.

Source: U.S. Department of Agriculture, Institute of Home Economics.

particular, can hardly fail to be impressed by the signs which indicate that a child is or is not well nourished. The two points of departure for observing general nutritional status are the child's growth record and his general appearance and behavior. The composite pictures of the well-nourished child and the malnourished child will bring out the outstanding differences between the two.

The Well-nourished Child	The Malnourished Child
Makes progressive gains in height and weight at his established rate of gain (see Plate 3), taking into consideration periods of decelerated and accelerated growth (see Stages and Rates of Growth in Chap. 3)	Fails to show measurable gains in weight and height over several months; or shows any sudden change in the rate of growth
Gives a general impression of physical fitness, vigor, and enjoyment of life (see Plates 4 and 16)	Has a strained, worried look (see Rosalie in Plate 4 and Plate 8)
Has an alert, happy facial expression (see Plate 1)	Is listless and inactive or high-strung and over-active
Has good skeletal and muscular development, a moderate amount of well-distributed fat (curves rather than angles) and good functional posture	Has typical fatigue posture: round shoulders, winged shoulder blades, protruding abdomen (see Freddie in Plate 16)
Enjoys good appetite, good digestion, good elimination, and restful sleep	Is excessively thin (angles rather than curves) or is excessively fat or has poor distribution of fat
	Is easily fatigued and possibly irritable and difficult to manage

General Appearance as a Guide

The pictures of ten-year-old Rosalie and six-year-old Jean shown in Plate 4 illustrate the differences that may be observed in the appearance of a child whose nutrition is good and a child whose nutrition is poor. Rosalie shows signs of being poorly nourished, not only because she is small and thin, but also because her face is pale, her hair dull, and her eyes ringed underneath with shadows. Her muscles, too, are very thin, and she has practically no fat between her skin and her bones.

The opinion of the teacher who referred Rosalie for a medical examination hardly differed from that of the physician. The teacher was going on her feeling for normality—her conviction that no healthy child should look the way Rosalie looked and get as tired as Rosalie got in the course of a school day. The physician based his opinion both on the teacher's observations and on his own findings during his examination of the child. Then he took the step the teacher could not take—he determined the cause of Rosalie's malnutrition and prescribed the measures necessary to correct it.

Skin Changes as a Guide

The skin pictures the nutritional status of the child much better than any other organ. The skin itself is nourished by food brought to it by the blood, and it is easy to tell whether it looks healthy and well nourished. We can tell, for example, whether there is enough fat in the lowest layer of the skin to fill out the upper layers so that the skin looks smooth and the body nicely rounded with curves rather than sharp angles. Observation teaches us that the aging process is reflected in wrinkled, thin, over-stretched, dry skin as opposed to the dewiness and bloom of youthful skin. Hence, the appearance in children of any of the skin conditions that are unnatural in youth—bagginess or flabbiness, wrinkles, cracks, extreme dryness, yellowish spots, for example—should make us suspect that all is not well.

The complexion is influenced by the skin's blood supply as well as the amount and distribution of pigment in the skin. A good supply of healthy blood depends upon good nutrition. One outward sign of a good blood supply is the pinkish color of the mucous membrane lining the mouth and eyelids, of the ears as seen against light, and of the fingernails. Whatever may be the natural color of the skin, the cheeks of healthy children will have a ruddy tinge after play outdoors.

In several nutritional deficiencies the skin or mucous membrane is involved (Table 12-4; also discussion in Chap. 15). When a physician suspects that a nutritional deficiency is to blame for a certain skin condition, he studies the child and his habits carefully before making his diagnosis. However, some children needing such careful study may not get to a physician unless teachers are quick to notice suspicious skin changes. A case in point is that of Anne (Plate 8). The teacher noticed a persistent cracking and slight redness at the corner of Anne's mouth. Also, Anne's general appearance and posture indicated chronic fatigue. The teacher referred Anne to the school physician for a medical examination. The physician discovered that Anne was suffering from inadequate nutrition, and more particularly from a riboflavin deficiency.

Screening Children for Medical Examination

It is seldom nowadays that school children show signs and symptoms of severe nutritional deficiency except in regions where the customary diet is completely lacking, or is seriously deficient, in one or more essential food elements. In mild form, however, nutritional deficiencies are not infrequent, and some severe cases still occur.

Nutritionally needy children may be suffering from an insufficient intake of one or more of the essential food elements or an all-round poor or unbalanced diet. If any of the essential food elements are lacking or supplied inadequately, the organs or tissues needing it in the greatest amounts will suffer most.

The chief food sources of the most important food elements and what may happen when a person does not get enough of each one are given in Tables 12-1 through 12-4. Teachers may use these tables as a guide in observing children. However, it must be remembered that while a diet supplying all essential nutrients in the right amounts is necessary for good nutrition, other causes may be responsible for poor nutrition; for example, acute or chronic illness, or an endocrine imbalance, or prolonged worry or other emotional disturbance, which may interfere with the consumption, assimilation, or utilization of essential food elements. Also, nutritional biochemists are now learning through animal experimentation that the requirements for specific nutrients can be changed with alterations in the amount consumed of other nutrients. It may be possible, for example, to show the signs indicating a particular vitamin or mineral deficiency not because one is not getting enough of that vitamin or mineral, but because one is getting too much or not enough of some other food element.

Another important thing to remember is that the screening out of nutritionally needy children is a highly technical procedure. Teachers and nurses can do no more than to call attention to the obvious warning signals that are commonly associated with malnutrition and specific nutritional deficiencies. In referring a child for suspected malnutrition, it will be helpful to the physician to know what the teacher and nurse can tell him about the child's living habits. This information provides a valuable supplement to tests made to measure nutritional status and may be used in planning the reclamation of children whose vitality has been allowed to burn low because of poor nutrition.

OVERWEIGHT AND UNDERWEIGHT

We are much more likely to associate poor nutrition with excessive thinness than excessive fatness. A common first reaction in observing a fat child is to think, "that youngster is certainly well fed!" And well fed he probably is, but not well nourished in the sense that we think of good nutrition as the outcome of getting enough of everything a person needs from food. Enough is enough—not too little and not too much. And by and large, obesity, that is, excessive overweight, is the result of eating more than enough to meet the body's needs for energy. The problem of overweight is in most cases a simple problem in arithmetic. If a child takes in 4,500 calories worth of food, let us say, and spends only 2,500 calories worth in growth and activity, he will have 2,000 left over to be turned into fat.

There is no question that in later life obesity is a distinct menace to health. There is agreement among medical authorities that obesity, if not strictly a disease in itself, in many cases contributes to the development of serious disease. Statistics show that hypertension, diseases of the heart, and diabetes are much more common in overweight persons than in those whose weight is normal or under the average. Also the length of life of obese persons as a group is shorter than that of lean persons.

Obesity in Childhood

Teachers and parents should be concerned about excessive overweight in a child because a pattern of obesity established in childhood is so often carried over into adult life. A well-known pediatrician has estimated that as many as 15 per cent of American children may be dangerously overweight, and that four out of five of them will grow up to be overweight adults. In one study fifty girls from ten to fourteen years of age, all of whom were 20 per cent or more overweight, were followed for twenty-one years. At the end of this period forty were still obese. In a group of average-weight contemporary controls, only nine were overweight twenty years later.

Many factors may contribute to the establishment of the obesity pattern. An inherited tendency to stoutness must be taken into consideration, but family eating and cooking habits often play an important role. Studies have shown that only 10 per cent of children from average-weight families become fat. In families with one overweight parent, 50 per cent of the children are likely to grow into fat adults. Among children with two obese parents, 80 per cent will be too heavy.

Why Some Children May Eat Too Much or Too Little

There are many different reasons why children may eat more or less than they need to meet their energy requirements. In some families children acquire the habit of overeating because good food and plenty of it is a family tradition. Children in other families may show little interest in food because eating is not considered to be important enough to have meals properly prepared and served at regular times.

Emotional Causes. Emotions often play a part both in overeating and in undereating. A child who feels unloved or unwanted, for example, may turn to food for comfort. Another child with unhappy feelings may react in just the opposite way and show an exasperating indifference toward food. Some parents, especially mothers, may interpret overfeeding as a sign of affection. Other mothers may overfeed a child to compensate for guilty feelings engendered by their unconscious rejection of the child. Emotional disturbances may also interfere with normal digestion or metabolism.

Helping the Too Fat and the Too Thin

Any child who is excessively fat or excessively thin should have a thorough medical examination to determine the cause. The physician will then evaluate any physical or emotional factors or individual living habits involved and work out the proper program of diet, exercise, and rest. Girls in their teens who are anxious to take off weight or to remain slender are likely to go in for drastic reducing programs without making provision for all the essential food elements required for growth and good health. They should understand that only a physician has the necessary skill and equipment to decide how much weight they can safely lose, how fast they can lose it, and with what diet.

Teachers can help older children on weight-reducing or weight-gaining diets to understand that taking off or putting on extra pounds is largely a matter of decreasing or increasing calorie intake. Extra sleep at night and rest before and after meals in addition to more food may help the underweight child to gain. But less rest and more activity cannot counter-balance the excessive storage of fat resulting from overeating.

Exercise is important, however, both in weight-reducing and weight-gaining programs. Inactivity is definitely a contributing factor in obesity at any age, and overweight children are inclined to compound their problem by shunning exercise. Underweight children may be restless and overactive but tend to tire easily. In both cases exercise is needed to get and keep the body in good condition (see Physical Fitness, in Chap. 18).

NUTRITION EDUCATION

Convincing children of the importance of good nutrition and helping them to learn how to attain it requires teachers who are well grounded in the subject. Although everyone knows that one must eat to live, no one knows intuitively what and how much one must eat to be as healthy as possible. That knowledge must be acquired. Many authorities believe that all teachers should receive adequate training in nutrition as part of their preparation for the teaching profession and also should be provided with consultation services in this field.

But no matter how skillfully nutrition is taught, school and home must work together if children are to get the full benefits of nutrition education. Guiding children in food selection requires an intimate knowledge of their food habits. Also what the children learn can be put into practice only when nutrition education is carried into the home and the cooperation of the parents obtained. Essential contact with the home may be made by encouraging parents to visit the school to observe the school lunch in operation or to talk over their children's eating problems, and to have a teacher or school nurse or school nutritionist visit the home for the purpose of giving guidance and help in the solution of family food problems.

Learning Experiences in Nutrition Education

Nutrition makes up a large part of the subject matter of direct health teaching. It also enters into the teaching of several other subjects and is intimately related to the school-lunch program. A well-integrated plan of nutrition teaching provides for the participation of all those in the school who can contribute learning experiences in this field.

In science teaching, for example, it may be possible to manage animal-feeding experiments. There is no better way of impressing young people with the value of good nutrition. Such experiments are fascinating to youngsters and furnish them with eyewitness evidence of the part played by food in growth, energy, and good looks.

Students who have opportunities to use the space and equipment for home economics classes will enjoy preparing meals. The meal may be a breakfast, a luncheon, or a party. Planning the menu, setting the table, serving the food, and washing the dishes afterward are good experiences in taking responsibility for arranging and carrying through a project. Having good table manners and being pleasant and courteous to one another and to guests can all be practiced. Parents may share in such experiences as guests or as instructors in the arts of cooking, table setting, dishwashing, and so on.

In schools where it is impossible for children to prepare and serve meals, parents may take turns giving this experience to small groups in their homes.

Educational Value of the School-lunch Program. The school-lunch program furnishes many opportunities for implementing nutrition education. Careful planning between those who are familiar with the food and eating habits of the children (teacher and parents) and those who are responsible for school lunches (the cafeteria or lunchroom manager and the nutritionist, if one is employed by the school) has resulted, in many instances, both in filling up the gaps in the daily meal patterns of individual children and in cultivating tastes for important foods with which some children are not familiar or which they have not learned to like. If the teacher eats lunch with her students, she will be able to plan many learning situations related to food choices and eating habits.

If the students are permitted to buy what they like in the school cafeteria or lunchroom, it is important to give them the knowledge and the incentives required for making good food choices. A youngster left to his own devices in buying his lunch is not likely to be concerned with choosing a well-balanced meal. It is helpful to have a classroom collection of separate pictures or models of basic foods which the class can use in arranging meal patterns for breakfast, lunch, and dinner.

If plate lunches are served to the students, the teacher may be faced with the problem of getting some boys and girls to try unfamiliar foods or to eat foods which they dislike. The home economics teacher may be able to encourage such children to branch out in new directions by helping them to cook unfamiliar foods or to prepare foods in new ways.

If any students bring their lunches to school, the teacher may unobtrusively observe the contents of their lunch boxes. Lunches brought from home or eaten at home may, in some cases, be inadequate. The teacher or school nurse may find it advisable to confer with parents about the type of lunch that all young people need so as to win their cooperation in providing lunches that will result in well-balanced meal patterns for each day.

Many young people have the habit of eating too fast so as to have more time for play before school begins again in the afternoon. Yet the students learn that adequate chewing, enjoyable talk, and relaxation for a while after eating are desirable health habits. They are not likely to give these habits much chance to form unless the teacher helps to make their lunchtime a pleasant time and gives them the experience of learning that they can have fun in quiet activities as well as in strenuous games.

FOR REVIEW AND DISCUSSION

1. Tell the difference between the following:

    a. Nutrition and malnutrition
    b. Energy metabolism and basal metabolism
    c. Glucose and glycogen
    d. Saturated fatty acids and unsaturated fatty acids
    e. Oxidation and hydrogenation

2. Match the word or term in Group A with the word or term in Group B that you associate with it.

Group A	Group B
5 Cholesterol	1 Vitamin A deficiency
Beriberi	2 Amino acids
10 Calorie	3 Iodine deficiency
8 Vitamin D	4 Vitamin C deficiency
2 Proteins	5 Atherosclerosis
3 Simple goiter	6 Thiamine deficiency
Xerophthalmia	7 Vitamin D deficiency
7 Rickets	8 Cod-liver oil
11 Pellagra	9 Indigestible food material
9 Cellulose	10 A unit of heat
4 Scurvy	11 Niacin deficiency

3. What deficiency or deficiencies in the diet would you suspect if a doctor told you that a poor or unbalanced diet was responsible for underweight and listlessness in a child? lowered resistance to infection? nutritional anemia? inflammation of the eyelid margins? constipation due to poor intestinal muscle tone? cracking of the corners of the mouth? spongy, bleeding gums?

4. What would you say or do if

    a. The mother of an excessively fat boy told you that she would far rather have a child nicknamed "Fatty" than a child nicknamed "Skinny"?

   b. A girl in her early teens who thought she was getting too fat told you that she had decided to try on her own a reducing program described in a magazine article?

   c. A child told you that he didn't see why he had to drink milk when his parents did not?

   d. You noticed that a child consistently left uneaten the vegetables included in the plate lunches served in the school lunchroom?

   e. You wanted to impress a youngster with the importance of eating a good breakfast?

SELECTED REFERENCES

Best, C. H., and N. B. Taylor: *The Human Body* (first mentioned as reference in Chap. 1). Part VI, *The Physiology of Digestion,* Chap. 24 (includes general description of types of food); Part VII, *Metabolism and Nutrition,* Chaps. 30–31.

Bogert, L. Jean: *Nutrition and Physical Fitness,* 7th ed., W. B. Saunders Company, Philadelphia, 1960.

Cooper, L. F., and others: *Nutrition in Health and Disease,* 13th ed., J. B. Lippincott Company, Philadelphia, 1958. (A classic college and professional text on nutrition.)

Keys, Ancel, and Margaret Keys: *Eat Well and Stay Well,* Doubleday & Company, Inc., New York, 1959. (Presents the scientific aspects of nutrition and the hazards of overeating.)

King, C. G.: *Personality "Plus" through Diet,* Public Affairs Pamphlet No. 290, Public Affairs Committee, Inc., New York. (Food lore for teenagers.)

McHenry, E. W.: *Foods without Fads,* J. B. Lippincott Company, Philadelphia, 1960. (Briefly and simply covers principles of nutrition, meal planning, weight control, vitamins and food fads.)

Maddox, Gaynor: *The Safe and Sure Way to Reduce,* Random House, Inc., New York, 1960. (A book praised by the medical experts as giving sound weight control and nutrition information in easy-to-read form.)

Nasset, Edmund S.: *Your Diet, Digestion, and Health,* 2d ed. rev., Barnes & Noble, Inc., New York, 1961.

Taylor, Clara Mae: *Food Values in Shares and Weights,* 2d ed., The Macmillan Company, New York, 1959. (Contains tables giving the nutritive value of about 500 foods.)

Organizations

American Home Economics Association
Bureau of Human Nutrition, U.S. Department of Agriculture
Food and Nutrition Board, National Research Council

Preparation of Food for the Body's Use
Waste Removal
Signs and Symptoms of Gastrointestinal Disorders
Gastrointestinal Infections

Health is profoundly influenced both by the adequacy with which the food needs of the body are met and by the efficiency with which the food eaten is digested and utilized. Many of the physical distress signals and complaints of school children are related to minor or major disturbances in digestion, metabolism, and excretion. As an aid to understanding why such disturbances may occur, some information is given in this chapter regarding the normal setup and operation of these processes.

PREPARATION OF FOOD FOR THE BODY'S USE

Foods, as we have seen, are complex substances made up of many different kinds of raw materials. Assuming that it were humanly possible to arrange these materials into the multifarious patterns characteristic of the different foodstuffs and then to combine them into the great variety of foods with which we are familiar, we should have to turn right around and break them all down again before they could even get into our bodies. As a matter of fact, we do just this every time we eat. It is the function of digestion.

Digestion

Digestion takes place in a long tube of varying diameters, open at both ends to the outside world (see Fig. 13-1). This tube is called the alimentary canal. In it complex foodstuffs are broken down into simple molecules and dissolved in water so that they can pass into the bloodstream and eventually into the cells.

It is illuminating to think of the alimentary canal as being outside the body in the sense that food, while it is in it, is not actually in the body. A potato as eaten, for example, could not get through the intestinal and capillary walls into the bloodstream, but a watery solution of glucose (the simple sugar into which all carbohydrates are changed during digestion) can. Similarly, fats like butter and oil, and the proteins of meat, eggs, milk, and so on must be broken down chemically into their soluble constituents before they can pass into the bloodstream.

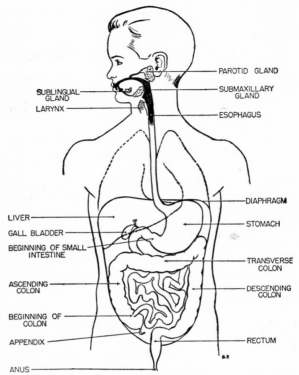

FIG. 13-1. Important points along the alimentary route.

Mechanical Digestion. Before solid foods can be acted upon by the enzymes, or digestive ferments, which change them chemically, they must be broken down mechanically and thoroughly saturated with water. The mechanical part of digestion consists (1) in breaking up the food into small pieces by the teeth and kneading it into a swallowable bolus by the tongue; (2) in mixing the food with digestive ferments, or enzymes, in the mouth, stomach, and small intestine; and (3) in moving the food along in the direction away from the mouth toward the anal canal.

The passage of food through the four large divisions of the alimentary canal—the mouth and esophagus, the stomach, the small intestine, and the large intestine—is regulated by ringlike bands of muscle called sphincters. When a sphincter contracts, it closes the tube at that point so that the food cannot pass onward. One of these sphincters is located at the place where the esophagus leads into the upper end of the stomach. Another guards the opening from the lower end of the stomach into the upper part of the small intestine (duodenum). Still another is placed at the point where the lower end of the small intestine (ileum) leads obliquely into the cecum, or blind beginning of the large intestine (colon). The vermiform appendix projects from the cecum (see Appendicitis, further on). Last of all come the anal sphincters, which guard the beginning and end of the short anal canal leading back from the lowest portion of the large intestine (rectum). Only the external anal sphincter is under voluntary control. It opens when we obey the urge to defecate, or "move the bowels."

All the other sphincters open and close automatically in response to stimuli which indicate that the food is ready to pass from one division of the alimentary canal into the next. The orifice leading from the esophagus to the stomach, for example, opens at the gentle tapping, or pressure, of a well-chewed food bolus after each swallow. Sometimes it stays open for two or three swallows when fluid is being drunk. The sphincter between the stomach and the small intestine opens at the touch of an acid morsel, that is, a morsel thoroughly saturated with the acid gastric juice on the stomach side, and closes behind it as the acid morsel comes in contact with the alkaline mucous membrane on the intestinal side.

Peristalsis. From the lower end of the esophagus to the anal canal, the kind of muscle responsible for moving the contents of the alimentary canal along is smooth muscle. This kind of muscle is involuntary; that is, it is controlled only by the autonomic nervous system. The smooth muscle of the alimentary canal is arranged in two layers—an inner circular layer and an outer longitudinal layer.

The pressure of food against the muscular walls of that part of the tube through which the food is passing is responsible for setting up the wave-like motions of the walls which force the food along. These waves are called peristaltic waves. As a wave of contraction passes along the intestinal tube, for example, it strips the contents of the tube before it, in much the same manner as a tube of toothpaste may be stripped by the strong pressure of fingers sliding along the outside surface. After the wave of contraction has traveled a short distance, a wave of relaxation spreads along the segment through which the food has just been propelled. This segment is now empty. Since its walls are relaxed, it can be filled with another load of food coming from the direction of the mouth. This process takes place repeatedly and rhythmically.

Normally peristaltic waves travel only in one direction, that is, away from the mouth and toward the anal canal. However, reverse peristalsis can and does occur. Many of the unpleasant sensations resulting from digestive misbehavior are caused by reverse wavelets and ripples passing upward toward the mouth.

Chemical Digestion. Chemical digestion is as different from mechanical digestion as is the burning of wood from the splitting up of wood into small fragments with ax or saw. In the latter case the wood remains wood, whether it is in the shape of logs, boards, kindling, chips, shavings, or sawdust, because its molecules remain intact. In burning, however, the wood ceases to be wood because the wood molecules are dismembered and their atoms recombined to form new and different molecules. The wood is gone—into the air as CO_2 (carbon dioxide) and H_2O (water vapor), and onto the hearth or the ground as the noncombustible minerals of which ashes are composed.

In essence, the purpose of chemical digestion is the breakdown of food into its basic elements so that it can be absorbed and used by the body cells (see Fig. 13-2). After the food mass has been ground into fine pieces mechanically, its large molecules are chemically taken apart so that the simpler molecules can pass by the process of osmosis through semi-permeable membranes from the small intestine into the blood and lymph streams and on into the cells.

Enzymes. We know that food substances are in themselves more or less stable compounds; that is, they will keep for a long time when dried or frozen or sterilized in cans. A lump of sugar (if protected from moisture) can be kept for centuries without undergoing any appreciable change. If a chemist wanted to split starch molecules into the small soluble sugar molecules of which they are composed, he would have to boil the starch

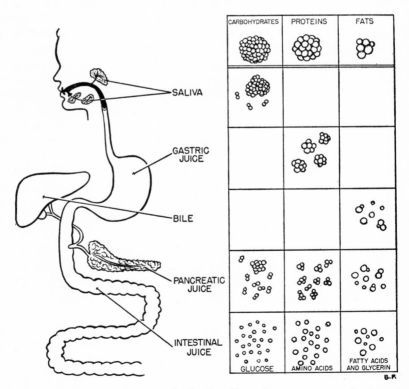

Fig. 13-2. Chemical digestion. The foodstuffs in the top row are broken down by enzymes in the digestive juices into the simple elements in the bottom row.

for many hours and add certain acids besides. But we change starch to sugar in a few minutes whenever we eat bread or potatoes or any other starchy food. We can do this because saliva—the digestive juice in the mouth—contains a powerful reagent which can quickly and expertly change starch into sugar. This reagent is ptyalin, a member of a large class of substances called enzymes.

Enzymes participate in practically all chemical wrecking and building operations that take place in living tissue. These extraordinary agents come on stage at the very beginning of life, since enzymes play an essential role in the formation in the fertilized egg of protein (the mother substance of protoplasm) from some twenty-odd amino acids.

Enzymes, like hormones, belong to the family of chemical substances known as catalysts. These substances change the speed of a reaction by their mere presence without taking part in it.

In the mouth, the salivary enzyme begins the splitting up of starch molecules into sugar molecules. In the stomach, pepsin, the chief enzyme in gastric juice, begins splitting up the giant protein molecules into smaller molecules. In the duodenum, or upper part of the small intestine, bile from the liver divides the large fat droplets into very fine droplets, that is, emulsifies them. Here, too, pancreatic juice and intestinal juice, each of which contains three different enzymes or ferments, finish up the splitting of all higher starches and sugars into simple grape sugar (glucose); all the large protein molecules into their constituent amino acids; and all the fats into fatty acids and glycerin. These three groups of substances are the end products of digestion; that is, they are the digestible portions of food as chemically split up into molecules small enough to be absorbed into the blood and lymph streams and used by the cells.

Absorption of the End Products of Digestion

Digested food is absorbed almost entirely from the small intestine (see Fig. 13-3). The lining of the small intestine is covered with millions of tiny fingerlike projections somewhat like the nap of velvet. These slender fleshy projections are called villi (singular, villus). Running through the center of each villus is a network of capillaries and a tiny lymph vessel.

The Absorption of Amino Acids and Glucose. Water and the soluble amino acids and glucose pass into the small veins leading out of the capillary networks of the villi and are carried first to the liver by way of the portal vein. In the liver the amino acids may be held for further chemical changes or may pass unchanged into the general bloodstream. The glucose also passes through the liver into the general circulation, but most of the excess that the body does not immediately require for energy is held back and stored in the liver as glycogen (see Carbohydrates, in Chap. 12).

The Absorption of Fatty Acids and Glycerin. Fatty acids and glycerin are absorbed into the epithelial cells covering the villi. Here they are re-

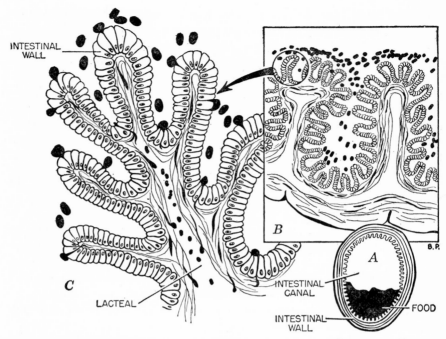

Fig. 13-3. How digested food is absorbed. *A*, cross section of intestine. *B*, cross section of intestinal wall showing food elements in canal ready for absorption. *C*, magnification of one fold of the intestinal wall showing lipoproteins passing through intercellular spaces into the lacteals (lymph vessels).

combined to form fats. As fats are insoluble in water, they are then combined with proteins which act as special vehicles to effect their transport in the bloodstream. The fats in association with their protein carriers are known as lipoproteins. The lipoproteins for the most part pass into the minute lymph vessels in the villi. When mixed with the lymph they form a milky-white fluid called *chyle* which makes the lymph vessels in the villi look white and glistening. Hence these lymph vessels are called lacteals (from *lac*, the Latin word for milk). The lacteals merge into larger lymphatic vessels that drain into a duct leading into a great vein (the subclavian vein) in the upper left part of the chest. In this roundabout way most of the fat in a meal reaches the general circulation to be carried to the tissues. A large part of it is taken up for further treatment by that busy chemical laboratory the liver, whence it is transported in the bloodstream to adipose (fatty) tissue in various parts of the body.

Nervous Control of Digestion

Throughout practically the entire length of the alimentary canal, networks of nerve cells in the walls act as local stations for the autonomic nervous system. One important service made possible by this innervation is the conducting of messages from one part of the digestive tract to another by way of local hookups. Thus widely separated portions can act together for the good of the whole. For example, the exit of food from the stomach into the duodenum signals the colon to get rid of its contents to make room for new waste material coming along. This signal stimulates peristalsis in the colon and explains the call to defecation (a bowel movement) following a meal.

The tone and motility of gastrointestinal muscle and the secretion of the digestive juices are controlled by impulses from the autonomic nervous system. Many of these impulses are psychic; that is, they are aroused by our feelings about food. If these feelings are pleasant, psychic impulses help to make the digestive mechanism ready for work. They increase muscular tone before or while eating food that is pleasant in odor and taste and start the secretion of the digestive juices. Almost everyone has experienced the watering of the mouth due to the psychic secretion of saliva at the smell, sight, or even thought of appetizing food. Psychic influences also start the secretion of gastric juice and pancreatic juice when we start to eat food that is palatable.

It has long been known that the stomach and intestines are extremely sensitive to intense or prolonged emotions such as fear, anger, and resentment. These emotions use the autonomic nervous system (predominantly the sympathetic division) to achieve their physical effects. Their influence is inhibitory; that is, they stop operations instead of starting them, as the pleasant impulses do. We have all experienced the disagreeable feelings that occur when the movements of the stomach and intestines and the secretion of the digestive juices have been brought to a standstill. They include the "all gone" feeling in the pit of the stomach at moments of impending disaster, the dryness of the mouth in moments of fear, the indigestion following intense excitement or worry or fatigue.

The moral of all this, of course, is that many of the digestive disturbances of childhood—and maturity, too—can be avoided by taking advantage of the beneficent influence of pleasant psychic impulses. That is why doctors tell us that it is important to have food pleasant in taste and smell at regular times each day, to eat with relish and enjoyment, to have cheerful, or at least interesting, table talk, and to avoid excessive exertion before or after a meal. If anything has made us angry or scared or excited, we should calm down before eating.

Metabolism

To the body cells the comparatively simple chemical compounds into which the various foodstuffs have been broken down by digestion are merely raw materials. The cells must reduce these raw materials literally to atoms in the process of using them and discard the parts they cannot use as by-products, or wastes. Thus the changes that foodstuffs undergo in digestion are only the overture to the more dramatic changes that take place during their metabolism.

Metabolism comes from a Greek word meaning "change." It is the sum total of all the chemical work involved in the utilization by living tissues of the food materials required for heat and energy production, growth, maintenance and repair, and the regulation of vital functions.

Metabolism is partly constructive and partly destructive. Constructive activities include the changing of food into energy, the building up of new tissue during growth, the repair of worn-out tissues, and the manufacture of complex substances out of simple ones. Destructive activities include the splitting up of complex substances into simpler ones and the breaking down of tissue.

WASTE REMOVAL

Two kinds of wastes are produced as a result of the processes of digestion and metabolism. The first kind is made up of the portions of food that cannot be digested. The second kind consists of the end products of metabolism, that is, the wastes produced in the various processes involved in the body's use of food.

Removing the Waste Products of Digestion

After most of the good, except water, has been absorbed from food in the small intestine, what remains passes onward into the large intestine for elimination from the body. Other names for the large intestine are the colon and the bowel.

The colon is shaped somewhat like the small letter n. It begins in the lower right segment of the abdomen, ascends to a point just below the stomach, crosses over to the left side, and descends to the rectum. Many of the feelings of fullness (distention) and rumblings of various kinds blamed on the stomach actually arise from the transverse colon.

The Makeup of Feces. Food residues as they pass into the ascending colon are in almost a liquid state. A little more than thirteen ounces of this liquid material passes into the colon in twenty-four hours; about five ounces are evacuated in the same length of time. The difference is made up mostly of water which is absorbed during the progress of the food residues through the colon to the rectum. The evacuated material is called feces.

The bulk of the feces is composed of a much smaller proportion of cellulose and other indigestible materials in food than is popularly supposed. In addition to food residues, the solids in feces consist of bacteria, material secreted through the wall of the intestine and in the bile, worn-out epithelial cells, and leukocytes.

Bacterial Decomposition. The bacterial flora of the colon is very luxuriant. The bacteria decompose cellulose (the woody, or fibrous, parts of vegetables, fruits, and grains) and other materials. The color of the feces normally comes from a substance produced by the action of bacteria on bile pigment. The odor of feces is due to the breakdown by bacteria of amino acids (proteins) into various aromatic substances. Some of these substances are highly toxic. It was once thought that their absorption into the bloodstream from the large intestine was responsible for many of the ills of mankind. It has been determined, however, that only insignificant amounts of such toxic products get through the intestinal wall into the bloodstream and those that do are detoxified in the liver. There is no truth in the idea that constipation (see further on) "poisons the system."

Defecation. Defecation is initiated by the propulsion of the feces into the rectum by peristaltic waves traveling across the tranverse colon and down the descending colon. When the pressure of the feces on the wall of the rectum reaches a certain height, the defecation reflex, consisting of a strong peristaltic contraction of the colon, occurs. The movements of the bowel wall are accompanied and helped by voluntary contractions of the diaphragm and the abdominal muscles. Relaxation of the sphincters at the beginning and end of the short anal canal permits defecation to take place. The external anal sphincter is under voluntary control; that is, under ordinary circumstances we can obey or disobey the urge to have a bowel movement.

The defecation reflex has a center of its own in the medulla oblongata not far from the respiratory and vomiting centers and a subsidiary center in the spinal cord. As we have seen, pressure on the rectal wall pushes the button, so to speak, which sets off this reflex. However, the rectum adjusts its capacity to the bulk of the feces, and when that happens the pressure stimulus is abolished (see Constipation, further on).

Removing the Waste Products of Metabolism

Metabolic wastes would be lethal if they were allowed to accumulate. They consist chiefly of the carbonic acid (carbon dioxide dissolved in water) and excess heat produced in energy metabolism, and the nitrogen wastes produced in protein metabolism.

As we have seen, the lungs excrete the carbon dioxide and the skin excretes the excess heat produced in the oxidation of glucose and fatty acids. We are now to consider the body's remarkable provisions for getting rid of the metabolic wastes produced through the breakdown of amino acids.

The Kidneys and Their Work

The water-soluble wastes produced in protein metabolism are excreted by the kidneys in urine. The kidneys are brownish bean-shaped organs, each of which is about as big as a fist. They hang loosely on the back wall of the abdomen, one on each side of the lower portion of the spine (lumbar region). The kidneys clear the blood of several end products of protein metabolism literally by filtering blood plasma.

The Nephron. The nephron is the functional unit of the kidney. In each human kidney there are about a million nephrons. Each nephron consists of a twisted skein of capillary loops called the glomerulus, and a tube leading from it called the renal tubule (Fig. 13-4). The glomerulus is thrust like a tiny clenched fist into the closed cuplike upper end of the tubule. This upper blind end is called Bowman's capsule after its discoverer, Sir William Bowman, an English physician (1816–1892).

Beyond Bowman's capsule the renal tubule pursues a tortuous course, including two series of snakelike convolutions and an abrupt hairpin turn, before it emerges to join a branch of the treelike system of urine-collecting conduits. The length of a single nephron, when strung out in a straight line, is between 1½ and 2 inches. The estimated total length of the nephrons of both kidneys is some 45 miles.

Under ordinary circumstances large numbers of the million nephrons in each kidney are not working. This luxurious surplus of labor is an indication of the importance to the body of urine excretion. One kidney can be removed if the other is uninjured, and the amount and composition of the urine remain practically unaltered. Indeed, two-thirds of the kidney substance can be put out of commission before there is serious impairment of kidney function.

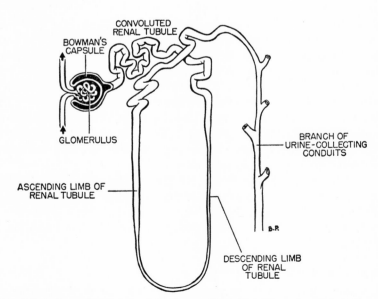

Fig. 13-4. A nephron, one of the two million filtering units of the kidneys.

How Urine Is Produced. Fluid containing everything in blood plasma except the plasma proteins passes from the glomerulus into Bowman's capsule and on through the capsular membrane into the renal tubule. About 150 liters of this filtrate is formed in twenty-four hours. This is more than fifty times the total volume of blood plasma. As this huge quantity of fluid drains through the tubules, from 98 to 99 per cent of the water together with relatively large amounts of sugar and mineral salts are actively reabsorbed, leaving between one and two liters of fluid to be excreted as urine.

The substances reabsorbed with water as the filtrate passes through the tubules are either absent from the urine or present in extremely small amounts. However, they appear in the urine in greater amounts if their concentration in the blood plasma is too high. The sugar found in the urine in diabetes is one example. Another is the more than usually large amount of salt present in urine when excess amounts are eaten. By removing surpluses of this kind, the kidneys help to offset harmful changes in the composition of the blood and body fluids.

The substances that are reabsorbed in very small quantities, or not at all, are the ones that are highly concentrated in the urine. As we should expect, they consist mostly of the metabolic wastes that it is the duty of the kidneys to excrete. Of these, urea is present in the urine in by far the largest amount. Urea is made from the basic nitrogen group which is split off in the form of ammonia from an amino acid during deaminization (see Proteins for Building and Repair of Tissue, in Chap. 12). Ammonia has a highly toxic effect on the nervous system. It must have its teeth pulled, so to speak, before it can be allowed to enter the bloodstream. This is done chiefly in the liver. There the poisonous ammonia is changed into urea, which is one of the least toxic of all nitrogenous compounds.

How Urine Is Removed from the Body. Drops of urine drip from the renal tubules into a system of collecting conduits, arranged like the spokes of a wheel, which convey the urine to the kidney pelvis. From this basin-like sac the urine enters a slender tube (ureter) which opens into the urinary bladder. The ureters (one for each kidney) contract rhythmically in peristaltic waves which squirt the urine into the bladder. The latter is a balloonlike muscular organ lined with mucous membrane. Sensory nerves of the autonomic nervous system end in the bladder wall in delicate little bulbs.

Distention of the bladder is responsible for the desire to urinate. Normally this stimulus acts on the sensory nerve endings in the muscular bladder wall when about half a pint of urine more or less (250 to 300 cubic centimeters) has collected.

Urination is essentially a reflex act, but after infancy and early childhood it is normally controlled by the will; that is, it can be voluntarily started, stopped, or interrupted. Ordinarily, the healthy child or adult can wait to empty the bladder until there is opportunity to do so. If the wait is too long, however, a feeling of fullness and discomfort culminating in pain results.

When the voluntary restraint on urination is lifted, the reflex operates automatically. The sphincter that guards the orifice leading into the urethra (the canal leading from the bladder to the outside) relaxes, and the urine is expelled with considerable force.

Normal Variations in Urine Excretion. The volume of urine excreted in twenty-four hours depends upon many different factors. Among them are diet, the quantity of fluid drunk, environmental temperature and humidity, posture, exercise, mental excitement, weight, age, and sex. The healthy adult usually excretes about 1½ liters of urine in twenty-four hours. Young children excrete three to four times more urine for their weight than adults. A diet high in protein results in a greater output of urine. The caffeine in coffee acts as a powerful diuretic, that is, a promoter of urine excretion. Drinking large quantities of water causes the urine output to increase manyfold. Copious sweating on warm days and exercise reduce the urine output. More urine collects when a person is lying down than when he is standing up. Exposure to cold constricts the blood vessels of the skin, causing more blood to flow through the kidneys with the result that the urine is increased in amount.

Abnormal Variations in Urine Excretion. There are several abnormal conditions that have an effect on the quantity of urine excreted. For example, the amount may be reduced below normal in fever and in acute nephritis (see further on). It is almost always increased in diabetes (see Diabetes, in Chap. 8) and often in nervous states.

Frequency of urination, regardless of the amount excreted, also may have significance. In diabetes and in some nervous disorders frequency of urination is increased. In pyelitis (inflammation of the kidney pelvis) the bladder is very irritable. A child with this condition may not be able to get to the toilet between the time he feels the need to urinate and the time he is forced to let go.

Unwise toilet training in early childhood may prolong involuntary urination beyond the time it usually stops (between the ages of 2½ and 3 years). In most cases this occurs at night (nocturnal enuresis, or bed wetting). Some children may "wet their pants" to get attention or to express resentment.

Observing Deviations from Normal in Kidney Function. The most valuable observations regarding kidney function which teachers can make are those that indicate a persistent change in a child's toilet habits. Requests to leave the room to go to the toilet which persistently occur more often or less often than usual should be reported to the nurse or physician serving the school. Repeated complaints of excessive thirst or mention of the need to urinate more often than usual also should be reported.

Acute Kidney Inflammation

Acute inflammation of the kidneys goes by the general name of nephritis, that is, inflammation of the nephrons. When the glomeruli are primarily affected, the inflammation is called glomerular nephritis. When the tubules are involved the condition is called tubular nephritis, or nephrosis.

Acute glomerular nephritis is usually preceded by a streptococcal infection, such as scarlet fever, streptococcal sore throat, or a streptococcal skin infection. The streptococcal toxin causes inflammatory changes in the glomeruli which produce the signs and symptoms of this form of nephritis. These changes permit serum albumin and red blood cells to escape from the blood into the kidney tubules. Hence the most reliable signs of acute glomerular nephritis are albumin and red blood cells in the urine. They can be detected only through urinalysis (see further on).

The onset of acute glomerular nephritis may be so slow that it is detected only through a routine urinalysis. Or the child may suddenly show signs of severe illness and have to be treated as an emergency case until arrangements can be made to have him taken home or to a hospital for medical diagnosis and treatment.

Edema and reduction of the urine output are characteristic of acute glomerular nephritis. The edema is caused by the loss of serum albumin from the blood plasma. This loss lowers the osmotic pressure of the blood (see The Circulatory System, in Chap. 10), with the result that large amounts of fluid escape from the capillaries into the tissues. The decrease in urinary output is caused by the inflammatory changes which put large numbers of the kidney filtering units out of commission.

If so many nephrons are incapacitated that kidney function is seriously impaired, urea may pile up in the blood and cause urea poisoning, or uremia. This unhappy event occurs very seldom in children. With proper treatment acute glomerular nephritis usually results in complete recovery. However, there may be relapses in some cases, and in others the acute form of the disease may progress to chronic glomerular nephritis (chronic Bright's disease). The chronic form, however, is rare in children. It is mostly a disease of middle and old age.

Nephrosis, or tubular nephritis, is usually not preceded by an infection. It may be the second stage of a transient glomerular nephritis so mild that it was not detected. Nephrosis is marked by degenerative changes in the mucous membrane covering (epithelium) of the renal tubules. The manifestations of nephrosis vary widely. Usually they include edema and albumin in the urine, but the urine output is not reduced. Many cases of nephrosis are very mild and clear up by themselves. However, there may be many recurrences marked by edema over a period of years.

Urinalysis. Because of the efficiency with which the nephrons in healthy kidneys act as selective filters, it is easy to see why a urinalysis is a valuable tool in diagnosis. For example, if serum albumin—which makes up about 50 per cent of the plasma proteins—is found in the urine in appreciable amounts, kidney damage is suspected because normally no plasma proteins are allowed to pass through the kidney filtering units. Other things looked for besides albumin and sugar (which may indicate diabetes) include the specific gravity of the urine (which indicates the quantity of solid substances contained in it), acid–alkali reactions, fragmented or whole red blood cells, white cells (pus), and bile pigment.

Children with a history of acute nephritis should have their urine examined periodically for red blood cells. This requires a microscopic examination of the sediment.

The physicians of an earlier day placed very great stress upon the appearance, odor, and volume of the urine. Sometimes they ventured to predict the outcome of a sickness (prognosis) simply by looking at and smelling the patient's urine. A flask of urine held aloft was the sign manual of the medieval physician, as the stethoscope around the neck is that of the modern physician.

Even now the physician can learn a great deal about the functioning of the kidneys by noting the amount, clearness or turbidity, and color of the urine.

SIGNS AND SYMPTOMS OF GASTROINTESTINAL DISORDERS

The term gastrointestinal is a combination of a Greek word meaning "stomach" and a Latin word meaning "intestine." Gastrointestinal upsets are extremely common in children, partly because the stomach and intestines are so sensitive to both psychic and physical stimuli.

Indigestion is practically the generic name for a set of symptoms which varies according to the ways in which digestion fails to proceed in a calm and orderly manner in different individuals. There are many different causes of gastric indigestion, or dyspepsia, which range all the way from hurried eating, indiscretion in eating, or eating when nervous or tired, to allergic sensitivity to certain foods, or organic disease of one kind or another.

The mechanism of the more common signs and symptoms associated with gastrointestinal disorders is described here.

Furred Tongue

"Stick out your tongue" is a command with which most youngsters are familiar. Furring of the back of the tongue, accompanied by bad breath and perhaps by loss of appetite and regurgitation of fluid into the mouth, is a common indication of an upset stomach or constipation. It is believed that reverse peristaltic wavelets or ripples are responsible for coated tongue and its accompanying signs. In constipation, according to this explanation, small waves of contraction originating in the loaded bowel travel in a reverse direction over the small intestine, stomach, and esophagus.

Halitosis

The disagreeableness to others of bad breath is a potent argument for the advertisers of products designed to sweeten the breath. It is possible to have bad breath without knowing it, because expired air flows along the floor of the nose, where there are no endings of the olfactory nerve (nerve of smell).

Halitosis may have any one of a number of causes, including stomach or intestinal trouble of one kind or another; infections of the sinuses, tonsils, and gums; and extensive decay or uncleanliness of the teeth. Malodorous breath also may be caused by the odors of incompletely digested fats and of volatile substances like garlic which have been absorbed from the large intestine by the blood and carried to the lungs where they are thrown off in expiration. Medical attention should be secured for a child who continues to have this affliction in spite of faithful brushing of the teeth after each meal and the use of a mouthwash.

Heartburn

A burning sensation in the esophagus which is often felt in the heart region is a common complaint. It is caused by the regurgitation of acid fluid from the stomach. The mucous membrane of the esophagus is very sensitive to acid but the gastric mucosa (mucous membrane lining the stomach) is not. Gastric juice contains hydrochloric acid, which is necessary for the activation of pepsin, its protein-splitting enzyme. Hence, anything regurgitated from the stomach after it has been mixed with gastric juice will have a sour acid taste and cause an unpleasant burning sensation in the esophagus.

So-called "acid indigestion," which is associated with excessive secretion of hydrochloric acid, may or may not be accompanied by heartburn.

Belching

Many healthy individuals have a tendency after a meal to expel small amounts of gas from the stomach by way of the esophagus and mouth. Normal belching has become associated with hearty eating and was once more polite than it is now when large meals are not in fashion. Among the Chinese, belching to this day is said to be a means of expressing appreciation for a good meal. Belching is brought about by peristaltic waves operating in reverse from the upper end of the stomach.

Although occasional belching after a meal is normal, the repeated belching of gas is considered to be abnormal. In repeated belching, the gas expelled is not produced by the fermentation of food in the process of digestion; rather, it is swallowed air, most of which collects at the lower end of the esophagus. We all know that babies swallow air in nursing and have to be "burped" or "bubbled." In older individuals the swallowing of air seems to be a trick to induce belching in order to gain relief from the sensation of "gas on the stomach." As a matter of fact, this feeling is not accompanied by increased pressure within the stomach, and the pressure within the stomach is not lowered after belching.

Children who belch repeatedly are likely to be of the nervous type. They may do it deliberately to attract attention, or they may actually have some gastric discomfort. In any event they need medical attention.

Lump in the Throat

The sphincter guarding the entrance to the stomach from the esophagus is sensitive to anything swallowed which might damage the stomach. If something large or hard like an unchewed piece of meat or a tablet is swallowed, the sphincter may not relax and open up until the substance has had a chance to dissolve or disintegrate.[1]

In hurried eating, food may pile up in the esophagus waiting its turn to go through the sphincter as it contracts and relaxes to let the food descend gradually into the stomach. As a result a feeling of fullness, or heaviness, of the throat or chest may persist for some time after eating.

Very rarely the sensation of "something sticking in the throat" is caused by the failure of the sphincter in the esophagus to relax properly during swallowing. Only a physician can detect and treat this condition.

The feeling of having a lump in the throat is quite often a psychogenic symptom. Probably most of us have experienced this sensation when we felt like weeping.

Vomiting

Vomiting is a reversal of the normal movement of food away from the mouth toward the stomach and intestine. A common prelude to vomiting is nausea or "feeling sick to the stomach" (see further on).

In order to vomit, the muscles of the stomach, esophagus, and abdominal wall must work together. This muscular mechanism is governed by a vomiting center located in the medulla oblongata close to the respiratory center. The vomiting center may be influenced by impulses coming in from the stomach and other organs in the abdomen or from

---

[1] If a child swallows a foreign body such as a piece of broken glass or a pin or a coin, the physician should be consulted at once. A laxative should not be given. (See Choking, in Chap. 11, for any object lodged in the windpipe.)

practically any region of the body. Consequently, almost any disorder may result in upheaval of the stomach's contents.

The act of vomiting is essentially a reflex act. Various mechanical and chemical irritants acting on the gastric mucosa may be responsible for pulling the trigger, so to speak. Among them are toxic substances in food or toxic products formed in the process of digestion. Certain chemical substances are very irritating to the endings of nerves running to the vomiting center. These substances are called emetics. Those most commonly used to induce vomiting are ipecac, mustard water, and salt water.

Impulses coming from structures other than the stomach also excite the vomiting center. It is well known that tickling the throat with a feather or pushing a finger into the throat will induce vomiting. Any inflammation or obstruction in the intestines, appendicitis, for example, may cause violent vomiting. Also irritation of any other organ, such as the kidneys, urinary bladder, or gall bladder, may initiate vomiting when nothing whatever is irritating the stomach.

Severe pain anywhere in the body; strong emotions such as disgust, fear, or anxiety; and unpleasant stimulation of the sense organs of sight, taste, or smell by greatly disliked or unappetizing foods may set off the vomiting reflex. Physical fatigue and mental stress may have the same effect. Also vomiting may be a neurotic sign if it recurs frequently for no apparent reason.

The motions of the stomach in vomiting are very interesting. In human beings, except babies, there are usually no reverse peristaltic movements of the stomach walls. However, there may be violent churning movements. Just before vomiting there is a sudden reduction in the tone of the stomach walls and the lower part of the stomach drops a couple of inches. This coincides with the sensation of nausea. That sinking feeling in the stomach has a sound physiological basis. Sharp pressure on the relaxed stomach by contractions of the diaphragm and abdominal muscles ejects the stomach's contents.

Nausea

Nausea may precede vomiting or occur alone. It is usually associated with pallor and sweating. The actual sinking of the stomach that takes place when a nauseous odor or some other stimulus is applied stretches the esophagus and stomach walls. It is thought that this movement exerts tension on the nerve endings and so induces nausea. The sensations experienced in the changes of speed of an elevator, or in the rolling of a ship at sea or in an airplane, or while riding in an automobile or train are probably the result of tension on the esophagus and stomach walls. However, the most powerful factor in the production of motion sickness, or "seasickness," as this sensation is popularly called, is the stimulation of nerve endings in the semicircular canals in the inner ear (see Motion Sickness, in Chap. 18).

Loss of Appetite

Appetite and hunger are different sensations, although they often occur together. In hunger a hollow or empty feeling in the stomach and contractions of the walls of the empty stomach (sometimes called "hunger pains") direct us to eat in order to "keep the home fires burning." Few persons in lands of peace and plenty experience the pangs of hunger caused by dire need for food. Usually there is plenty of unabsorbed food in the small intestine when an empty stomach causes the sensation of hunger.

It is common knowledge that the more active a child is the hungrier he is at mealtime. An active child eats more than the child who is temperamentally inclined to lead a quiet existence, because he spends more energy which must be replenished by food. Eating meals at the same time each day tends to establish the periods at which a child begins to feel hungry. Appetite is connected with pleasure in eating. It may coincide with hunger, but it also may exist independently. The habit of "nibbling" or consuming sweet foods or drinks between meals, which most children fall into if they are allowed to, is one of the chief causes of lack of appetite at mealtimes in healthy children.

Happy memories of the taste of certain foods, appetizing odors, and foods pleasing to the eye normally stimulate appetite; fatigue and emotions like worry, fright, and sorrow normally banish it. The smell or even the thought of disgusting or unpleasing food will, as we have seen, cause nausea, which is the exact opposite of appetite.

Poor appetite or loss of appetite (anorexia) may be associated with lowered tone in the stomach walls. As gastric tone is low in various disorders, poor appetite or loss of appetite in children whose appetite has hitherto been good may indicate the onset of illness.

In some cases lack or loss of appetite is an expression of resentment caused by adverse attitudes of the parents toward the child or toward each other or by some psychological shock connected with food or with the mouth. Very often the child gets extra and gratifying attention from his parents because of his lack of appetite, and this so-called "secondary gain" must be removed before steps can be taken to find and remove the underlying cause through psychiatric treatment.

Pain

Several different types of pain are among the most common symptoms of gastrointestinal disturbances and diseases. Yet the organs of the abdomen (and of the chest, also) are not sensitive to the various stimuli that arouse the sensation of pain in the skin, muscles, and other superficial structures of the body. The stomach, intestine, and heart, for example, can be touched, cut, pinched, burned, or frozen without immediately causing pain. Food or drink would have to be very hot or very cold indeed before the stomach would "feel" it. The sensations of heat and cold aroused by the temperature of what we eat and drink originate for the most part in the lower portion of the esophagus. The stomach, as we have seen, is also insensitive to acid.

What then does give us a stomachache or some other kind of abdominal distress? The answer to this question is highly controversial. It is safe to say, however, that the pain felt as a result of a disease process or disturbance in any organ of the chest or the abdomen may be referred pain (see Referred Pain, in Chap. 7) or pain localized in or near the organ itself. In the case of stomachache, for example, the pain is usually referred to the superficial structures overlying the stomach; in coronary heart disease, to the left arm; in gall-bladder disease, to the right shoulder. If the pain is localized in the organ itself, the stimulus is thought to be tension. Pain may be felt in any hollow organ if it is distended by its contents (an overstuffed stomach or too-full bladder, for example) or by inflammation or obstruction of any part. The pain impulses arise in response to the stretch stimulus acting on the nerve endings in the organ's walls.

Jaundice

The yellowish tinge of the skin which goes by the name of jaundice is caused by the presence in the blood of an excess amount of bile pigment. The pigment escapes from the blood into the skin, mucous membrane, and conjunctiva of the eyes, which then become stained a yellow tint.

The chief bile pigment is bilirubin, the iron-free fraction of the red-blood-cell pigment, hemoglobin. When the red cells fall apart as a result of bumping around at great speed through the blood vessels, their hemoglobin is set free. This liberated hemoglobin is in turn broken up. Part of it is used to produce new hemoglobin and the other part—bilirubin—is carried in the bloodstream to the liver, whence it is excreted in bile. Besides serving as a vehicle for the excretion of bilirubin and other waste products, bile also is essential for the emulsification of fat during digestion.

Bilirubin will accumulate in the blood and produce a yellowish skin discoloration in the following conditions:

1. When red blood cells are destroyed faster than the liver can excrete bilirubin. The excess pigment then piles up in the blood. Any illness in which the destruction of red blood cells is a pronounced feature may produce this type of jaundice.

2. If the bile duct through which bile passes from the liver to the small intestine is obstructed (by a gallstone, for example).

3. If for some reason the liver itself cannot excrete bilirubin in normal amounts, as, for example, in infectious hepatitis (see further on).

In any given case of jaundice, two or all three causative factors may, and frequently do, exist together. The important point is that a pronounced yellowish tinge of the skin and eye whites is not normal and should always be brought to the attention of the doctor or nurse. A period of observation and tests of various kinds are required to determine the cause of the jaundice.

Constipation

Constipation (from a Latin word meaning "crowding together") is the term used in referring to the retention of feces for a longer period than is normal for a particular individual. Children—and adults, too—differ from one another in their bowel habits. It may be usual for an individual to have one bowel movement in twenty-four hours; for another to have two or three movements in the same time; for still another to have one movement every two or every three days. The average is once or twice in twenty-four hours.

Occasional constipation is rarely harmful. Its worst feature is the anxiety it rouses in worried parents or in others who have been conditioned—largely by advertising—to look upon a daily bowel movement as essential. Chronic constipation, however, is difficult to correct. The habit of "cleaning out the bowels" by taking cathartics or purgatives which stimulate peristalsis penalizes the whole digestive tract for the sluggish action of only one part. It is like burning down the house to roast a pig, as Charles Lamb tells us the Chinese did before they learned a better way. Moreover, depending upon purgatives or laxatives (which are mild purgatives) is likely to make the colon lazy and hence to prolong the very condition that they are supposed to correct.

Aside from mechanical obstruction the chief causes of constipation are:

1. *Irregular toilet habits.* We have seen that defecation is on the borderline between a voluntary and an involuntary act. The sensation of a full rectum automatically arouses the urge to defecate, but the act can be inhibited voluntarily. Refusal to respond to this sensation and failure to acquire the habit of clearing the bowels at a regular time each day (for example, after breakfast) are common causes of constipation. The tone of the muscles in the colon and rectum will suffer, and the nervous impulses responsible for the call for defecation may cease to be given if it is persistently disobeyed. This means that the rectum has become resigned to the increased bulk of feces and has made the neces-

sary adaptations. Also more fluid is absorbed from the retained feces. As a result, they become hard and dry and difficult to expel. It is very important to make it easy for youngsters to have a regular time for moving their bowels. Once the colon has established the habit, it usually continues to function automatically at that time throughout life.

2. *Too little roughage and water in the diet.* Indigestible materials, especially cellulose, increase the bulk of the feces and stimulate intestinal activity. Water is an aid to elimination, as to many other body functions.

3. *A misbehaving colon.* In some individuals the colon may be too tense (hypertonic or spastic) or too slack (atonic or weak) or too absorbent ("greedy" or "thrifty"). These conditions can be detected and treated only by a physician.

Diarrhea

In diarrhea the bowels move much more frequently than usual and the feces have a watery consistency. Feces may be hustled through the colon before the normal amount of water can be absorbed (premature evacuation) for many reasons besides the irritation of the intestinal wall by the action of transient bacteria (not normal inhabitants of the colon) or their toxic products.

Psychic influences, such as excitement or fear, may speed up peristaltic movements in some individuals, with the result that diarrhea persists until the exciting cause is removed.

In severe diarrhea caused by bacteria or their toxins, such as cholera or bacillary dysentery (see further on), water is drawn into the intestine from the tissue spaces to aid in flushing out toxic substances. As a result, dehydration of the body occurs and weight is lost.

GASTROINTESTINAL INFECTIONS

Infectious diseases of the gastrointestinal tract are much less common than formerly, chiefly owing to the successful efforts of public health officials in our country to safeguard our water, milk, and solid-food supplies and to ensure the sanitary disposal of human and animal intestinal wastes.

The average American family and its members and the American school also may take part of the credit. An important part of the health education of children and their elders has been, and still is, concerned with sanitary food handling, sanitary dishwashing, fly and rodent control, and similar measures in the home, and with personal habits, such as hand washing before eating and preparing food and after toilet, which make it difficult for germs to gain access to the body by being swallowed alive.

Bacterial Infections

Typhoid Fever. The classic water-borne, milk-borne, fly-borne disease is typhoid fever. Its control in our country has been called "perhaps the greatest triumph of organized preventive medicine." Since the beginning of the twentieth century the annual death rate from this disease has been reduced by almost 100 per cent. It now occurs in the United States chiefly in sporadic cases and in small outbreaks which can be traced to a single polluted well or other source of drinking water, or to a single unknown carrier concerned with milk handling or with the handling of food in a home, camp, or eating establishment. The typhoid carrier (a person who harbors and spreads the bacilli of typhoid without himself being ill) has always been a great problem in typhoid control.

The bacillus of typhoid fever (*Salmonella typhosa*) belongs to the same species of bacteria as those which we shall meet later on in this chapter as the bacteria responsible for salmonellosis, a form of food infection.

It is not necessary for teachers to be on the lookout for early signs and symptoms of typhoid (see Sec. 3, Appendix B) except during an epidemic in their own locality and during floods or other disasters that threaten the purity of communal or family water supplies.

Active immunization with typhoid fever vaccine is not considered necessary in the United States and Canada except in the presence of a typhoid epidemic or for persons living in rural areas where typhoid fever is prevalent. Vaccination is often recommended for campers. When travel outside the continental United States and Canada is anticipated, immunization with a combined typhoid-paratyphoid vaccine is considered advisable.

Dysentery. Dysentery is a common disease among children, especially children under the age of five. Since the decline of typhoid fever, it has assumed a greater relative importance as a cause of gastrointestinal infection. Bacilli belonging to the *Shigella* group are the most frequent cause of dysentery. Amebas (*Endamoeba histolytica*) are responsible for another fairly common form of the disease.

Bacillary dysentery (shigellosis) is spread in the same way as is typhoid fever. However, it is much more difficult to prevent by public health measures because most measures are ineffective against the hand-to-mouth transfer of contaminated material through direct or indirect contact with infected persons or carriers which plays a large part in epidemics of dysentery.

The hallmark of dysentery is diarrhea (see Sec. 3, Appendix B, for signs and symptoms at onset). Attacks differ in severity with different individuals. Some children may have only mild discomfort with a few loose bowel movements. Others may be extremely ill with severe prostration and colic. In severe cases the diarrhea begins with a thin watery discharge, which later contains blood and pus.

Contact with a mild case of bacillary dysentery may result in severe cases in older children. All children who complain of diarrhea in school should be referred to the nurse or physician serving the school. Laboratory examination of the stools (bowel movements) is the only sure means of detecting whether a child has dysentery and, if so, what type is present.

Food Poisoning. Gastrointestinal upsets caused by "something we ate" usually are referred to indiscriminately as "food poisoning." We hear of food poisoning chiefly as occurring simultaneously in large numbers of persons who have eaten the same food at a picnic or church supper or school cafeteria or some other eating establishment. Probably it is more common than reports of outbreaks of this kind lead us to believe, because many cases of "common diarrhea" or dysentery are in reality caused by the presence in food of bacteria or bacterial toxins (poisons).

There are two forms of so-called food poisoning. One form is salmonellosis, or salmonella infection; the other is staphylococcal food poisoning.

Salmonellosis. This form of food infection is caused by members of the *Salmonella* group of pathogens, of which there are numerous species. However, only seven members of the *Salmonella* group are common in the United States.

The salmonella organisms are very widely distributed in nature. They are present in the feces of infected human beings and convalescent carriers, especially mild and unrecognized cases. Also they are present in the intestinal droppings of domestic and wild animals and in the eggs of infected ducks and hens, including dried egg powders. Rodents are dangerous sources of infection because they often contaminate food both before and after it has been prepared for the table. Perhaps the most common source of salmonellosis, however, is the infected food handler who handles food with soiled hands during its preparation or serving.

Epidemics of salmonellosis usually are traced to insufficiently cooked foods, especially meat pies and roast fowl, and foods containing dried or frozen hen or duck eggs; unpasteurized milk or dairy products; pastries contaminated by rodent feces possibly through the medium of cockroaches; and food prepared by an infected food handler.

Salmonella organisms, taken into the body in food or drink, lodge in the intestinal tract where they grow rapidly. In epidemics people who have eaten the offending food become ill with diarrhea, abdominal cramps, and vomiting in from six to forty-eight hours. The usual incubation period is twelve hours. Most victims of salmonella infection recover.

Staphylococcal Food Poisoning. This gastrointestinal illness is a poisoning, not an infection. Staphylococcal food poisoning is caused by toxins preformed in food by certain strains of our ubiquitous foe, the staphylococcus. Staphylococci may be planted in food by food handlers with staphylococcal skin infections (such as boils and pimples) on the hands or wrists, or in milk from the udders of infected cows. Dried milk powder has been involved with increasing frequency in recent years.

When the contaminated food stands at room temperature for several hours, the staphylococci produce enough toxin in the food to poison those who eat it. The foods in which these bacteria grow best are those with custard fillings—for example, eclairs, cream puffs, and layer cakes.

The poison works quickly. Usually persons who have eaten food containing it become acutely ill (see Sec. 3, Appendix B) in two to four hours. Recovery usually takes place in twenty-four to forty-eight hours.

Undulant Fever (Brucellosis). Three closely related bacilli of the genus *Brucella*—one infecting goats, one infecting cows, and one infecting swine—are responsible for the animal disease known as brucellosis. Reservoirs of infection are cattle, swine, sheep, goats, and horses. The family name *Brucella* was bestowed in honor of the British army surgeon, Sir David Bruce, who first isolated the goat-infecting species (1887) from British soldiers on the island of Malta. The name undulant fever was given to brucellosis in human beings because of the characteristic up-and-down—wavelike—nature of the fever.

Human beings catch undulant fever by direct contact with infected animals or their carcasses, or by consuming the raw milk or dairy products from infected goats, sheep, and cows. By far the most common route of infection in our country is direct invasion of the intestinal tract by living *Brucella* bacilli present in unpasteurized cow's milk or milk products. Undulant fever is rare in cities and larger towns, where most of the milk supply is pasteurized. However, these city dwellers are more susceptible to the disease than are country dwellers, who have had a chance to build up immunity by repeated slight infections. There have been many cases in which city dwellers on vacation have contracted undulant fever by drinking a single glass of raw cow's milk.

The acute form of the disease usually begins insidiously (see Appendix B, Sec. 3). Treatment with antibiotics and sulfadiazine combined usually is effective in controlling the fever and symptoms within several days. The relapse rate, however, is high. Undulant fever may last for several days, many months, and occasionally for several years. Recovery is usual, but disability often persists.

Vaccines are available for immunizing stockyard workers, farmers, veterinary surgeons, and laboratory workers who handle cultures of *Brucella* bacilli. As for the rest of us, the best preventive is to make sure that we and our children use only milk and milk products that have been pasteurized.

Infectious Hepatitis. This inflammation of the liver (Greek *hepar,* meaning "liver," plus *itis*) has been known for generations under the name of catarrhal jaundice. It is now known to be caused by a specific virus (IH virus). The disease occurs most commonly in children and young men. It spreads in epidemic form among children who are gathered together as in schools, summer camps, and institutions. Extensive outbreaks have occurred among military forces during wars.

The disease appears to be spread by intimate person-to-person contact, with respiratory spread possible. Experimental evidence shows, however, that the circuit consisting of intestinal discharges contaminated with IH virus→ to food, water, or fingers→ to mouth is the most important method of transmission. It is of great importance during epidemics to emphasize personal cleanliness, especially after toilet and before eating or handling food.

The onset of infectious hepatitis (see Appendix B, Sec. 3) is similar to that of many other so-called digestive upsets in children. The jaundice usually does not appear until five to seven days after onset.

Gamma globulin obtained from pooled adult blood plasma (see Passive Immunity, in Chap. 7), administered promptly after exposure to infectious hepatitis, gives passive protection lasting for from six to eight weeks. It is considered especially important for exposed susceptible adults to be given this protection because the disease may be more severe and more prolonged than in young children.

Serum Hepatitis. Another form of hepatitis is known as serum hepatitis. The chief differences between serum hepatitis and infectious hepatitis are (1) a longer incubation period; (2) greater severity; and (3) lack of direct transmission from man to man. The virus of serum hepatitis is probably related to the IH virus, but its only known source is the blood or blood products of an infected person. It is transmitted by the inoculation of infected human blood or blood products (except gamma globulin and heat-treated serum albumin) or by the use of syringes, needles, or lancets contaminated with traces of blood from an infected person. The incubation period is from two to six months, usually from twelve to fourteen weeks. Except for the greater severity of the illness, serum hepatitis is clinically indistinguishable from infectious hepatitis.

The danger of serum hepatitis has led doctors to exercise great caution in prescribing the transfusion of whole blood and particularly of pooled blood plasma or serum. No person known or suspected to have had infectious hepatitis is permitted to be a blood donor. Scrupulous heat sterilization of all syringes, needles, lancets, and dental instruments is a necessity.

Appendicitis

The appendix is a small wormlike (vermiform) pouch composed of lymphoid tissue which projects from the cecum like one finger of a glove. The cecum itself is the closed lower portion of the ascending colon (see Fig. 13-1). This blind alley extends some 2½ inches below the juncture of the small and large intestines, low down on the right side of the abdomen. Opening from a cul-de-sac as it does, with no outlet at its other end, the appendix has poor drainage.

The inflammation of the appendix known as appendicitis probably starts in most cases as a result of the blocking of the appendix by foreign matter entering it from the large intestine. Blockage of the appendix interferes with its drainage, injures its walls, and permits bacteria present in the intestinal tract to set up an infection.

Children and young adults are unsually susceptible to appendicitis, but it may occur at any age.

Pain in the abdomen is the earliest sign of acute appendicitis. Frequently it starts with generalized pain or pain in the upper part of the abdomen which shortly becomes localized in the lower right side. The pain may be severe and cramplike, or it may be a dull ache. Occasionally it may let up, but this does not mean that the attack has passed.

Soon after the pain sets in, nausea and vomiting usually, but not always, begin. The temperature usually rises slightly above normal; and the abdomen, especially over the appendix, becomes increasingly tender and painful.

Any child who complains of pain or tenderness in the abdomen, with nausea and vomiting, should have medical attention as quickly as possible. He should be taken home from school, not sent home by himself, and his family should be impressed with the importance of (1) sending for a physician without delay; and (2) doing nothing except to keep the child lying down and quiet until the doctor gets there.

It is especially dangerous to give the child a laxative or an enema. The action of the laxative or enema increases the pressure in the appendix and may cause it to rupture or "blow out" and spread the infection. This may be followed by the serious condition called peritonitis. The sulfonamides and penicillin are now often used successfully in the treatment of peritonitis, but peritonitis may cause death.

Appendicitis is sometimes difficult to diagnose. The physician may need to take several blood counts and make other tests. Surgical operation after the diagnosis of appendicitis is made results in recovery of the great majority of children in whom the appendix has not ruptured.

Sometimes a child has an attack of acute appendicitis in which the inflammation subsides without an operation but never entirely clears up. Mild attacks may recur from time to time, and between attacks the child may be troubled with spells of indigestion or have rather constant pain or discomfort soon after eating. Any child complaining of such symptoms should be referred for medical attention.

Intestinal Parasites

Several species of worms are parasitic in the intestines of human beings. Three of these, the pinworm (*Enterobius vermicularis*), the roundworm (*Ascaris lumbricoides*), and the hookworm (*Necator americanus*), are the ones most likely to be found in children.

Infection with any of these worms may not produce symptoms. In that case, the discovery that the child has "worms" may be made only by having the stools examined by a physician. Ordinarily, however, the child shows that something is wrong by losing weight, by becoming paler than usual, or by complaining of dizziness, headache, nausea, abdominal pain, diarrhea, constipation, or feeling tired all the time. He may lose his appetite or have an increased appetite. Of course this bewildering array of signs and symptoms will not occur in any one child. Moreover, any of them, either singly or in combination of two or more, may be present in a great variety of conditions. Parents used to suspect "worms" more often than they do now when any child seemed "out of sorts" or not like his usual self.

Pinworms (Enterobiasis). Other names for these tiny, white, threadlike intestinal worms are "threadworms" and "seat worms."

Infection occurs when pinworm eggs from the anal region are transferred directly to the mouth of the same host by way of the fingers or indirectly to the mouth of the same host or to new hosts by contaminated foods or other articles. Frequently a child with pinworms reinfects himself by scratching the anal region, thus getting eggs on his fingers, and then putting his fingers in his mouth.

After being swallowed the eggs hatch in the stomach and small intestine. The young worms reach maturity in the lower part of the small intestine, the cecum, and the upper part of the large intestine. They then migrate to the rectum and deposit their eggs on the skin in the anal region.

The presence of pinworms in the rectum and anus (and sometimes in the vagina and urinary bladder of girls) causes intense itching. This constant irritation makes the children restless and interferes with their sleep and appetite. Infection with pinworms is one possibility when a child continually squirms in his seat and acts irritable and tired. Appendicitis in children is sometimes caused by pinworms which get into the appendix from the cecum.

Pinworms can usually be cured quickly by appropriate chemotherapeutic drugs given under medical direction. Improvement in the child's health after cure is often dramatic.

To prevent reinfection and spread to new hosts, the strictest hygienic measures must be observed. Children must be impressed with the necessity for washing their hands with soap and water after going to the toilet and before eating and for not putting their fingers in their mouths (as in nail-biting, for example). Toilet seats in the home and the school should be washed daily with a disinfectant. The bed linen and underclothing of members of an infected household should be changed daily and boiled to kill the eggs.

Roundworms (*Ascariasis*). Roundworms are large and resemble earthworms. They lead a parasitic existence in the small intestine, which they reach by a circuitous route. Eggs containing the embryos are present in soil or on various articles in and about the house which are polluted with the intestinal excreta of infected persons. When taken into the mouth, the embryonated eggs travel to the intestinal canal, where they hatch. The larvae penetrate the intestinal wall and reach the lungs by way of the bloodstream. Thence they pass through the air passages into the throat and are again swallowed. Upon reaching the small intestine they settle down and develop into mature worms.

Roundworm infection is most prevalent in families where standards of hygiene are low and essential toilet facilities are either lacking or so poorly constructed that the soil can be polluted by excreta containing the eggs. Preschool children and children of early school age are likely to be more frequently and more heavily infected with roundworms than are older children and adults.

Children infected with roundworms may show no symptoms other than vague indications of poor health. When heavily infected, however, they usually have colicky pain and diarrhea and are nervous, restless, and tired because of disturbed sleep.

Roundworms can be readily eliminated by medical treatment. To prevent infection and reinfection in homes and neighborhoods where ascariasis is prevalent, measures must be taken to avoid soil pollution by the construction of sanitary toilets or privies; and the children, especially, must be encouraged to use their toilet facilities and to wash their hands thoroughly before handling food and after toilet.

Hookworm (*Ancylostomiasis*). Full-grown hookworms are small whitish worms not quite half an inch long and as thick as an "invisible" hairpin. In most cases they enter the body in the larval stage by penetrating the skin, usually of the feet. The larvae pass by way of the lymphatics to one of the big veins leading into the right heart. Thence they travel in the bloodstream to the lungs, whence they pass through the capillary walls into the alveoli. From there they pass up the bronchi and windpipe to the throat and are swallowed. Eventually they reach the small intestine, where they develop into adult worms. Infection can take place by mouth from water, food, or fingers contaminated with larvae, but the most common avenue is through the skin.

Hookworm disease is endemic in regions where soil pollution is favored by inadequate facilities for disposing of human intestinal wastes and where the temperature does not get low enough in winter to destroy the larvae in the soil by freezing. The practice of going barefoot is an important factor in its spread. Hookworm disease is widely endemic in the southern United States although its prevalence has been greatly decreased in recent years by determined efforts to control it.

The signs and symptoms of hookworm disease vary greatly according to the degree of infection. Inflammation of the skin of the feet or of other parts of the skin coming in contact with polluted soil may be the first sign. The itching sore spots are called by various names— "ground itch," "dew itch," "cow itch," "foot itch," or "toe itch." If only a few worms are present, there may be no general symptoms. In mild infections the person may seem merely listless or lazy. Moderate to severe infections are marked by great depression, indigestion, and diarrhea or constipation. There may be severe anemia and swelling (edema) of the abdomen and legs. The skin is harsh and dry, and the gums and lips pale. Children infected with hookworm may be retarded physically and mentally. They may crave unusual things to eat such as paper, chalk, dirt, or clay—hence the name "dirt-eater's disease" which is sometimes used.

All that is necessary to cure hookworm disease is to get the worms out of the small intestine. Physicians have effective drugs for accomplishing this. In a section where hookworm is endemic, any child who shows signs or symptoms of having the disease should be referred to a doctor, or a clinic, for a stool examination. If the child has the disease, eggs will be found in the intestinal discharges.

The prevention of hookworm disease depends primarily upon keeping human excreta containing hookworm eggs off the ground. This may be accomplished by the construction of sanitary privies in communities not served by communal sewerage systems and by teaching children—and their elders—never to defecate on the ground. Hookworm disease also may be prevented by wearing shoes so that the larvae cannot bore their way through the skin of the feet. But the most effective measure is to keep intestinal discharges off the ground.

FOR REVIEW AND DISCUSSION

1. Suppose you were correcting the papers of high school students who had been given a "supply the missing words" test on the digestive system and you found the following mistakes. Make the corrections.

   a. The contraction and relaxation of ~~peristalsis~~ sphincters regulates the passage of food through the alimentary canal.

the walls
peristalsis

   b. The wavelike motions of ~~sphincters~~ are responsible for pushing food along the digestive tract away from the mouth toward the anal canal.

   c. Large food molecules are chemically taken apart during digestion by ~~hormones.~~ *enzymes*

   d. The ~~pepsin~~ *amylase* in saliva starts the digestion of starch.

   e. The enzymes of ~~pancreatic juice~~ *gastric juice* begin the splitting up of protein molecules into ~~grape sugar.~~ *amino acids*

   f. Chemical digestion is completed in the ~~large~~ *small* intestine.

   g. Pressure on the walls of the ~~duodenum~~ *external anal sphincter* gives the stimulus for defecation.

   h. The end products of the digestion of proteins are ~~lipoproteins.~~ *amino acids*

   i. The end products of the digestion of fats pass into the *capillary* ~~networks~~ *epithelial* of the villi.

2. Select the correct ending for each of the following incomplete sentences:

   a. The waste substance into which the nitrogen-containing factor of amino acids is changed is (1) chyle, (2) urea, (3) feces.

   b. Peristaltic waves operating in reverse from the upper end of the stomach cause (1) halitosis, (2) belching, (3) anorexia.

   c. Hunger is caused by (1) an empty stomach, (2) a good appetite, (3) smelling appetizing odors.

   d. Water-soluble protein wastes pass into the kidney tubules from (1) the ureters, (2) the glomeruli, (3) the urinary bladder.

   e. Jaundice is caused by the presence in the blood of an excessive amount of (1) hemoglobin, (2) ptyalin, (3) bilirubin.

   f. Infectious hepatitis is spread by (1) intimate contact with infected persons, (2) transfusion with whole blood from an infected person, (3) staphylococci planted in food by an infected person.

   g. The most important factor in the spread of undulant fever in our country is (1) failure to wash the hands before eating, (2) drinking raw milk, (3) drinking polluted water.

   h. The most effective method of preventing hookworm infection is (1) to keep intestinal discharges off the ground, (2) to wash the hands after toilet, (3) to drink only pasteurized milk.

3. Have class discussions on ways of helping a child who is known to have:

   a. Constipation due to irregular toilet habits

   b. Lack of appetite at meals due to the habit of eating between meals

   c. Loss of appetite due to overconcern on the part of his parents

   d. Frequent spells of vomiting before schooltime

SELECTED REFERENCES

American Medical Association: *The Digestive System,* Part 7 of *The Wonderful Human Machine* series, The Association, Chicago. (The workings of the human body in words and pictures.)

American Public Health Association: *Control of Communicable Diseases in Man* (first mentioned as reference in Chap. 7).

Best, C. H., and N. B. Taylor: *The Human Body* (first mentioned as reference in Chap. 1). Part VI, *The Physiology of Digestion,* Chaps. 24–27; Part VII, *Metabolism and Nutrition—Renal and Cutaneous Functions,* Chap. 32.

Cannon, Walter B.: *Digestion and Health,* W. W. Norton & Company, Inc., New York, 1936. (A classic on digestion by a distinguished physiologist.)

Chapter 14   THE MOUTH AND TEETH

The Mouth
The Salivary Glands
Teeth, First and Last
The School Dental Health Program

In the mouth both the mechanical and the chemical processes of digestion begin. Here the food is tested by the taste buds on the tongue and the olfactory (smelling) apparatus of the nose, masticated by the teeth, mixed with saliva, and rolled into a swallowable bolus by the tongue. From the portals of the mouth to the base of the tongue there are several lookout points of importance in child-health observation.

THE MOUTH

The portals of the mouth are the lips. They are covered with mucous membrane which is an extension of that which lines the mouth and throat. In healthy children the lips, mouth lining, and gums are pink, smooth, and firm.

Chief Disorders of the Lips and Mouth

Cheilosis. Scarring, cracking, or sores at the angles of the lips (see Plate 8) should be called to the attention of the physician, as it may indicate cheilosis, a riboflavin deficiency. Cheilosis is usually associated with inflammation of the tongue (see further on).

Herpes Simplex. Practically everyone is familiar with the appearance on the lips or skin of the face of the superficial watery blisters called cold sores or fever blisters. Their scientific name is herpes simplex. Herpes simplex is an infection caused by a virus. The frequent recurrence of cold sores in persons subject to them was something of a puzzle until a satisfactory solution was proposed as a result of studies made several years ago. According to this explanation the primary infection occurs during infancy (before the age of three), and after recovery the virus remains permanently implanted in the skin. At any time thereafter the virus may be called into activity by the appropriate stimulus. This may be exposure to sunlight, weather changes, menstruation in girls and women, or a variety of other conditions, including certain infectious diseases (colds, for example) which lower body resistance.

If a primary infection with the virus does not take place in infancy,

334

the person seems to acquire a nonspecific immunity. Hence, with reference to herpes simplex, the population may be divided into two classes —the nonherpetic, those who never have cold sores, and the herpetic, those who frequently do.

Cold sores ordinarily are a minor affliction and dry up within a few days if they are let alone. Camphorated ointment or an astringent like powdered alum may be helpful. With children, the trick is to keep them from touching or picking at the sores so as to avoid secondary infection or delay in healing.

Stomatitis. A sore, inflamed mouth may be the sign of any one of several different conditions including infections and nutritional deficiencies. Inflammation of the mouth is known medically as stomatitis (from the Greek word meaning "mouth," plus "itis").

Canker Sores. Sometimes children are bothered with canker sores— small white spots on a red base—which appear on the inner lining of the lips or cheeks or on the tongue. If they do not clear up spontaneously within a week or if they recur frequently, the child should be referred for medical attention.

The Tongue

The tongue is an organ of many functions. It assists in the formation of many of the sounds of speech (see The Tongue in Speech, in Chap. 17). By means of the taste buds on its surface, it cooperates with the olfactory nerve endings in the nose to give us information about each mouthful of food. What we like and what we dislike in the way of food and drink depends very largely upon whether this information is pleasing or not pleasing according to the associations connected with it. Finally, the tongue kneads food, after it has been cut and ground by the teeth, in much the same way that a baker kneads dough.

The surface of the tongue is rough, as we can easily see by inspecting it in a mirror. As the saliva-moistened food is kneaded by the tongue against the hard palate, it is pulverized, frayed, and rolled into a lump that can be swallowed.

Beefy Tongue. Redness and soreness of the tongue (glossitis) are associated with B complex vitamin deficiencies. A beefy red or magenta tongue accompanies the dermatitis and digestive and nervous disorders of pellagra (see Niacin, in Chap. 12). The particular nutritional deficiency or other condition responsible for a beefy red or sore tongue calls for medical attention.

Other conditions that require medical attention include a furred or coated tongue (see Furred Tongue, in Chap. 13); a tongue marked by deep depressions or furrows; and a tongue with denuded patches surrounded by thickened areas in its top covering, or epithelium (geographic, or mappy, tongue).

THE SALIVARY GLANDS

The parotids are the largest of the three pairs of glands that manufacture and secrete saliva into the mouth through ducts. They are situated one in front of each ear. The next largest salivary glands are the submaxillaries, located one on each side below the angle of the jaw. The smallest are the sublingual glands, one on each side beneath the tongue (Fig. 13-1).

The discovery of the parotid duct was made by Niels Stenson (1638–1686), a Danish physiologist, while he was still a young medical student. One morning when he was dissecting the head of a sheep, the instrument he was using was inserted by chance into the opening of the parotid duct and slipped down to strike with a sharp clink against the teeth. Stenson knew at once that he had discovered the duct of the gland.

The salivary glands, particularly the parotids, are open to attack by a specific virus. This virus is the cause of mumps, or infectious parotitis.

Mumps

Primarily, mumps is a disease of childhood. The greatest incidence is between eight and fourteen years. However, mumps is not nearly so communicable as are measles and chicken pox. As a consequence many individuals escape infection in childhood. In males who catch mumps after puberty a painful inflammation of the testes, called orchitis, frequently develops as a complication. More rarely, in adolescent girls the ovaries may be involved.

Generally, prolonged and intimate contact is required for the transmission of mumps. The virus is present in the saliva of the infected person. Airborne droplets probably play an important part in the transmission of mumps in schools.

In children mumps is ordinarily a mild disease—so mild, in fact, that a private New York school once made the experiment of not attempting to control an epidemic, on the principle that it was far better to gain immunity from mumps in childhood than to take the risk of contracting it later, when it would be more likely to have serious consequences. The experiment was abandoned, however, when it was found that the free spread of mumps among the children resulted in the exposure of more adults than would have been the case had the usual isolation procedures been set up at the beginning of the epidemic.

Mumps is characterized by swelling and tenderness in front of the ear, extending down the neck behind the angle of the jaw. One or both parotid glands may be affected. The other two pairs of salivary glands also may become inflamed either at the same time or in rotation. Before the swelling develops the child may have slight fever and sometimes earache, sore throat, or vomiting. He may complain of pain.

For his own sake a child with mumps should stay home in bed until the swelling subsides. For the sake of adolescent boys and girls and adults, he should be isolated during the period of communicability (see Sec. 2, Appendix B).

When a boy after puberty has been exposed to mumps it may seem advisable to the physician to give him temporary passive immunity by the injection of gamma globulin prepared from the pooled blood serum of persons convalescing from mumps (hyperimmune gamma globulin). Before doing this, however, the physician may perform a skin test to determine whether the boy is already immune as a result of previous unrecognized infection with mumps virus.

A vaccine is available for active immunization from mumps. However, the course of mumps in children who have not reached puberty is usually so mild that it is not recommended for routine use in healthy children. The degree and duration of immunity conferred by mumps vaccine have not been clearly established.

TEETH, FIRST AND LAST

Mastication involves biting off pieces of food of the right size to fit the dimensions of the mouth, tearing these pieces apart into smaller fragments, and then grinding them into bits. To perform these functions we have biting teeth (incisors), tearing teeth (cuspids and bicuspids), and grinding teeth (molars). The location of these teeth in the permanent set and the ages at which they erupt are shown in Fig. 14-1.

How Teeth Grow

Teeth begin to develop within the jaws in little sacs which are filled with a jellylike substance composed of dentin-forming cells, enamel-forming cells, blood vessels, and nerves. Enamel (the hard substance that covers the crown of the tooth as a thimble covers a fingertip) and dentin (the ivorylike substance that makes up the principal body of the tooth) are deposited in layers until the crown is completed and root formation begins. As the crown grows larger, the sac in which it started shrinks to form the pulp of the tooth (see further on). After the enamel is completely formed, the enamel-making cells disappear. Hence, there is inadequate provision for self-repair. The margin of safety for the teeth is narrow compared with that of other body structures. However, a few dentin-forming cells remain after the dentin is completed and can deposit additional dentin as long as the tooth remains alive and healthy.

The root of each tooth is fixed in the jaw in its own individual socket. It is coated with cementum, a slightly less hard substance than the enamel which coats the crown. An outer sheath called the periodontal membrane, or dental periostium, cushions the tooth root in its socket. The neck of

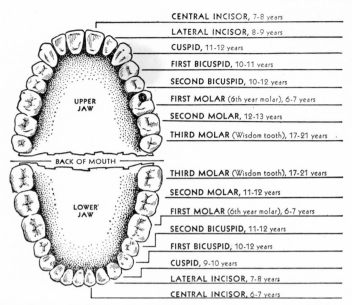

FIG. 14-1. The teeth of the permanent set and the ages at which they erupt.

the tooth is at the gum line; that is, it forms the transition area between the crown above the gums and the root below. (See Fig. 14-2.)

Children from the age of six onward are shedding their first, or deciduous, teeth and acquiring the teeth of the permanent set. It is a sad fact that a very large percentage of these newly acquired teeth are doomed to early decay.

Dental Caries

Conceivably the coating of the crowns of the teeth with enamel, the hardest substance in the body, might be sufficient protection if the teeth had nothing to contend with except the wearing down of the enamel over a lifetime of chewing or the accidental cracking or chipping of the crowns. Unfortunately, teeth are subject to a very common disease which attacks the enamel. This disease is dental caries. The damage done by dental caries steadily mounts through the entire period of youth and early maturity. In middle age the pace of the caries process slackens and, for this reason, prevention during youth is of particular value.

The discovery of the precipitating cause of dental caries was made in 1882 by W. E. Miller, an American dentist. Dr. Miller found that tooth enamel is readily dissolved (decalcified) by acids produced in the fermentation of carbohydrates by bacteria (notably the lactobacilli) normally present in the mouth. Decalcification of the calcified tissues by these acids (usually lactic acid) accompanied or followed by disintegration of the organic substance of the tooth, is now widely accepted by dental authorities as the cause of dental caries. Enough acid to carry on the decay process is held in contact with the enamel by firmly adhering gelatinous plaques containing multitudes of acid-forming bacteria.

Although we know the cause of dental caries, several other factors enter the picture.

Susceptibility. It has long been common knowledge that some persons are more susceptible to tooth decay than are others, although very few are immune. Probably many teachers have observed that some youngsters who do not take care of their teeth have perfect ones, while others who follow the rules about diet and toothbrushing have many dental defects. Inherited differences in the ability to resist caries may account for a great many of these variations in susceptibility.

Solubility of the Enamel. At one time it was believed that a daily diet containing all the essential food elements in the right amounts would result in the development of caries-resistant enamel. It appears now, however, that nutritional status has little or no bearing on the caries process. It has been shown that well-nourished children may have as many cavities as poorly nourished children, or more. And well-calcified teeth may develop many cavities, whereas teeth with gross defects in

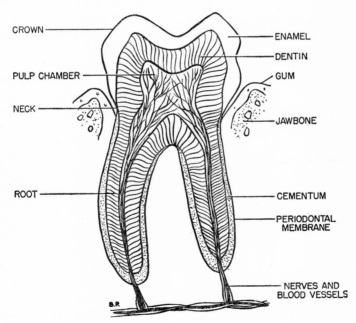

Fig. 14-2. Cross section of a tooth showing its structure.

the structure of the enamel may not develop any cavities at all. It appears that differences in the solubility of the enamel account largely for variations in the number of cavities in different individuals.

The Oral Environment. Individual differences in the environment of the mouth seem to account for many variations in susceptibility to dental caries. One of the most important factors is the number of acid-forming bacteria, particularly lactobacilli, present in the saliva. Persons highly susceptible to tooth decay have a high lactobacillus count, but persons in whom caries is inactive or absent have few or no lactobacilli.

The Role of Saliva. Another factor in the oral environment, besides the bacterial count, is the biochemical nature of saliva. It has been shown that in persons with rampant caries the composition of the saliva differs from that of persons free of caries. This becomes understandable when we realize that twelve or thirteen enzymes and coenzymes are essential to the production of lactic acid from sugar (sucrose) and that the presence or lack of certain substances in the saliva seems to inhibit or encourage the action of one or more of these ferments.

Some persons are immune from dental caries because they have the ability to develop ammonia compound naturally in their mouths. Not only does the ammonia interfere with the production of lactic acid by the lactobacilli, but also it serves to neutralize the acid produced.

Our National Sweet Tooth. Since lactobacilli produce acids by the fermentation of carbohydrates, especially sugar, most dental authorities now believe that our national "sweet tooth" is very largely responsible for our high caries attack rate. Sweets are good sources of energy and make some foods more tasty. The fact that they appear to play an important role in the process of tooth decay, however, leads dental authorities to recommend temperance—not total abstinence—in the consumption of sweets. It is especially important to encourage youngsters to cut down on the amount of sweets they eat between meals when few people bother to brush their teeth or rinse their mouths afterward.

The Role of Toothbrushing. It would seem that the removal of tough patches of mucin, mouth debris, and bacteria (bacterial plaques) which readily form on the surface of tooth enamel and provide feeding grounds for lactobacilli and other acid-forming and acid-tolerating bacteria would be an important factor in preventing tooth decay. However, these plaques adhere firmly, especially on surfaces that cannot be reached by toothbrush bristles or even by the instruments used in prophylactic cleansings. It has been shown that within a few minutes of being bathed in a sugar solution (as happens in eating candy or drinking highly sweetened beverages, for example) the acidity of dental plaques in caries-susceptible mouths becomes high enough to dissolve tooth enamel and remains so for thirty to ninety minutes. The feltlike consistency of the plaque keeps

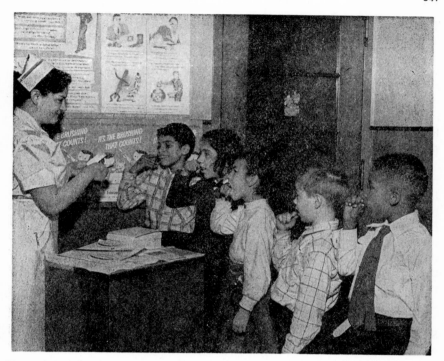

FIG. 14-3. School nurse demonstrates proper toothbrushing technique. (*Courtesy of the New York City Department of Health.*)

this acid from being neutralized by the saliva, which normally maintains a nice balance between acidity and alkalinity.

Toothbrushing and mouth rinsing, therefore, if given a sporting chance, may be of great help in reducing the caries rate by getting rid of fermentable carbohydrate residues. The old admonition regarding toothbrushing ran something like this: Brush your teeth after each meal, if possible, or at least twice a day—in the morning and before going to bed. However, the usual thirty-second brush-offs the first thing in the morning and the last thing at night accomplish little except to make the mouth and teeth feel pleasantly clean. Thorough brushing within ten minutes after eating does give the teeth some protection from decay. If brushing immediately after a meal or between-meal snack is not possible, thoroughly rinsing the mouth with water will do some good.

Fluorides in the Prevention of Dental Caries

The most important development in preventive dentistry in this century has resulted from the discovery that fluorides (compounds of the chemical element fluorine) are helpful in controlling dental caries.

The investigation of the use of fluorides in preventing dental caries had its beginning when the mottling of tooth enamel observed among children living in certain geographical areas was traced, first, to the drinking water and, later, to the presence in the water of unusually large amounts of fluoride. It was then learned that the prevention of tooth mottling depends upon measures taken to provide drinking water with a fluoride content below the threshold at which mottling appears. This threshold has been established as one part of fluoride to one million parts of water (abbreviated as 1 ppm).

After fluoride was recognized to be the cause of tooth mottling, a still more striking discovery was made. It was found that persons who have lived all their lives in areas in which the drinking water contains fluoride, or who have lived in such areas at least during the period of enamel formation (from birth to eight or ten years of age), experience a dental caries incidence only one-half or one-third as much as that of persons living in areas where the drinking water contains no fluoride. Whether the influence of the fluoride is helpful in that it gives relatively high protection from caries, or unsightly in that it causes tooth mottling, depends upon the amount ingested.

Long-term controlled experiments were begun in 1944 in the United States and Canada to determine whether the fluoridation of communal water supplies in localities where the drinking water is not naturally fluoridated would result in a reduction in the incidence of dental caries. The reports from these experiments are so favorable that all dental, medical, and public health authorities have endorsed water fluoridation as a practical, economical, simple, and safe approach to the overwhelming problem of dental caries. The latest reports from the Newburgh-Kingston (New York) fluoridation experiment, for example, indicate that the number of teeth with new cavities found among Newburgh children whose drinking water is fluoridated is less by an average of two teeth per child at each year of age than among children of the control city of Kingston. The bar chart shown in Fig. 14-4 gives a picture of the results in the two cities in terms of the average number of decayed, missing, and filled permanent teeth per child at the ages of six to sixteen years.

The American Dental Association has indicated that the total number of cavities resulting from dental caries in children's teeth is so high (285 million is the nationwide figure) that if all the dentists practicing now were to devote all their time to children, they could not hope to be able to fill all the cavities. "From the dental public health point of view, the benefit to the community of a decrease in caries experience of two teeth per child per year is significant." [1]

An increasing number of towns and cities whose water is not naturally

[1] *Health News,* New York State Department of Public Health, Vol. 32, No. 1 (January), 1955.

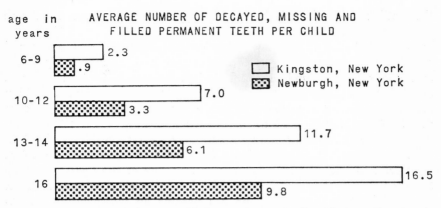

FIG. 14-4. Results of the controlled experiment in fluoridation of water in Kingston and Newburgh, New York.

fluoridated are now adding fluoride to the communal drinking water supply. In communities without fluoridated water the application of a solution of sodium fluoride directly to the teeth at ages three, seven, ten, and thirteen is giving good results. This treatment will prevent nearly 40 per cent of the cavities which otherwise might be expected to occur. Beneficial results also have been reported in the use of dentifrices containing stannous fluoride.

Devitalized Teeth

The end result of unchecked dental caries is the death of the tooth. When alive each tooth is supplied with the necessities of life by blood vessels and nerves which run up through canals in the roots. The spongy mass of blood vessels and nerves which forms the pulp of the tooth occupies a central chamber within the tooth called the pulp chamber. Minute tubes filled with pulp material ramify into the dentin to nourish it.

As the processes of decay extend inward toward the pulp cavity, its ivory walls become so thin that heat and cold can penetrate them more readily. Sensitivity to hot and cold foods and liquids is an alarm signal transmitted by the nerves in the pulp. Toothache may begin even before the dentin wall finally breaks down, thereby exposing the soft pulp to bacterial action. Possibly a dentist may be able to save a tooth's life after it starts to ache. But when the pulp has been invaded, the fate of the tooth is generally sealed. After the spongy pulp collapses under bacterial attacks the tooth is devitalized—dead. The pressure of the pus and gas that form during the process of destruction makes the tooth feel very sore. If at this point the dentist can successfully clean out all the infected pulp and sterilize and plug the pulp chamber and the root canals, the tooth may last for a long time without giving trouble. But if the tooth is still neglected, the tragedy may, and usually does, close with a final act that is very painful for its owner.

The infection in the pulp chamber extends down the root canals and collects at the ends of the roots. The pus may push through the jawbone and gum to form a gumboil and drain into the mouth. Or it may remain concealed as an abscess at the roots of the tooth. Sometimes a hidden abscess may not cause pain or swelling of the face. It is, however, a focus of infection which drains into the blood and lymph vessels (like chronically infected tonsils or sinuses) and may be responsible, at least in part, for lowered physical resistance to arthritis or some other condition.

Referral to a dentist for an X-ray examination of the teeth is usually included in any thorough medical checkup of a child whose health is substandard. The X-ray machine has become an indispensable instrument in dental practice because it often shows up hidden abscesses, decay under fillings, impacted teeth, and many other abnormal dental conditions that can be detected in no other way.

Malocclusion

In looking at the picture of Evelyn (Plate 9) it is easy to see that she would be a pretty little girl if only her teeth came together properly. Malocclusion—the condition in which the upper and lower teeth do not occlude, or meet, correctly—may spoil a child's looks and interfere with happy adjustment to life. Also it may make adequate chewing and proper cleansing impossible and as a result favor tooth decay and gum inflammation.

Heredity plays an important part in determining the size and shape of the jaw, which in turn may influence the size, shape, and position of the teeth, and the relation of one jaw to the other. One often hears of a certain type of jaw as "running in the family." The best known example is the famous "Hapsburg jaw." In many cases there is not enough room in the jaw to accommodate all thirty-two teeth of the permanent set. Hence they erupt in a crooked position or become shifted from their normal places in the jaw during the growth period. If a tooth in the lower jaw is not in its proper place, the opposing tooth in the upper jaw also gets out of line.

The conditions under which the jaws develop and the teeth erupt may also favor malocclusion. Bad influences on growing jaws and teeth include:

1. Thumb-sucking, or biting the tongue, lips, or cheeks, if continued during the time that the permanent teeth begin to erupt
2. Failure to take proper care of the primary teeth
3. Losing the primary teeth too soon or keeping them too long; this often results in an irregular lineup of the permanent teeth
4. Failure to replace permanent teeth that have been extracted

The teacher who notices that a child has malocclusion and encourages the parents to get dental advice may make a valuable contribution to the child's future health and happiness. Besides checking faulty habits and giving needed dental care, the dentist may advise taking the child to an orthodontist, that is, a specialist in preventing and correcting malocclusion and irregularities of the teeth. The corrections may take some time and cause some inconvenience, but they are well worth while, because they will eventually give the child a normal chewing surface and at the same time greatly improve his appearance.

Gum Inflammations

Gingivitis is the general term used in referring to an inflammation of the gums (*gingivae*, in Latin). It is characterized by tender, inflamed spongy gums that bleed easily (the "pink toothbrush" syndrome). An inflamed condition of the gums can readily be observed and ought always to be brought to the attention of a physician.

One form of gingivitis is caused by a vitamin C deficiency. Although most dental authorities are now of the opinion that no single nutrient has more than a very small role in controlling the caries process, there is no question that ascorbic acid (vitamin C) is essential for healthy gums. Probably George (the boy shown in Plate 10) has not been getting enough Vitamin C.

Tartar. Another common cause of gum irritation is a deposit of tartar around the necks of the teeth. Tartar is a brownish or greenish incrustation formed by a mixture of calcium carbonate (chalk) and organic matter derived from saliva. It most often collects on neglected teeth, that is, teeth that are not brushed daily and are not given thorough prophylactic cleansings by a dentist or dental hygienist at regular intervals. Although tartar is not known to favor tooth decay, it does affect the health of the gums.

Other possible predisposing factors in the development of gingivitis include persistent wedging of food in crevices between the teeth, poor mouth hygiene, and defective dental fillings, crowns, and bridges.

Pyorrhea. A possible complication of neglected gingivitis is pyorrhea, a much more serious condition. The word pyorrhea is derived from the Greek words for "pus" and "flow," and means literally "a discharge of pus." It is now used almost exclusively to refer to an infection of the periodontal membrane, that is, the elastic tissue that connects the roots of the teeth with their bony sockets. If not checked, the infection spreads to the sockets themselves and the teeth become loosened and finally lost.

Gingivitis favors the development of pyorrhea because any gum inflammation, if neglected, spreads deeper into the tissues, becomes chronic, and provides a fertile field for the growth of the pus-producing germs. Active pyorrhea can be checked successfully by a dentist if it has not progressed too far, but some permanent damage to the tissues will result in almost every case. That is why prevention is doubly important.

Vincent's Infection. Vincent's infection is a fairly common infectious disease which most often attacks the gums but may also attack other parts of the mouth and throat. Its frequency among soldiers engaged in trench warfare in World War I gave it its popular name, trench mouth. Dental scientists now believe that Vincent's infection is caused by germs that are present even in healthy mouths. Anything that lowers the resistance of the mucous membrane, such as poor diet, loss of sleep, or uncleanliness of the mouth, paves the way for an attack by these germs.

In Vincent's infection the gums become swollen and sores covered with a whitish membrane appear. Children with this infection are usually referred to a dentist for treatment. The treatment may take some time but it usually ends in a cure. The patient should be impressed with the fact that he can help the dentist to get good results by following the diet and using the mouthwash that the dentist prescribes.

THE SCHOOL DENTAL HEALTH PROGRAM

Dental disease is almost universal, and no infallible means of preventing it have been found although the fluorides are proving helpful (see Fluorides in the Prevention of Dental Caries, in this chapter). Regular examinations by a dentist and dental treatment of the defects found hold out the best hopes at present for the control of serious tooth decay, malocclusion, and the premature loss of teeth. Observations by teacher and nurse will aid in the detection of gross dental defects, and inspection by a physician who uses a throat stick and flashlight in examining the mouth during a medical examination will reveal many that are less obvious. Experience has shown, however, that a high proportion of caries will be missed unless all children regularly receive a dental examination with mirror and explorer, supplemented, when advisable, by dental X rays. The American Dental Association recommends that each child be given such an examination by a dentist at least once a year.

The dental hygienist has a strategic place in the school health program. She is trained to make preliminary inspections of the teeth which are of great value in case finding. Her work of prophylactic cleansing, although it may not have much effect in reducing the incidence of caries, does help greatly in preventing gum troubles of various kinds and in improving personal appearance. Furthermore, she acts as liaison officer between the dentist and the classroom teacher in providing the teacher with information about the condition of the teeth of individual children and with material for dental health education.

The dental hygienist, the nurse serving the school, and the teacher working together can be of great service in promoting corrections through follow-up procedures. However, the teacher's most important job in the school dental program is that of presenting the story of what good dental care is and its importance in growth and development in ways that will motivate the child and his parents to go to the dentist regularly for dental examination and needed corrections.

FOR REVIEW AND DISCUSSION

1. Match each word or term in Group A with the word or group of words in Group B you associate with it:

Group A	Group B
Cheilosis 1	8 Gum inflammation
Herpes simplex 2	3 Salivary-gland infection
Mumps 3	9 Periodontal-membrane infection
Enamel 4	
Malocclusion 5	11 Living part of a tooth
Dental caries 6	4 Body of a tooth
Lactobacilli 7	2 Cold sores
Gingivitis 8	7 Production of enamel-dissolving acids
Pyorrhea 9	
Dentin 10	5 Failure of upper and lower teeth to meet properly
The pulp 11	1 Riboflavin deficiency
	6 Tooth decay
	10 Crown of a tooth

2. Select the correct ending for each one of the following incomplete sentences:

   a. The fluoridation of drinking water is valuable in preventive dentistry because it (1) destroys harmful bacteria in the water, (2) completely prevents dental caries, (3) reduces the incidence of dental caries.

   b. The factor chiefly responsible for the high incidence of dental caries in our country is (1) excessive consumption of sweet foods and drinks, (2) neglect of tooth brushing, (3) poor nutrition.

   c. Tooth decay begins (1) when bacteria reach the pulp of a tooth, (2) acids produced by lactobacilli dissolve the enamel of a tooth, (3) chewing hard foods wears away the dentin of a tooth.

3. Suppose you are on the affirmative side in debates on the following propositions:

   a. Resolved: that our community should fluoridate its water supply.

   b. Resolved: that our school system should employ a dental hygienist.

   Make an outline of the arguments you would use in favor of each proposition.

SELECTED REFERENCES

Best, C. H., and N. B. Taylor: *The Human Body* (first given as reference in Chap. 1). Part VI, *The Physiology of Digestion*, Chap. 25.

Dublin, Louis I.: *Water Fluoridation; Facts, Not Myths*, Public Affairs Pamphlet No. 251, Public Affairs Committee, Inc., New York.

Stoll, Frances A.: *Dental Health Education*, 2d ed., Lea & Febiger, Philadelphia, 1960.

Yahraes, Herbert: *Your Teeth—How to Save Them*, Public Affairs Pamphlet No. 147, Public Affairs Committee, Inc., New York.

Organizations

American Dental Association

Chapter 15   THE BODY'S ENVELOPE

Topography and Functions of the Skin, Hair,
*   and Nails*
Troublesome Conditions of the Skin, Hair,
*   and Nails*
Allergic Skin Reactions
Skin Infections
Skin Infestations

Normally the skin presents a relatively smooth, dry surface to the naked human eye. But an account of the travels of a mythical, ultramicroscopic pygmy wandering over the skin would include descriptions of mighty mountain ranges and deep valleys filled with pitfalls, of vast forests, of a wet, slippery terrain subject to sudden floods and quick unpredictable changes of climate, and of a highly varied fauna and flora. Some knowledge regarding the structure and functions of healthy skin will help teachers to understand what they see in observing various deviations from normal.

TOPOGRAPHY AND FUNCTIONS OF THE SKIN, HAIR, AND NAILS

The skin has three major jobs. First of all, it forms a tight-fitting elastic protective envelope for the body. When unbroken and healthy, it serves to keep blood and other essential body fluids in and foreign substances, including bacteria, out. The second job is the regulation of body temperature. The skin forms an essential part of the mechanism by which wanted heat is kept inside the body and excess heat is permitted to escape. The third job is to act as a receiving set for the stimuli that evoke the sensations of touch, pressure, stretch, pain, heat, and cold.

"Upon the Skin"

The part of the skin we see is the extremely thin top sheet of the epidermis. Strictly speaking, the epidermis has no proper name of its own, since its name means simply "upon the skin." From the top downward, the epidermis is built up of a horny layer and a layer of living epithelial cells sometimes called the germinative layer (see Fig. 15-1).

The horny layer consists of sheet upon sheet of flat, dry, inert scales closely packed together and overlapping like the shingles of a roof. As the existing top sheet is rubbed or scrubbed off, the one next below takes its place and so on while life lasts.

The horny layer never wears out because it is continually being re-
newed from its underside with new sheets formed of cells pushed up from
the germinative layer. The deepest row of cells in this living layer is attached to the dermis or true skin underneath. The cells of the germinative
layer are perpetually dividing. In this process the daughter cells are
crowded upward. During their upward journey the strong, living nucle-
ated cells become less and less virile as they get further away from their
source of nourishment. Finally they undergo a process of hornification
which changes their protoplasm into keratin, the substance of which the
sheets of the horny layer are composed.

The Coloring Matter of the Skin. The natural inherited color of the
skin depends upon the amount of pigment it contains. This pigment, or
coloring matter, is found chiefly in the germinative layer of the epidermis.
The amount of skin pigment is greater in some persons than in others and
also varies greatly in different races. The Negro's skin has a high concentration of pigment. The skins of American Indians, East Indians,
Chinese, and Japanese have less. The skins of the white races have the
least pigment, that of albinos none at all. The amount of skin pigment
varies not only in different people and in different skin areas of the same
person, but also from time to time.

Suntan and Freckles. In late spring, summer, and early fall light-
skinned children who have had a
chance to play outdoors in the
sun and wind will have coats of
tan or crops of freckles. Exposure
to the ultraviolet rays in sunlight
increases the deposits of pigment in the epidermis. These deposits act as a screen to protect
the more delicate structures underneath from further action of
the ultraviolet rays. In blond
children, especially redheads, the
pigment in the skin is unevenly
distributed. These children usually freckle instead of tan. They
are much more susceptible to
sunburn than are children whose
skins tan evenly. The redness of
sunburn is caused by the dilation
of the blood vessels of the skin by
histamine, which is released under the influence of ultraviolet
irradiation.

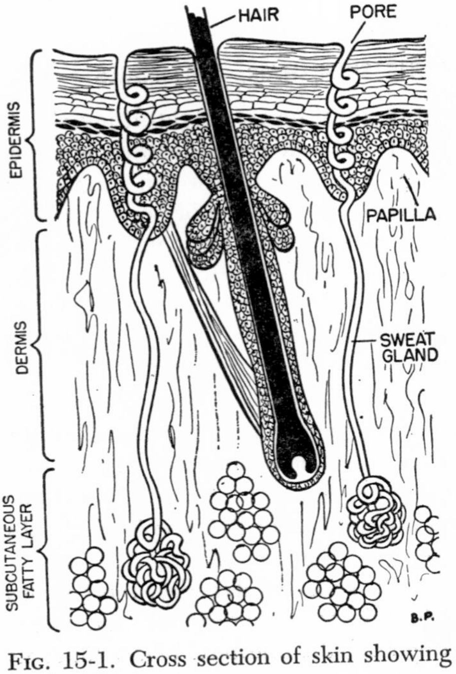

FIG. 15-1. Cross section of skin showing
its three layers.

True Skin

The dermis, or true skin, contains blood vessels, nerves, muscles, connective tissue, in short, all the structures that go to make up what we call "flesh." The surface of contact between the epidermis and the dermis is undulating rather than flat and smooth. Miniature conical peaks called papillae project upward from the upper face of the dermis and fit into corresponding hollows in the underface of the epidermis. This arrangement locks the two surfaces together so that the epidermis cannot easily be rubbed off.

Blisters. Sometimes fluid collects between the horny top layer of the skin and the layer underneath. When this occurs, the one is lifted away from the other. This is called a *blister.* Blisters frequently develop as a result of burns or mechanical rubbing or pinching. If the blister is filled with clear fluid—a water blister—the injury is confined to the epidermis. If it contains bloody fluid—a blood blister—we may be sure that the dermis also is involved, because there are no blood vessels whatever in the epidermis.

Unless there is danger that a blister may be accidentally ruptured, it is best to leave it alone until it dries. The intact horny layer of epidermis is the best protection from infection while a new horny layer is being manufactured to take its place.

Bruises. A bruise is caused by a fall or blow which ruptures the capillaries in the dermis without breaking the epidermis. The bruised area first looks red and swollen because the blood has oozed into the tissues. It becomes discolored—"black and blue" and later "green and yellow"—as the blood clots and is eventually absorbed.

Fingerprints. Minute ridges that are seen on the palms and the soles owe their existence to the fact that the papillae of the dermis are most prominent in these locations and are arranged in parallel rows. On the undersurfaces of the fingers and toes the papillary ridges form whorls which are peculiar for each individual. That is why the fingerprints are a valuable means of identification.

How the Skin Is Fed. The skin is nourished with materials brought to it by the blood circulating through the networks of capillaries enmeshed in the dermis. It is impossible to puncture the dermis anywhere without drawing blood. The living cells in the lower layers of the bloodless epidermis are nourished with food materials in the lymph or tissue fluid, which percolates up from the dermis. We are all familiar with the dewiness and bloom of well-nourished youthful skin as distinguished from the thin, dry, splotchy skin often associated with illness or aging.

Mucous Membrane. In the soft, moist skin that lines the eyelids, the lips and mouth, and all body tubes and cavities, the dermis is thinner and more loosely built than elsewhere, and the epidermis has no horny surface layer. Hence the red color from the underlying blood vessels shows through more clearly. This modified skin is called mucous membrane.

Observing Changes in Skin Color

Normally, there is a wide variation in skin color apart from that due to pigment. There is a tendency amounting almost to an obsession in some of us to think of rosy cheeks in white-skinned children as denoting good health and of pale cheeks as indicating poor health. Yet many healthy children in whom the epidermis is comparatively thick or heavily pigmented may have a naturally creamy, sallow, or olive complexion with little or no pink in the cheeks. The color of the skin in any individual is not a static thing, however. It registers the play of emotions and of physical ups and downs as the color of water registers the effects of sunshine or shadow or the ruffling wind.

Influences of Blood Circulation on Skin Color. Changes in skin color depend largely upon changes in the circulation of blood in the skin. The skin's blood supply (see Fig. 15-2) is influenced by the number and arrangement of the blood vessels in the dermis, the amount of blood in the blood vessels, and the character of the blood itself.

As the arterioles approach the bases of the papillae in the topmost layer of the dermis, they shed their muscle coats and form capillary loops. The arterial branch of each capillary loop ascends into a papilla, makes a hairpin turn, and descends as the venous branch. Upon reaching the base of the papilla the venous branch joins with the venous branches of other capillary loops in the neighborhood to form a venule. The venules unite with one another to form a rich network which runs horizontally beneath the bases of the papillae. The venous networks drain into deeper veins.

When the blood vessels of the skin are dilated or widened, they can hold far more blood than when they are constricted or tightened up. Hence the intensity of the skin color will be deeper when the blood vessels are dilated, lighter when they are constricted.

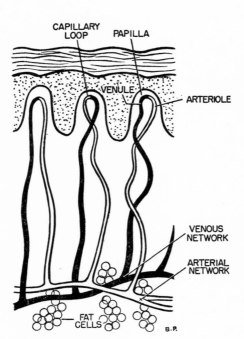

Fig. 15-2. The arrangement of blood vessels in the dermis.

The red color of the blood is intensified when the hemoglobin in its red cells is rich in oxygen. After the hemoglobin has given up part of its oxygen in the tissues, the blood takes on a bluish shade—becomes duskier. When the flow of blood through the blood vessels near the surface of the skin is rapid, there is not so much chance for the hemoglobin to give up its oxygen. Then the hue of the skin will be reddish. When the flow is slow, the amount of oxygen given up will be increased considerably. Then the hue will be slightly bluish. Hence the hue or tint of the skin at any time will depend upon the rapidity with which the blood is coursing through the cutaneous blood vessels.

Formation of Wheals. The small blood vessels of the skin are extremely sensitive to stimulation by mechanical and other agencies. If a blunt-pointed instrument is drawn lightly over the skin of the forearm, a white line will quickly appear along the path taken by the instrument. This "white reaction," as it is called, is caused by the contraction of the capillary walls. If the instrument is drawn more firmly over the skin a red line instead of a white line appears. This "red reaction" is caused by the dilation of the capillaries. An unusually strong stimulus, like a slap, calls nervous mechanisms into play and the arterioles dilate, with the result that there is a spreading flush or flare surrounding the path of the stroke.

A still more intense stimulus, like severe whipping, raises wheals on the skin. Wheals are white elevated patches that follow the red reaction in two or three minutes and are surrounded by the red flare. They are due to increased permeability of the capillary walls which permits fluid from the blood to seep into the tissues. Hence wheals are a localized edema. They disappear as the fluid disappears into wider areas of the skin. The stimulus of an allergen from within may raise wheals similar to those caused by a strong mechanical stimulus from without (see Scratch Tests and Intradermal Tests—for allergy—in Chap. 7; and Urticaria further on in this chapter).

Normal Temporary Changes in Skin Color. Almost everyone has had the experience of temporarily "changing color"—flushing with embarrassment or getting red from exercise, or white with rage or fear, or blue with cold. These temporary changes in skin color take place, as we have seen, when the blood vessels in the dermis dilate or contract in response to temperature changes, increased physical activity, or strong emotions.

Observant teachers will notice that there are wide temperamental variations in the rapidity with which different white-skinned children change color in response to emotional stimuli. Some children normally change color very little or not at all. At the other extreme is the occasional child who changes color rapidly. He blushes at the slightest compliment or criticism, or turns pale when only mildly annoyed or frightened. Such a child may have "nervous blood vessels." He is likely to suffer from temperature changes and have frequent colds.

Abnormal Changes in Skin Color. The observant teacher quickly becomes familiar with normal skin color and tone in her children. Reference has already been made to several common changes in color, such as unnatural pallor, blueness, and a yellow hue which are associated with illness. Abnormal color is rarely the only sign of trouble. Almost always it is accompanied by other signs and symptoms, such as lassitude or drowsiness, complaints of feeling ill (malaise), circles under the eyes, sore throat, excessive underweight or overweight, and fatigue posture. The skin of a child returning to school after an illness is quite likely to look pale or sallow and flabby or doughy, both from the effects of the illness and from the confinement indoors (see Plate 2).

Feverish Flushing. Besides the healthy flushing of the skin on a hot day or during vigorous exercise or as the result of embarrassment, the skin is usually flushed when any form of fever is present. In a number of acute infectious diseases—scarlet fever and measles, for example—the skin becomes red in patches. Such patchy flushing is called a rash. Rashes typical of different acute infections (see Sec. 1, Appendix B) rarely appear at the onset of the disease. The teacher is much more likely to be alerted to the need for medical attention by earlier signs and symptoms than to be presented with a rash as the first warning that something is wrong.

The Skin's Secretory Apparatus

In looking at the skin through a powerful magnifying glass, it is possible to see small openings known as pores. The pores are the outlet of deep-rooted sweat and oil glands.

The Sweat Glands. The total number of sweat glands is about two million. From each one a long duct, which is spirally twisted like a corkscrew as it passes through the epidermis, leads to the surface of the skin. Although the secretion of sweat is continuous, it is seldom noticed because it evaporates faster than it is produced (insensible perspiration). Either increased heat production within the body or a rise in environmental temperature calls for increased sweating as a means of stepping up the amount of body heat lost through evaporation (see Reaction to Internal Temperature Changes, in Chap. 7). When sweat does not evaporate as fast as it is secreted, it becomes visible in the form of drops standing on, or running off, the oily surface of the skin (sensible perspiration).

The Sebaceous Glands. The oily coating of the skin comes from sebaceous (fat) glands lodged in the dermis, or true skin. Occasionally their ducts open directly upon the surface of the skin. More frequently they open into the hair folliciles, and their secretion passes out to the skin surface along the hairs. The fat glands connected with the hair follicles are called pilosebaceous glands (*pilo*, meaning "hair," plus *sebaceous*, meaning "fatty"). Sebum, as the secretion of the fat glands is called, is squeezed slowly out of the glands by pressure exerted across them by minute strands of the "hair-raising" muscles, much as toothpaste is squeezed out of a tube by the pressure of the fingers on the tube. The function of sebum is to keep the skin and hair soft, pliable, and waterproof. In smooth velvety skins the amount of sebum, or oil, secreted is just about right—not too little, not too much. But many individuals have skin that is either too dry or too oily. Fair, "thin-skinned" children are the ones who are most likely to have dry skin. Also dryness of the skin is sometimes associated with a nutritional deficiency.

The Fatty Layer of the Skin

The subcutaneous, or fatty, layer of the skin serves as the connecting link between the dermis above and the tissues below. It acts as a shock absorber against possible injury caused by falls or blows and as an insulating material. It furnishes rotundity to body contours, which is considered advantageous or disadvantageous depending upon its quantity and its distribution.

The tone of the skin—its firmness and texture—depends partly on the cushion of fat below the dermis and partly on the elastic fibers in the skin itself. The elasticity of the skin can easily be observed by pinching up the skin between thumb and finger and then releasing it. This elasticity is not so great, however, that it can accommodate itself to considerable variations in tension. If a plump person loses a great deal of weight, for example, his skin does not retract, or shrink, and become as smooth and tense as it was before. Hence, it tends to look baggy or wrinkled.

The wrinkled, thin, overstretched skin in old age is usually due both to the depletion of subcutaneous fat and to loss of elasticity from the skin. In healthy, well-nourished children the skin looks smooth and firm, and the body is pleasantly rounded, with curves rather than sharp angles.

The Hair

Hair and nails are appendages of the skin. Hair is found in all regions of the skin except that of the palms, the soles, the lips, and the backs of the fingertips and toetips. There are three kinds of hair: (1) the short, soft, downy hairs usually seen on the face, trunk, and limbs; (2) short, strong, or bristly hairs such as those of the eyebrows and eyelashes; (3) and the long hairs of the scalp, beard, armpits, and pubic region.

How Hair Grows. The follicles, or sockets, out of which hair grows are formed by a dipping down of the epidermis into the dermis (see Fig. 15-3). The part of the hair showing above the surface of the skin is the hair shaft and the part contained within the follicle is the hair root. The lower end of the root, which is thicker than the upper part, is the hair bulb. The bottom end of the hair bulb fits like a snug cap over a tiny mound containing blood vessels which is called the hair papilla. For a short distance above the hair papilla the hair is a mass of succulent living

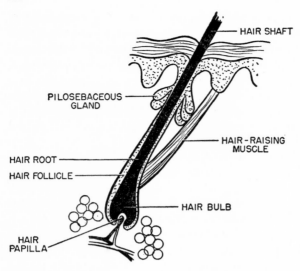

PILOSEBACEOUS GLAND

HAIR-RAISING MUSCLE

HAIR ROOT

HAIR FOLLICLE

HAIR BULB

HAIR PAPILLA

HAIR SHAFT

FIG. 15-3. One hair and the structures that oil and move it.

cells similar to that of the surrounding dermis. The cells in dividing and multiplying push upward. As they move farther and farther away from the papillae from which they get their nourishment, they become horny like the upper layer of the epidermis.

Gooseflesh. A tiny muscle is attached to each slanting hair follicle. As we have seen, the pressure of strands of this muscle upon the sebaceous gland draining into the hair follicle distributes sebum over the hair shaft. When stimulated by cold or fear, the muscle pulls the slanting hair follicle erect. The result is the puckering of the skin known as gooseflesh.

Gooseflesh is a survival from a time when human beings had more body hair than they do now and could increase their protection from cold by erecting it. Many mammals and birds can do this. For example, the sight of sparrows perched with their feathers ruffled is a familiar one in city parks on a cold day. The sensation of the hair lifting on the scalp at moments of extreme fright gave rise to the expression, "his hair stood on end," in describing terror-stricken behavior. Gooseflesh is a common accompaniment of the shivering and chattering of the teeth which occur when the body is chilled as a result of very cold atmospheric temperature or in a disturbance of the body's heat-control mechanism at the onset of an infectious fever (see Fever, in Chap. 7).

Shape, Color, and Texture of Hair. The natural shape and color of each person's hair are determined by heredity. The narrow slanting follicles mold the hair into shape as the roots push up through them. If the follicle is cylindrical, the hair will be round and straight; if the follicle is oval or flattish, the hair will be flattened and curly, kinky, or wavy.

The color of the hair is due mainly to varying amounts of pigment granules present in the hair shaft. The pigment granules are deposited in the hair as pigment-containing cells in the hair bulb wander upward and die. The color of the horny substance of the hair itself is yellow. According to the amount of pigment mixed with it, hair color will range from platinum blond to coal black. Light hair tends to grow darker after childhood. The presence of tiny air bubbles in the central portion of the hair shaft also may affect hair color, especially in contributing toward "platinum blond," gray, or white hair. How air bubbles get into the hair shaft is not yet known. It is presumably owing to a rapid evolution of air bubbles that "sudden graying of the hair" is produced.

Hair varies in texture as well as in shape and color. Hair texture may be as coarse as a horse's mane or as "fine as silk." Redheads have the coarsest hair, and blonds the finest.

In addition to noting inherited differences in the shape, color, and texture of hair, we see also the effects of variations in grooming and in style of hairdo on appearance. But whatever may be the normal variations on the theme of hair, all healthy, well-cared-for hair has something in common. It is clean and glossy; it has a shine; it looks alive. Many departures from good health may be first evidenced by changes in the texture and amount of hair because the nutrition of the hair, like that of the skin, depends upon the adequate functioning of other organs of the body. (See Troublesome Conditions of the Skin, Hair, and Nails further on.)

The Life Span of Hair. The hair of the scalp grows about 4 or 5 inches a year. There is a very wide variation in the length of life of individual hairs—from six months to four years. When a hair reaches the end of its life span it becomes detached from the papilla and falls out, to be replaced by a new one growing from the same papilla.

Fingernails and Toenails

Nails protect the tips of the fingers and toes, and fingernails help in the picking up of things. The growth of fingernails and toenails is much like that of hair. At the base of the nail the epidermis folds under to form a slot which corresponds to the hair follicle. Out of this slot the nail grows from a collection of living cells called the matrix. The half-moon at the base of the nails represents the upper limit of the matrix. The cells of the matrix are continually being pushed outward by new cells forming behind them. Gradually their food supply is cut off, with the result that they are changed to horny plates. Beyond the matrix the nail rests on the nail bed, over which it is pushed as the cells in the matrix divide and multiply.

TROUBLESOME CONDITIONS OF THE SKIN, HAIR, AND NAILS

The skin, at least of the face and hands, and its appendages, hair and fingernails, are practically always open for observation. What can be learned from the skin and its appendages depends upon observing them from several different points of view. This section is devoted to various conditions and defects more or less closely associated with their structure or function.

Skin Troubles

Vesicles and Pimples. Small blisters, not larger than a split pea, are called vesicles. Usually the skin around a vesicle is red, in which case it may look like a small dewdrop on a rose petal, but occasionally the red area is lacking. The formation of vesicles is associated with many different conditions—for example, small burns, sunburn, chicken pox, and ivy or oak poisoning or other forms of dermatitis.

Pimples are small, solid elevations of the skin, sometimes called papules. Pimples usually begin as a result of irritation and pressure from the waxy plugs obstucting the flow of sebum from the fat glands. These plugs have much the same effect as any foreign body in the skin, a splinter, for example. It is easy for germs to get in under the plugs of sebum and start an infection. When infected pimples or vesicles become filled with yellowish pus, they are called pustules.

Blackheads and Whiteheads. Blackheads, or comedones, are simply hard plugs of sebum and other debris protruding from blocked fat-gland ducts. Their blackness is caused by oxidation of that portion of the plug which is exposed to air and not by negligence in face washing as is popularly supposed. A whitehead, or milium, is white because the gland involved has no excreting duct and so the tip of the waxy plug is not exposed to oxidation.

Oily Skin. In oily skins the texture of the skin is usually coarse, the pores large, and the face and hair greasy. Hence, an oily skin is a handicap because it detracts from personal appearance and predisposes the skin to many troublesome conditions such as acne and boils.

Young people who have excessively oily skins should learn that they cannot change the texture of their skins, but they can do a great deal to improve their appearance by proper care of the face. Following the directions for cleaning the face given below in the section on adolescent acne will be helpful for young people troubled with an oily skin.

Acne. The signs of acne—blackheads, whiteheads, oily skin, distended pores, pimples, and scars of healed pimples—singly or all together make up the picture of acne. No wonder that boys or girls troubled with acne may be left with worse scars on the psyche than on the face!

Unfortunately acne disfigures the complexion at the very time when an attractive appearance counts the most. Young people afflicted with it worry inordinately about their bumpy, pimple-studded faces and are likely to pick at or squeeze blackheads and pimples in an attempt to get rid of them. Understanding teachers can do a great deal to help these troubled young people by giving them the facts about acne.

During adolescence, hormones secreted by the gonads or sex glands activate the pilosebaceous glands (see The Sebaceous Glands in this chapter) of the face, chest, and back which are relatively inactive during infancy and childhood. While this is going on, the ducts of the pilosebaceous glands and their external outlets may not enlarge fast enough to take care of the increased production of sebum. Or the hair-raising muscles may be too weak to squeeze out the sebum fast enough. Or an alteration in the viscosity of the sebum itself may contribute to its stagnation within the glands or their ducts. As a result, at least some breaking out of the face, if only an occasional pimple, is common during adolescence. That is why this skin condition is often called "adolescent acne."

It may be of some comfort to young people to learn that acne is a temporary condition in the great majority of cases. Just as soon as the fat-gland ducts and their outlets grow large enough to take care of the increased secretion of sebum, the acne will clear up. But it is not necessary to wait for that happy event. A young person should know that his regular doctor or a skin specialist can do much to improve his present appearance and spirits and to prevent permanent scars. Also there are many things he can do to help himself.

One of the most important helps is to keep the hands away from the face at all times except when washing it. In persons with acne who sit with the face resting on the hand, it has been observed that the acne is most pronounced where the hand touches the skin, because the heat of the hand increases sebaceous secretion. Also contact of the fingers with the face leads to picking at or squeezing pimples until they break. This practice serves to spread the infective matter with which they are filled. Wherever this material is "planted"—on the skin near the original pimple or on some other part touched with soiled fingers—another pimple may grow. Also squeezing fingers may serve to spread infective material into the surrounding tissues. When this happens the pimple may become larger and harder to get rid of and eventually leave an ugly scar. As a means of breaking the habit of picking at the face, physicians often tell their young patients to avoid looking into a mirror until the face has improved.

Another great help is to keep as healthy as possible. If there is any condition that is keeping a youngster below par, sinusitis or infected tonsils, for example, a doctor should be consulted. Also vigorous outdoor exercise, adequate sleep, fresh air, and sunshine are all important. Acne nearly always improves in the summer time. This improvement is supposed to be due to the action on the skin of the ultraviolet rays in summer sunlight.

Making sure that the daily diet contains enough of all the essential food elements is another thing young people can do. No special vitamins, however, will prevent or cure acne; *all* are important for the health of the skin.

Certain foods have a bad effect on acne in some individuals but not in others. For some, the greatest offender is chocolate. This means chocolate in any form—in ice cream, cake, pastry, candy, and beverages (chocolate malteds, hot chocolate, chocolate ice cream sodas, and cola drinks). A young person troubled with acne should be encouraged to "swear off" chocolate for a trial period anyway. Other prime offenders are nuts, sharp cheese, and rich fatty foods. It seems logical to assume that, if more oil than usual is being formed by the fat glands of the skin, it is wise to decrease the amount of fat in the food eaten. The only way a young person can tell whether a particular food is making his acne worse is to stop eating it for a week or two and see whether any improvement takes place.

Skin cleanliness is the third great help in controlling acne. It stands to reason that keeping the pores and hair-follicle openings cleared of debris will promote better drainage of sebum. A young person troubled with acne should wash his face, using soap or a detergent, for as many times a day as is necessary to keep it free of oiliness. He may need to do this three times a day, or six, or even more. A dry, oil-free skin recovers from acne much more quickly than does an oily one.

A doctor can be of great help when acne is especially bothersome. He may prescribe a lotion or ointment to be applied to the face after a cool rinse. If he wishes the patient to keep the lotion on his face night and day he may prescribe one that matches the color of the skin. Cosmetics especially prepared for cases of acne are available, but a doctor should specify which one to choose. Ordinary face powders and creams or face lotions containing fat or oil should be avoided because they may further clog the oil-gland ducts.

Warts. A wart is an overgrowth of epidermal cells which does not break through the thin dividing line between the epidermis and the underlying true skin. It is roughened, like a cauliflower, and grayish or blackish in color. Warts are much more common in girls than in boys. The reason for this is unknown. Two-thirds of the cases occur in girls and boys from eleven to fifteen years of age.

It has been known for some years that warts are caused by a virus. They often appear in crops. Also, one or two warts may be followed by others through self-inoculation. For example, a row of warts sometimes develops along a scratch on the hand on which other warts are present. Combing the hair, shaving, and similar acts also may transplant the virus from one location to another.

The question, "How easily can the virus of warts be spread from one person to another?" has not been satisfactorily answered. Dermatologists report, however, that they often see several members of one family with warts. Also warts on the soles of the feet sometimes occur among school children almost in epidemics. Warts in this location are very painful because of the pressure exerted on them in walking.

The peculiar thing about some warts is the suddenness with which they appear and disappear. This has led to innumerable superstitions regarding their treatment. Any hocus-pocus may seem to succeed in a condition that naturally disappears as if by magic.

Warts are not dangerous except in the rarest instances. If they are uncomfortable or unsightly, medical treatment will give relief.

Moles. Moles belong to a class of skin blemishes called nevi (singular, nevus). Actually they are small birthmarks consisting of collections of densely packed skin cells which are brown or black in color because they contain more pigment than ordinary skin cells. Almost everyone has one or more moles. In the great majority of cases they are not dangerous or disfiguring—indeed, they were once called "beauty marks." The custom of wearing tiny black patches to accentuate some alluring facial line or dimple may have had its origin in observations of the pleasing effect of fortunately placed moles.

There are, however, many kinds of moles, and some of them may constitute cosmetic blemishes that will worry youngsters as they grow up, or may develop later into malignant growths. Any mole, but more particularly the black or blue-black variety, is potentially dangerous if it is located in a place where it is subject to frequent irritation. Young people should learn to leave moles alone—not to pick at them or try to remove them with caustics. If they wish to get rid of a mole or birthmark because of its unsightliness, they should be advised to consult a physician—preferably a dermatologist—not a beauty specialist. When a mole, either spontaneously or as a result of friction or other injury, shows signs of irritation, or change of color, or further growth, competent medical advice and care should be sought at once.

Chapping. In dry-skinned children, especially, chapping in cold weather is often troublesome. Chapping is a familiar form of inflammation of the skin, or dermatitis, to give it its technical name. It does not ordinarily occur in warm weather because at that time the sebaceous and sweat glands are most active and keep the skin thoroughly oiled.

In chapping, the skin first gets red and tender with some scaling, and then develops painful cracks and fissures. Like leather, skin cannot stand up when dry under conditions that it easily endures when properly oiled. Failure to dry the skin throughly after washing and before going outdoors favors chapping, because the rapid evaporation of the water by the dry cold air of winter causes sudden dryness of the skin.

To prevent or relieve chapping, children susceptible to it should learn to dry their hands and faces thoroughly and then to rub in cold cream, petroleum jelly, or any other bland oil such as olive oil or mineral oil. The use of superfatted toilet soap instead of ordinary soap may be suggested.

Chilblains and Frostbite. Exposure to cold damp weather also may produce chilblains on the fingers, toes, heels, or ears of some children. Chilblains are painful red spots which itch intensely, especially in a warm room. The redness is due to congestion of the skin capillaries. Chilblains sometimes develop when the frozen area of the skin is thawed out too quickly in frostbite.

In case of frostbite the frozen part should be warmed quickly by immersing it in lukewarm (*not hot*) water. Outside heat from a hot-water bottle, heat lamp, or radiator should *not* be applied as this may result in the rupture of blood vessels and the development of gangrene. After thawing occurs in frozen fingers or toes, the child should be encouraged to exercise them.

Hair and Fingernail Troubles

Dry Hair and Oily Hair. Dry, lusterless hair is due to a lack or shortage of oil deliveries from the pilosebaceous glands of the scalp. This condition may be natural in dry-skinned children. But it is important to observe and report changes from customary sleekness or glossiness to a condition of dryness, coarseness, brittleness, and lack of luster. Vitamin A deficiency and an acute or chronic illness are among the factors that may be responsible for producing these changes.

Flat, greasy hair is due to an overproduction of natural hair oil. This condition is often seen during adolescence as an accompaniment of acne. Frequent shampoos are necessary to remove the excess oil.

Simple Dandruff. Both in excessive dryness and in excessive oiliness of the scalp, dandruff may be especially bothersome. Simple dandruff is the constant scaling off of the topmost horny layer of the epidermis of the scalp. It is the same sort of scaling as that which goes on less noticeably from other areas of the skin. Almost everyone at one time or another has been annoyed by the showers of untidy little dandruff flakes that are so noticeable on the collars and shoulders of dark-colored coats and dresses. If the scalp is very oily the flakes are usually moist and sticky and hence difficult to brush off. Aside from appearance, there is nothing to worry about in simple dandruff of the dry or sticky variety. Usually it can be controlled by keeping the hair clean and well brushed. However, a persistently greasy, scaly scalp which itches constantly calls for medical investigation.

Falling Hair. The normal cycle of hair growth (see How Hair Grows earlier in this chapter) may be interrupted by sickness or complications resulting from neglect or abuse. Excessive falling out of a child's hair should always be brought to the physician's attention. However, a moderate amount of hair shedding is to be expected. Normally, one may lose as many as fifty to one hundred hairs a day.

Fingernail Defects. The white spots that sometimes appear in the fingernails are usually formed by bubbles of air between the cell layers. They may have no significance or may be caused by injury to the nail or by a nutritional deficiency. Severe injury to the matrix may cause loss of the nail, but if the lower layers of living cells are not destroyed, a new nail will be formed.

Any abnormal brownish or whitish discoloration or grooving or pitting of the fingernails, or nails that curve over the ends of the fingers, should be called to the attention of the nurse or physician.

Hangnails. The thick skin around the nail is called the cuticle. It is imperfectly oiled and for this reason cracks easily. The urge to pick at or bite a cracked or rough cuticle is hard to resist, and that is why hangnails are such common afflictions.

Children should learn how to care for their nails, both for the sake of appearance and to prevent the formation of hangnails. A little cold cream or oil rubbed into the cuticle from time to time helps to keep it soft and smooth. It is also helpful to keep the cuticle pushed back from the nail. This may be done easily with the blunt end of an orange stick when the cuticle is soft after a bath. If hangnails form they should be removed with sharp, clean manicure scissors, taking care to cause no bleeding.

Nail-biting. It has been found that nail-biting, far from being just a bad habit, is often used unconsciously by a child as an outlet for some suppressed emotion—aggression, for example. Also, nail-biting has frequently been observed in irritable, restless children whose trouble is a nutritional deficiency. Children who persistently bite their nails need thorough medical study.

ALLERGIC SKIN REACTIONS

The skin or the walls of the skin capillaries is the shock tissue in many forms of allergy (see Allergic Reactions, in Chap. 7). Any child who is subject to skin inflammations, puzzling rashes, hives, and so on, which suggest sensitivity to one or more substances, needs careful study by a physician to determine the cause or causes. Besides taking the child's history and giving a complete and thorough physical examination, the physician will perform a series of skin tests for the purpose of determining sensitivity to various suspected substances.

The most common forms of allergy involving the skin are contact dermatitis, eczema, and urticaria (hives).

Contact Dermatitis

The form of allergic skin reaction known as contact dermatitis takes place when a substance to which a person is sensitive comes in contact with the skin. The cells of the epidermis swell and fluid forms between them. The characteristic manifestations are redness, vesicle formation, and itching. "Weeping" occurs as the vesicles break. Itching leads to scratching and further skin injury.

A great many different substances which are harmless to most people cause contact dermatitis in some people. Examples are clothing dyes, cosmetics, toilet preparations, matches, newsprint, shoe polish, insecticides, materials used in cleaning or dyeing furs, and materials used in stuffing mattresses, pillows, and upholstered furniture. Plant oils such as those of poison ivy, poison oak, and poison sumac cause contact dermatitis in most people.

Eczema

The term *eczema* comes from a Greek word meaning "boiling out." The allergen, or causative agent, responsible is brought to the skin by the blood. Fluid seeps into the tissues through the capillary walls. The signs of eczema are redness, papule formation, itching, and a watery discharge which tends to dry into scales and crusts. These signs are so much like those of many other skin diseases, however, that actually no form of dermatitis is called eczema unless similar conditions have been ruled out by painstaking medical examination.

The allergens in eczema are usually various proteins present in eggs, milk, cereals, and other foods rich in proteins. Less commonly they are inhalants, such as pollens, animal danders, house dust, and other airborne substances. Many other factors, besides specific allergens, may be involved both in predisposing a person to eczema and in perpetuating it. That is why eczema may persist even when an offending substance (or substances) has been discovered and removed.

Urticaria

The term *urticaria* is derived from the Latin word for "nettle," probably because grasping a stinging nettle results in the raising on the skin of lumps or wheals similar to urticaria.

As in eczema, the shock tissue is the walls of the skin capillaries. The allergen is brought to the skin by the blood, and fluid seeps into the skin tissues through the capillary walls. Urticaria is characterized by the sudden development of wheals ranging in size from a dot to a dime or larger. The wheals may run together forming huge irregular welts. They are usually whiter than the surrounding skin, but may be pink in color, and itch, sting, or burn intensely. They usually last for only a short time— from several minutes to a few hours—and disappear as rapidly as they appeared.

The allergen responsible for the development of hives is usually a food, such as shellfish, pork, cheese, butter, eggs, strawberries, mushrooms, and tomatoes. Less frequently it may be a drug, especially opium, morphine, or penicillin; a serum injection if the person has been sensitized to the animal serum used; or an inhalant.

SKIN INFECTIONS

The outermost horny layer of the skin of every human being at any one time is covered by a vast flora and fauna in the form of microorganisms, or germs, of various families. Some are transients picked up on things touched with the bare hands or other exposed areas of the skin; others are more or less permanent residents. Some families are harmful; others are not. Some are harmful only when they are present in unusually large numbers, or when one group gangs up with another group, or when the previously established balance of one group with other groups is upset. Some germs are able to do harm only when the biologic defenses of the skin falter, or when the epidermis is broken, as in a cut or raw blister, or when its impenetrability is weakened.

The acidity of the skin is disagreeable to many bacteria and fungi which do not thrive in an acid medium. Sebum, which gives the skin its oily coat, and perspiration, which gives it its moist one, are responsible

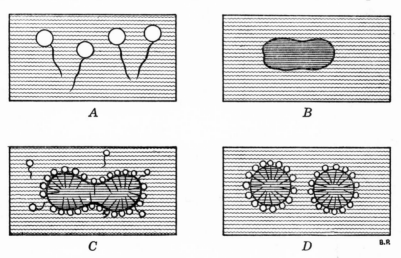

FIG. 15-4. The emulsifying action of soap.

A. A soap molecule. Its head dissolves in water but not in oil. Its tail dissolves in oil but not in water.
B. A drop of oil surrounded by water.
C. The tails of the soap molecules dissolve in the oil and split it into droplets.
D. The heads remain on the outside of the droplets and keep them from coalescing.

for the fact that the surface of the skin has an acid reaction. Perspiration is in itself slightly acid, and the decomposition of sebum, which is continually going on, yields acids.

Skin-dwelling microorganisms lead a precarious existence. They barely get established when the terrain that they occupy lifts, separates from the new horny layer next below, and is shed. With the constant scaling off of the epidermis, myriads of germs are removed from the skin. This process is expedited considerably whenever the skin is washed with soap and water (see Fig. 15-4). The rubbing and scrubbing mechanically loosens the dirty worn top sheet of the epidermis, and the warm soapy water breaks up its oily coating into tiny oil droplets and keeps them from coalescing again. The latter process is called emulsification. The oil droplets containing tatters of skin and the particles of dirt and germs adhering to them are held in the lather or suds and can be easily flushed off.

Although soap in itself may kill several different kinds of harmful germs, everyone seems to agree that the principal way in which soap and water help to fight them is by the ability of this combat team to reduce their numbers simply by loosening and rinsing away the top sheet of the epidermis upon which they have established themselves.

Staphylococcal and Streptococcal Skin Infections

Of all the bacterial families that pick quarrels with the skin, the staphylococci and streptococci (see Classes of Pathogens, in Chap. 7) are the most frequent offenders. More than any other bacteria, streptococci have a tendency to act as accomplices of other pathogenic (disease-causing) microorganisms; that is, they often help, or are helped by, some other family of bacteria or viruses in setting up infection. On the skin the favorite allies of the streptococci are the staphylococci. There they live in such close harmony that whenever one is caught in the act of doing mischief, the other is almost sure to be found also. Injury to, or lowered resistance of, the skin greatly favors the development of infections caused by this infamous team.

Successful invasion and effective occupation of the skin at various levels by streptococcal-staphylococcal troops result in a great variety of skin infections. The two that are most commonly found in children of school age are impetigo contagiosa and furunculosis.

Impetigo Contagiosa. The name *impetigo* comes from the Latin verb meaning to "attack," and *contagiosa* is added to signify that impetigo is highly contagious, or "catching." In most cases the infectious agent is *Staphylococcus aureus,* but in some cases hemolytic streptococci alone or in combination with staphylococci may be responsible. Although impetigo may affect persons of any age, children seem to be most susceptible to it.

The lesions, or sores, of impetigo appear mostly on the face (especially at the corners of the mouth, nose, and ears) and on the hands. Occasionally they are widely scattered over the body. Any break in the continuity of the skin, including a scratch or an area from which adhesive tape has been removed, may become infected.

The lesions arise on highly inflamed skin areas from which a thick, sticky yellow or brown liquid oozes (Plate 11). Scabs or crusts are built up as this purulent liquid dries on the sore and on the surrounding skin. As the lesions cause intense itching, the crusts may contain blood drawn in the act of scratching to relieve the itch. The dried blood gives the crusts a black or dark-brown discoloration. Eventually the epidermis of the affected areas is lifted completely off its base, as in blistering, and the crusts are shed. The naked dermis thus exposed looks painfully red and "weepy."

It is important for teachers to know that impetigo is spread not only by direct contact with the lesions but also indirectly by handling anything that the infected child has handled. "Anything" includes pencils, paper, schoolbooks, doorknobs, desk or table tops, towels, and many other objects touched or handled in the course of the school day. Whether the child evidently has a skin infection or not, he should learn to be careful about keeping exclusively for his own use all articles that he personally owns. If he has impetigo or some other infectious skin disease, he should know that it is necessary to keep his fingers away from the lesions both to prevent spread of the infection to other regions of his own body and to protect others.

In some school systems children are excluded from school until the sores have healed. Usually healing occurs after only a few days of vigorous treatment. Red spots may remain on the skin for some time after the sores have healed and the danger of infection is past. Such spots disappear gradually as the epidermis returns to its normal thickness.

A child with impetigo should be under the care of a physician. Neither the parents, the school nurse, the teacher, nor any other lay person should attempt to treat this disease without medical advice. There are several reasons for this:

1. Other more serious skin infections or serious systemic diseases may be accompanied by lesions similar to those of impetigo. The sooner such conditions are recognized by the physician, the better are the chances of successful treatment.

2. Long-lasting impetigo may sensitize the child to staphylococci. Since these bacteria are very prevalent, heightened susceptibility to them may have serious consequences.

3. The physician is best able to teach the child and his parents what they must do to lessen the danger of spreading the infection.

In this connection it is worth saying that impetigo is a medical problem and not a socioeconomic one. No one in any status of life is immune from it, and no child who has it should be made to feel that it is disgraceful.

There are very effective ointments for the treatment of impetigo. The choice of ointment and the method of removing the crusts should be left to the physician in each case. For cases that appear to be alike, directly opposing measures may be indicated.

Furuncles. Practically everyone at one time or another has had a boil. The scientific name for boil is furuncle (from the Latin *furunculus,* meaning "petty thief"). Properly speaking, every localized staphylococcal infection that starts within the tiny openings of the sweat gland ducts or sebaceous gland ducts is a furuncle. Names vary, however, according to the size or locality of the furuncle. A boil on the eyelid margins, for example, is called a sty (see Sties, in Chap. 16); a very small furuncle is usually called a pimple; a large and extensive one, including several hair follicles, is called a carbuncle (from the Latin *carbunculus,* meaning "little coal"). Since the ducts of most sebaceous glands drain into the hair follicles, boils occur most commonly on hairy areas of the skin.

A furuncle, be it lowly pimple or arrogant carbuncle, is an excellent example of one of the body's most important and interesting defense mechanisms. As soon as boil-producing staphylococci (frequently accompanied by streptococci) establish a beachhead in a pore or hair follicle opening or in a practically invisible break in the skin, two things happen almost simultaneously. Cells in the neighborhood start multiplying to wall off the theater of operations from the rest of the body, and shock troops consisting of great numbers of white blood cells, or phagocytes, are rushed into the area by the blood.

The redness and tenderness of the spot in the skin where a boil is forming is explained by the rush of blood to that spot and by the pressure of the white cells, the extra blood, and the rapidly multiplying bacteria against the delicate nerve endings in the dermis. The pus which forms as the boil "comes to a head" is made up of phagocytes that have "mopped up" the bacteria by engulfing them and have thereby lost their lives on the field of battle. The liquefaction of the dead phagocytes softens up the area of operations and the overlying layer of skin. Eventually the skin breaks and lets out the pus. As soon as this occurs, pain is relieved by the removal of pressure. Eventually the core of the boil, consisting of the protective wall and the closely packed white cells and bacteria not yet dissolved, is discharged or slowly absorbed.

The drama of phagocytosis, if successfully confined to one small walled-off theater in the skin, saves the body as a whole from bacterial invasion. But if the protective wall is broken down and the bacteria escape into neighboring tissues or into the lymph and blood streams, a very serious infection—even septicemia, or blood poisoning—may be the outcome.

Squeezing or pinching a boil to evacuate the pus, or amateur attempts to open it, may very well break down the wall. That is why children should learn that "hands off" is the only safe policy in dealing with any boil, small or large.

Some individuals seem to be especially susceptible to boils. Why this should be so is not always clear. In some cases the skin may harbor a particularly tough family of staphylococci; in others, the chemical reaction of the skin itself may favor the multiplication of the bacteria responsible. Also several different systemic diseases may be accompanied by outcroppings of boils.

Any child who has one boil after another or crops of boils should certainly have a complete medical checkup. The treatment of the boil itself should be carried out by a physician. The use of the sulfas and penicillin or other antibiotics has largely displaced the slow, painful, and sometimes hazardous treatments of the past. However, the drug must be given properly—that is, in the proper doses, by the proper method, and at the proper times. Otherwise, the patient may have a serious reaction, or the bacteria may build up resistance against the drug.

Infectious Dandruff. There is one form of dandruff that is infectious, although this form is not so common as advertisers of antiseptic hair lotions would have us believe. It is caused by an infection of the sebaceous glands of the scalp. The discharge from the infected glands collects in yellowish, greasy, thick scales which adhere rather closely to the scalp. When the scales become loosened and fall off, the skin beneath looks red and sore. Usually there is considerable itching. This form of dandruff, if allowed to continue, results in gradual thinning of the hair and possibly even in baldness. It is spread by hats, combs and brushes, and unsterilized barbershop or beauty-parlor instruments.

Ringworm Infections

Ringworm is a widespread infection of the skin, hair, and nails caused by microscopic fungi called dermatophytes. Three groups of ringworm fungi are recognized—the microsporums, the trichophytons, and an epidermophyton. Some of these fungi usually affect only human beings (the human types) whereas others affect both human beings and animals (the animal types). For convenience, ringworm infections are subdivided according to the sites of infection as follows: ringworm of the body; ringworm of the scalp; athlete's foot; and ringworm of the nails.

Many skin conditions resemble ringworm and are confused with it. For that reason a teacher should not state that a child has ringworm even though she strongly suspects it. The diagnosis in each case should be left to the physician. Prompt referral to a physician of children who have skin sores of any description will help greatly in checking the spread of ringworm as well as other skin infections.

The diagnosis of ringworm infection is made by the microscopic examination of specially prepared skin scrapings or hairs followed by laboratory culture of the fungi to identify the genus or species. The presence of certain ringworm infections of the scalp can be detected in their early stages with the use of a special type of lamp called "Wood's light." The light from this lamp, which was invented by Robert William Wood, an American physicist, is obtained by passing ultraviolet light rays through a special glass filter. The hairs of a child infected with ringworm fungi of the microsporum group fluoresce, or glow, in a characteristic manner when the scalp is exposed to the filtered ultraviolet light in a darkened room.

Griseofulvin. Treatment for ringworm in the past largely consisted of the application of ointments and lotions, known as fungistatic agents, which restrain or inhibit the growth of fungi. These agents are still used in general, or nonspecific, treatment but the treatment of choice for all ringworm infections is now the oral administration in tablet form of a drug known as Griseofulvin.

Griseofulvin was first known in 1939. Originally it was used on farms for the prevention of fungus diseases of plants. It was then shown to be effective in the treatment of guinea pigs infected with fungi. The effectiveness of Griseofulvin in the treatment of human ringworm was announced in 1958. Griseofulvin is an antibiotic derived from a species of the mold *Penicillium* from which penicillin is derived. However, there appears to be no cross sensitivity in persons allergic to penicillin. Side effects of the drug are few and mostly minor. As with any new therapeutic agent, however, medical authorities say that all patients receiving the drug should be under careful supervision, and appropriate laboratory studies should be made at regular intervals.

Ringworm of the Scalp. Various species of microsporum and trichophyton are responsible for ringworm of the scalp. The source of infection may be either human or animal. Epidemics caused by *Microsporum audouini* (a human-type fungus) have involved great numbers of school children in North America, especially in urban areas. *Microsporum canis* (an animal-type fungus) occurs in children both in rural and urban areas wherever infected cats and dogs are present. Trichophyton infections are less common but one type known as *Trichophyton tonsurans* is epidemic in the southwestern United States, Puerto Rico, and Mexico. The incidence of this type of ringworm of the scalp is increasing in the southern United States and New York City.

Nearly all ringworm infections of the scalp infect preadolescent children almost exclusively. The theory has been advanced that the increased activity of the sebaceous glands associated with adolescence has some power to kill the fungus responsible.

The fungus of human-type ringworm of the scalp (*Microsporum au-*

douini) invades the hair and the hair follicle, multiplies, and travels down the walls of the follicle and the hair root to the point where the hair bulb begins. The hair breaks off at the weakest point, which is just above the surface of the scalp. As long as the bottom end of the infected hair remains in its follicle, the infection goes on. However, the hair papilla, which is responsible for the reproduction of new hair, does not become involved.

The onset of the human-type infection is gradual and is seldom noticed by the child's parents or teachers until the infected areas are at least as large as a half-dollar. A typical fully developed patch of ringworm of the scalp in the majority of cases is rounded, grayish, somewhat scaly, and slightly but often imperceptibly elevated. It is covered with the stubs of broken-off hairs. In some cases the patch may have a puffed or goose flesh or plucked-fowl appearance. (See Plate 12.)

Adults as well as children are susceptible to the animal-type fungus (*Microsporum canis*), which is spread by contact with the lesions, or hairs from the lesions, of cats and dogs. An infection caused by animal-type fungus results in a much more inflammatory reaction than does that caused by human-type fungi. At first the appearance of the child's scalp is the same as that of a child infected with *Microsporum audouini*, but the infection progresses more rapidly. Occasionally, a painful, boggy raised mass, called a kerion, develops on the scalp. Animal-type infections, even when untreated, may clear up quickly largely because there is a great deal of inflammation and the fungi cannot tolerate this environment. Because there is little inflammation with human-type infections, this rapid recovery usually does not happen in children who are untreated or who have only topical (local) treatment.

The specific treatment for ringworm of the scalp is the administration of griseofulvin by mouth for thirty days. Nonspecific treatment must be prolonged and diligent to be successful. A daily shampoo and a vigorous application of fungistatic ointments or liquids form the basis of treatment. Plucking out the infected hairs by the roots (manual epilation) is generally necessary. Treating the scalp with X rays so that the infected hairs fall out by the roots (X-ray epilation) may be considered if the infection persists after three months.

X-ray epilation makes the child's hair fall out in about three weeks. He will be bald temporarily, but new hair will begin to grow back in about two months. Because of the great danger that the reproductive portion of the hair may be destroyed by inexpert treatment, X-ray epilation, when advised, must be done by, or under the supervision of, a competent dermatologist or radiologist. The oral use of griseofulvin will probably make X-ray treatment of ringworm of the scalp unnecessary.

The spread of ringworm infection of the scalp from one child to others is easily brought about. The fungi and their spores are transmitted by direct contact during play; by the interchange of caps, mufflers, combs, and brushes; by unsterilized barbershop instruments; and by the backs of seats in movie theaters, public conveyances, classrooms, and so on, which have been previously used by infected youngsters.

When ringworm of the scalp appears in a community, it almost always spreads rapidly and is extremely difficult to check. Specific methods of control usually recommended are as follows:

1. *Detection of cases.* Authorities agree that it is very important for teachers, school nurses, and parents to be familiar with the appearance of ringworm of the scalp, so that the first case, or cases, can be spotted in time to put into operation the measures required to prevent its spread.

2. *Preventive measures.* The exclusion of infected children from school is not considered to be practical, as recovery in many cases may require months. Such children should be under medical treatment, however, with periodic visits to a physician or clinic. The schools in some epidemic areas provide separate isolated classrooms for infected children. Young children in epidemic areas should be surveyed by a Wood's light before entering school. Special measures during epidemic outbreaks include the education of parents and children and the enlistment of the services of doctors and nurses for diagnosis.[1]

3. *Supervision of children.* Each infected child should wear at all times a cotton stocking cap, or other type of tight-fitting head covering, which must be sterilized by boiling after each wearing. The public health authorities may advise the wearing of such caps by all children under fifteen (infected and noninfected alike) when playing with others, and while at school, in the movies, on public conveyances, in children's clinics, and so on.

The nurses serving the school and, when appropriate, the teachers should help to educate the parents regarding the ways in which this highly communicable infection is spread, and the reason for the adoption by the school administrators of measures for its control. Parents should be warned of the danger of acquiring infection from infected children as well as from infected dogs, cats, and other animals. Effective control of animal ringworm is essential to control of the infection in man.

Ringworm of the Body (Tinea Corporis). The fungi responsible for ringworm of the body are in most cases various species of *Microsporum* and *Trichophyton*. The source of infection may be either human or animal. Human ringworm is usually caused by *Microsporum audouini*. The infection begins as a rounded, sharply limited, slightly elevated, red patch on the skin. It creeps out from its center in concentric circles. As

[1] *Control of Communicable Diseases in Man,* American Public Health Association, 9th ed., New York, 1960.

the patch tends to heal in the center, its periphery has the appearance of a reddish, vesicular, or pustular ring, thus giving the disease its name.

The fungus causing human-type infection is spread from one person to another by direct skin-to-skin contact and indirectly by clothing and by any surface on which scales from the lesions, or sores, have been shed. Children usually catch animal-type ringworm from infected cats or other pets.

The specific treatment is the administration of griseofulvin by mouth for thirty days. If the fingernails or toenails are involved the treatment is usually extended for from three to six months. Nonspecific treatment consists of the vigorous application of fungistatic ointments or liquids after thorough bathing with soap and water and the removal of scales and crusts.

Athlete's Foot. Cases of fungus infections of the feet are best known under the name of "athlete's foot." A fungus called *Epidermophyton floccosum* and various species of *Trichophyton* are responsible for this infection. A case of athlete's foot is not likely to be observed directly by the teacher. However, a child may tell the teacher of symptoms suggestive of this infection before medical attention has been obtained. Also, the health education of all children should include precautions to be taken in preventing it and the importance of medical care in its treatment.

Conditions of the skin between the toes of which a person with an early ringworm infection of the feet may complain are itching and slight redness, slight scaling, and perhaps some cracking. More severe cases are characterized by intense itching, deep fissures or cracks, and blisters that weep or ooze moisture when broken. Raw red places are left as the blisters dry up and scale off. Any child who reports troubles of this kind should be referred to the physician. If the diagnosis is ringworm of the feet, the teacher should be given any information that will help her to supervise the child properly and to guard others from the infection.

The sources of infection for athlete's foot are the skin lesions of infected persons, contaminated floors and shower stalls, and articles used by infected persons. Walking barefoot on wet or damp floors or pavements, where it is customary for many people to go barefoot, is a wide-open invitation to infection. Such places include swimming pools and gymnasium showers. For that reason children should learn to protect their feet with bathing slippers or sandals immediately after taking off their ordinary footwear in the locker room or dressing room before taking a swim or a shower. They should also be warned against the danger of swapping towels and bathing slippers, socks, and other footwear.

The fungi that cause athlete's foot are so widespread, however, that practically everyone gets them on his feet at sometime or other, no matter how careful he may be. When that happens the fungi may do no harm unless conditions are favorable for their growth. It has been discovered experimentally that it is impossible to give athlete's foot to some people even when the fungi are applied in large numbers to the skin of their toes. This has led to the conclusion that the condition of the skin has a great deal to do with whether or not athlete's foot will develop after exposure.

Exactly what it is about the skin of one person that makes it more resistant to ringworm fungi than the skin of another person is not known. It is known, however, that the fungi grow best when they are supplied with darkness, warmth, moisture, and food. Shoes that completely cover the foot provide the darkness and warmth and the skin between the toes provides the food and moisture. In warm weather, wearing sandals or shoes with open toes or other openings in the leather lets air reach the toes and may be helpful in preventing athlete's foot.

Keeping the feet clean and dry helps to eliminate some of the conditions which favor fungus growth between the toes. The skin between the toes should always be dried thoroughly after bathing or getting the feet wet in any other way. Talcum powder sprinkled between the toes helps to dry these areas and to keep them dry. Changing into clean socks or stockings every morning and giving shoes a good airing after each wearing will also help.

The specific treatment of athlete's foot, as of other ringworm infections, is griseofulvin administered in tablet form. The physician will prescribe the fungistatic powders and ointments and soaks for the feet which will be most helpful for the individual case.

Medicines advertised, or recommended by friends, as effective in the treatment of so-called "athlete's foot" may irritate the skin of some individuals and prolong the condition rather than cure it. Hence, any abnormal condition of the skin between the toes should be seen by a physician for diagnosis and treatment.

SKIN INFESTATIONS

Infestation means an invasion of the surface of the body with animal parasites that are not microscopically small and that produce mechanical effects. It differs from the term infection, which is reserved for an invasion

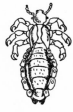
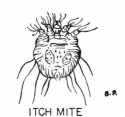

HEAD LOUSE   ITCH MITE

FIG. 15-5. The two chief offenders in skin infestations (highly magnified).

of the tissues by infectious agents (pathogenic microorganisms) that produce chemical and toxic effects within the body. Itch mites and head lice (see Fig. 15-5) are responsible for the skin infestations most often found in American school children.

Mites

Long before medical scientists made the acquaintance of microscopic skin dwellers, practically everyone was familiar with a family of living skin irritants that affected high and low alike until modern facilities for cleanliness and modern methods of treatment became generally available. These barely visible, less than pinhead-sized parasites are the itch mites that cause scabies (Latin for "itch").

Mites are the smallest members of one of the great divisions of the animal kingdom, the *Arthropoda*. They belong specifically to the order *Acarina*, which includes both ticks and mites. The itch mite has an important place in medical history. It was first discovered by Avenzoar, a great Jewish physician of the twelfth century; rediscovered in 1687 by Cosimo Bonomo, an Italian physician; and finally and permanently connected with the itch in the first half of the nineteenth century. In modern times, where there are ample facilities for bathing with soap and water, "the itch" (scabies) practically disappears. It becomes widespread, however, under insanitary conditions brought about by war, poverty, and social upheaval.

Scabies. Infestation with the itch mite occurs during a period of close bodily contact with already infested persons or with their clothing or bedding. The female itch mite burrows molelike in the skin, producing a minute, slightly elevated, black trail. These burrows are located most commonly on the inner sides and webs of the fingers, the wrists and back of the hands, the armpits, the abdomen, and the inner sides of the thighs. Scratching inflames the infested areas and may produce signs mistaken for those of eczema, poison ivy, "stomach rash," or almost any other form of dermatitis.

The female mite burrows in the horny layer of the epidermis, immediately starts laying her eggs there, and dies after six or seven weeks. Baby mites hatch out of the eggs in three to five days and excavate their way into the sides or floor of the burrow. When grown up they crawl over the skin, and the females make other small burrows. Itching is caused by the irritation of stout spines, or bristles, on each of the eight legs of these parasites, and in addition, by a highly irritating fluid released from their skin.

When it starts the itching is so intense as to be almost unbearable, especially at night. Scratching, scratch marks, or raw red patches in the areas where the burrows are most commonly located should suggest the possibility of scabies. Casual diagnosis of scabies, however, is impossible because there are probably a thousand-odd causes of itching and certainly the itch mite is not always the culprit. In dealing with children found by a physician to be infested with the itch mite, the safest procedure is to exclude them from school until disinfested. Several satisfactory ointments and lotions for external application make the cure of scabies relatively easy when carried out faithfully under medical supervision.

Harvest-mite Infestations. Close relatives of the itch mite are the harvest mites. Probably the best known harvest mite is the chigger (chigo, chigre, jigger), which is found in the southern United States. Other common types are the harvest bug and the red bug. Harvest mites burrow into the skin and cause itching as itch mites do, but their reproductive cycle is not so efficient and they tend to die out rather promptly. Their disappearance is hastened by medical treatment. A history of being in harvest fields or in underbrush during the season in which harvest mites are prevalent in a locality will help the physician to make a diagnosis of harvest-mite infestation in children suffering from it.

Lice

The Latin name for louse is *pediculus.* Hence, the medical term for infestation with lice is pediculosis. There are three kinds of lice for which man is the natural host—body lice, head lice, and pubic lice (crabs). Of the three, head lice are by far the most common in American school children.

Body Lice. Body lice really should be called clothing lice, because they live and lay their eggs in the seams of clothing and come out on the skin only when they want a meal of blood. Like other skin parasites, they cause intense itching and scratching which often lead to a dermatitis, or skin inflammation, of one kind or another. The possibility of body lice infestation is another good reason for never ignoring complaints of itching and the act of scratching in school children. Fortunately, treating clothing with 10 per cent DDT powder now makes delousing a comparatively simple procedure.

Body lice are responsible for the spread of epidemic typhus fever wherever conditions favor outbreaks of the vriulent European type of this dangerous rickettsial infection. Fortunately, epidemic typhus is now nonexistent in our country.

Head Lice. Head lice are rarely involved in the spread of communicable disease from one person to another. However, they are excedingly unpleasant, if not dangerous, guests and by their bites may cause considerable irritation of the scalp. Also, as a result of scratching the head, the germs responsible for folliculitis of the long hairs (a form of impetigo) and carbuncles may gain a foothold.

Head lice usually stay on the head, but they may wander all over the body, infecting other hairy parts. The nits, or lice eggs, are seen as tiny glistening lumps connected rather firmly to the hair a short distance from the scalp. The nits hatch in about ten days.

One child harboring head lice may be responsible for the infestation of large numbers of his schoolmates unless he is discovered and speedily disinfested. Children literally "put their heads together" so often in school and at play; so freely borrow and lend their combs, brushes, caps or hats, mufflers, coats or sweaters; and so frequently hang their outdoor clothing cheek by jowl in cloakrooms, that there is little wonder that head lice have always been one of the most vexatious school health problems.

One of the chief objectives of formal morning inspections was, and in some schools still is, the discovery of children with head lice. However, an effective search involves the use of a fine-tooth comb and, if this seems advisable, should be done by the school nurse or teacher in privacy, or at home by the parents, to avoid embarrassment for the child. Persistent scratching of the head should be a signal for this thorough inspection. In boys, especially, the nits may sometimes be seen on the hair behind the ears.

The insecticide DDT makes it much easier than formerly to get rid of lice. The preparation usually recommended by physicians is 10 per cent DDT dusting powder. This powder is perfectly safe when dusted into hair, garments, or on the skin. It may be applied with an ordinary shaker-type container. After the hair has been dusted, the head should be kept covered for several hours with a towel or cap. The hair should then be combed with a fine-tooth comb. After a week has passed, without washing the hair, the dusting should be repeated to destroy lice that have hatched from nits in the meantime. The parents of a child who has lice should be given instructions for applying DDT powder.

Like impetigo, pediculosis has often been looked upon as a disgrace. Actually it is a small part of the bitter that goes with the sweet of communal living.

FOR REVIEW AND DISCUSSION

1. If you were exploring the skin from the top downward, in which layer should you expect to find keratin? papillae? sweat glands? hair bulbs? sebaceous glands? the topmost layer of living cells? fat cells? blood vessels and nerves? pigment? pores?

2. What would you say to a child who asked you

   a. Where do freckles come from?
   b. Why can't I have curly hair like Jane's?
   c. What makes me break out in goose pimples when I'm cold?
   d. Why do I get red and sweaty after playing hard?
   e. What makes my hands get rough in cold weather?

3. From the three structures named after each of the key words given in the list below, choose the one you associate with it.

   a. Wheals: sweat glands, capillaries, arterioles
   b. Blackheads: pores, papillae, fat-gland ducts
   c. Acne: pilosebaceous glands, hair bulbs, venules
   d. Dandruff: hair follicles, horny layer of epidermis, germinative layer of epidermis

4. In each of the following groupings of diseases or conditions, there is one that does not belong with the group. Select the one that is out of place and tell why.

   a. Warts, moles, athlete's foot
   b. Impetigo, ringworm of scalp, furunculosis
   c. Scabies, acne, pediculosis
   d. Eczema, hives, comedones

5. Tell the difference between:

   a. Infection and infestation
   b. Dermis and epidermis
   c. Cutaneous and subcutaneous
   d. Griseofulvin and penicillin

6. Discuss in class ways in which you would help a child who:

   a. Has adolescent acne
   b. Has chapped hands in cold weather
   c. Has excessively oily skin and hair
   d. Is being taunted for having head lice
   e. Is worried about a noticeable skin blemish

7. Discuss from the point of view of disease control the admonition: "Always wash your hands with soap and warm water before eating or preparing food and after using the toilet."

SELECTED REFERENCES

American Medical Association: *The Skin,* Part 6 of *The Wonderful Human Machine* series, The Association, Chicago. (The workings of the human body in words and pictures.)

American Public Health Association: *Control of Communicable Diseases in Man* (first given as reference in Chap. 7).

Best, C. H., and N. B. Taylor: *The Human Body* (first given as reference in Chap. 1). Part VII, Chap. 32 (contains a section on the skin).

Goldsmith, N. R.: *You and Your Skin,* Charles C Thomas, Publisher, Springfield, Ill., 1953.

Lawrence, Herbert: *The Care of Your Skin,* Little, Brown & Company, Boston, 1955.

Levin, Oscar L., and Howard T. Behrman: *Your Hair and Its Care,* Emerson Books, Inc., New York, 1945.

Yahraes, Herbert C., Jr.: *Caring for Your Feet,* Public Affairs Pamphlet No. 345, Public Affairs Committee, Inc., New York.

Organizations

Allergy Foundation of America

Chapter 16 LET'S SEE

The Eyeballs and Their Setting
Seeing Right
Seeing Wrong
Vision Screening
Eyesight Conservation

Those of us who can see rely so much upon vision in all our dealings with the outside world that it is easy to take eyes for granted. There they are—one on each side of the nose—the most delicate yet the least protected of all our body organs. By means of these sensitive light receptors on the surface of the body we are able to become acquainted with all sorts and conditions of things in our surroundings, from a book held in the hands to the twinkling of stars hundreds of thousands of light-years away.

School children acquire most of their learning through the sense of sight. If a student has poor vision, and this fact is not known, the difficulty affects his entire adjustment to school. If for no other reason than this, education in eye health, periodic vision screening, and the provision of a good visual environment should be an integral part of the overall school health program.

THE EYEBALLS AND THEIR SETTING

Looking at her own eyes in a mirror will give the teacher a good idea of what she can observe in looking at the eyes of children. All that can be seen of the eye itself is the front curve of the eyeball. The normal eyeball is a small globe about an inch in diameter and slightly longer from front to back than from side to side, which fits snugly into a depression of the skull called the orbit, or eye socket. The size of a person's eyes—large, small, or medium—depends not upon the size of the eyeball, which is about the same in everyone, but rather upon the length of the slit between the edges of the eyelids.

The eyeball is well protected in its bony socket. The cheekbone and forehead guard it against blows, and through reflex action the eyelids snap shut involuntarily when anything comes toward the eye. The eyelashes filter dust and foreign bodies from the air, and the eyebrows keep perspiration from running into the eyes from the forehead.

The Eyelids and the Skin below the Eyes

The eyelids are two movable folds of skin from the margins of which the eyelashes spring. Both the eyelashes and the margins of the eyelids are kept oiled with secretions from fat glands.

Eyelids cover the eyes in sleep and during the daytime protect them from external injury, foreign bodies, undue exposure, and bright lights. They also serve to spread over the surface of the eyeball the tears and other lubricating secretions that keep it moist and clean.

The Sandman. Waking up with tiny, gritty particles in the corners of the eyes is such a common experience for practically all children that it gave rise to the legend of the sandman who sprinkles children's eyes with sand to put them to sleep. What really happens is that during sleep some of the fluid normally present in the eyes dries on the eyelid margins at the inner corners of the eyes. This dried secretion has the appearance of yellow or greenish specks. Its presence in a child's eyes in school usually means that the child either has not washed his face that morning or has been careless about washing it.

Inflammation of the Eyelid Margins. Some children may have persistent redness and swelling of the eyelid margins, accompanied by the appearance of scaly yellow crusts around the eyelashes. This may become a chronic condition, especially in children suffering from a nutritional deficiency (Table 12-4) or living in insanitary surroundings.

Children with inflammation of the eyelid margins (*blepharitis marginalis*) will probably say that their lids are stuck together when they wake up in the morning. They may also say that their eyes feel tired after a period of reading or other close eye work. The teacher may notice that such children frequently rub their eyes during the day.

If the condition is allowed to continue, it may result in loss of eyelashes or in drooping eyelids caused by thickening of the eyelid margins. Hence early medical attention is important both for preventing disfigurement and for determining and removing the underlying cause or causes of the condition.

Sties. A sty is an infection of one or more of the glands connected with the roots of the eyelashes. The sign of a beginning sty is a red swelling at the margin of the lid accompanied by pain and tenderness. Soon pus gathers to form a yellow spot at the summit of the red swelling. Shortly after the sty has come to a head, it breaks and the pus runs out. The application of hot compresses hastens the gathering and evacuation of the pus. Amateur attempts to prick open a sty with an instrument or to squeeze it may result in a dangerous infection.

The recurrence of one sty after another at frequent intervals means that medical attention is needed. Sties often appear in crops in children whose general health is poor or who are suffering from eye fatigue. A child with any eye difficulty is likely to rub his eyes frequently and may thus infect the eyelid margins with germs from his fingers.

Black Eye. The eyelids are easily bruised by blows on account of the looseness of their subcutaneous connective tissue. The common name for bruised eyelids is "black eye." The characteristic discoloration, which is due to the escape of blood into the tissues from ruptured capillaries, may not appear for several days after the injury. Usually it is of no importance and clears up in one or two weeks. However, a certain number of black eyes are associated with damage to the skull or eyeball. To be on the safe side, all black eyes should be examined by a physician. Cold compresses applied immediately after the injury will help to lessen the subcutaneous bleeding.

Circles under the Eyes. Of themselves, circles under the eyes have no significance. In some children, however, fatigue may produce changes in the skin below the eyes which result in the formation of shadows. These shadows may be most noticeable in children with fair complexion. Loss of skin tension in this region may be the cause in some cases; in others an actual change in skin color occurs. This change may be due to congestion in the small blood vessels close to the surface of the skin, and is not necessarily a sign of ill health.

Shadowy circles under the eyes are most likely to be observed at the end of the day. When seen occasionally they are of no particular significance other than to suggest temporary fatigue. Children who have persistent circles under the eyes combined with evidences of chronic fatigue should have medical attention. Among the possible causes of fatigue are increased nervous tension at home or in school, loss of sleep, poor nutrition, or a beginning illness.

Puffy Lids. This condition may be seen in some children, especially in the morning, when it is usually due to congestion in the nose. It may have no particular significance if seen occasionally. But if this sign appears in a child who has never shown it before, together with other signs, such as pallor, sudden increase in weight, and a tendency to tire easily, he should be referred to the nurse or physician.

The Conjunctiva and Tear Glands

The inner surface of the eyelids is covered with a delicate membrane called the conjunctiva. At the upper edge of each upper eyelid and at the lower edge of each lower eyelid the membrane folds over to pass from the inner surfaces of the lids onto the front of the eyeball, which it completely covers. When the lids move up and down, the two surfaces of the membrane slide over each other. The surfaces are kept lubricated by a small amount of tear fluid.

Tears. It is not necessary to weep to observe that the eyes are always kept comfortably moist by tears. Tears consist of a slightly salty fluid which is manufactured and secreted by small almond-shaped glands (lacrimal glands) located in the outer angle of each eye socket. The tears are piped from these glands to the eyeballs, across which they are conveyed by winking into the minute openings of ducts, or tubes, that drain into the nose (see Fig. 16-1). If it were not for the constant washing of the surfaces of the conjunctiva by the tears, this delicate covering membrane would soon become dry and inflamed and the eye would eventually be destroyed (see Vitamin A, in Chap. 12).

"Running" Eyes. Emotions that arouse the impulse to weep and irritations of the eyes cause a flood of tears which the drains are too small to handle. Hence the tears overflow their banks and roll down the cheeks. Watery, "weepy" eyes are a common occurrence in inflammation of the eyes due to mechanical irritations such as wind, smoke, bright sunlight, or foreign bodies in the eye.

Redness of the eyes and puffiness of the eyelids, accompanied by watering of the eyes and sneezing, are usually associated with the onset of communicable diseases affecting the upper respiratory tract, especially measles and the common cold (see Plate 7). The communication between the nose and the eyes by means of the tear ducts explains the frequent occurrences of eye symptoms and disturbances as a result of infections that involve the upper respiratory tract.

Bloodshot Eyes. In weeping or in irritations of the eyes, the normally colorless whites of the eyes become streaked with red wavy lines and the normally pale pink lining of the eyelids becomes red and swollen. The eyes are then said to be "bloodshot" or inflamed. This bloodshot appearance is caused by a temporary increase in the blood supply of the conjunctiva.

Sometimes after whooping cough or after bouts of violent sneezing one or two red spots may appear in the white of the eye. Such a spot is

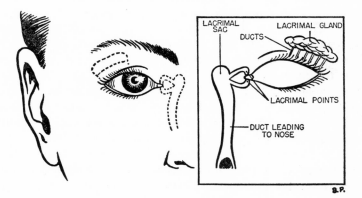

Fig. 16-1. Where tears come from.

caused by the rupture of a small blood vessel in the conjunctiva as a result of the strain of coughing or sneezing. It is usually of no importance and will clear up gradually in a week or ten days.

Exposure to wind, strong sunlight, smoke, dirt, and so on may make the eyes look bloodshot, but this effect usually clears up within twenty-four hours. In eye disturbances the conjunctiva, as well as the eyelid margins, may look inflamed, largely because the child is likely to irritate the conjunctiva by constant rubbing.

Infectious Conjunctivitis. Conjunctivitis, or inflammation of the conjunctiva, may have any one of a number of causes including mechanical irritation, an infection, a nutritional deficiency, or an allergic reaction. Cases of infectious conjunctivitis may be caused by a number of different bacteria and viruses.

Acute bacterial conjunctivitis is popularly called "pinkeye." In pinkeye the conjunctiva is red, swollen, and watery, and later there is a copious discharge of pus. As the eyes itch and smart in pinkeye, it is difficult for the child to keep from rubbing them. Pinkeye is very contagious and may occur in epidemic form in school, especially during the spring and fall. It is caught by touching the eyes with fingers, towels, washcloths, handkerchiefs, in short, with anything soiled with discharges from the eyes of persons suffering from the infection.

More than twelve different types of adenovirus, as well as several other viruses, may be responsible for nonbacterial conjunctivitis. (See also Conjunctivitis, and Keratoconjunctivitis, in Chap. 11.) Some of these virus infections also may occur in epidemics.

It is important for a doctor to see all children who show signs of acute inflammation of the conjunctiva. Only a physician can determine the cause and prescribe the proper treatment. Local application of an antibiotic or sulfa drug is effective in treating bacterial conjunctivitis. There is no specific treatment for viral conjunctivitis.

To prevent the spread of infection, as well as for their own sakes, children suffering from infectious conjunctivitis should not attend school during the acute stage. As part of their education in eye hygiene, all children should be impressed with the importance of keeping their fingers away from their eyes and with the dangers of using common towels and toilet articles.

"Something in the Eye." Pain and an increased flow of tears follow quickly after a particle of dust or other foreign body has lodged in the eye. *First aid is confined to removing particles on the conjunctiva of the eyelids.* Removing a speck on the eyeball should be done only by a physician.

It is best to send a child who complains of "something in the eye" to the nurse serving the school. But if professional help is not immediately available, instruct the child not to rub the eye and then try one or more of the following measures:

1. Inspect the conjunctiva of the lower lid by placing the thumb a little below the eye and pressing gently downward while the child looks up. If the speck can be seen, remove it from the lid with the corner of a clean handkerchief or a twist of sterile cotton moistened with water.

2. Grasp the lashes of the upper eyelid gently while the child looks upward and pull the eyelid forward and downward over the lower lid. This may dislodge the particle so that the tears can wash it out.

If the child is nervous and resists inspection, or if the speck cannot be located or removed by the simple procedures described, arrangements should be made to have him taken to a physician. It is important that foreign bodies be removed promptly to prevent serious inflammation of the eyeball.

The Wall of the Eyeball

The wall of the eyeball is built up of three layers or coats—an outer coat, a middle coat, and an inner coat. (See Fig. 16-2 for a cross section of the eyeball.)

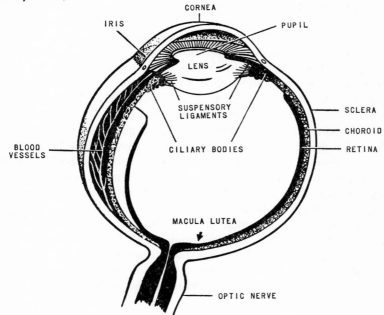

FIG. 16-2. Cross section of the eyeball with coats peeled at left to show the structure of the eye and its focusing apparatus. The macula lutea contains the fovea centralis, the point of clearest vision on the retina.

The White of the Eye. The tough outer coat of the eyeball is called the sclera or "white" of the eye. The sclera is tough, opaque, and supplied with very few blood vessels. Its functions are to keep the eyeball in shape and to protect the delicate structures within. The sclera is comparatively thin in childhood. Hence the "whites" of a child's eyes are often bluish-white in color, owing to the showing through of the dark pigment of the middle coat of the eyeball. A yellowish tinge is not normal, however, and should be called to the attention of the physician or nurse.

The Window of the Eye. Looking closely at the eyes, the observer sees a slightly bulging, clear, colorless disk covering the colored disk in the center of the white of each eye as a watch crystal covers the dial of a watch. This is the cornea, or "window" of the eye. It is the transparent part of the sclera, or outer coat, and its function is the same as that of a window in a house, that is, to let in light. There are no blood vessels in the cornea, but it is richly supplied with nerves, as anyone knows who has ever had it hit by a speck of dirt. Any cloudiness or opaque spots in the cornea call for immediate attention. If the surface of the cornea is injured in any way a scar will form which, if large and in the line of vision, will cause blindness.

Keratitis. Among the possible causes of keratitis, or inflammation of the cornea, are nutritional deficiency (Table 12-4), infection, and allergy. The cause in a particular case can be detected only by ophthalmic examination. Some forms of keratitis are accompanied by pain (as if there were "something in the eye") and blurring of vision. Such symptoms are associated with several other forms of eye trouble. Needless to say, any child who complains of them should have immediate medical attention.

Epidemic Keratoconjunctivitis. This eye infection involves both the conjunctiva and the cornea. Its most common cause is type 8 adenovirus. As already pointed out, it occurs chiefly among adults who work in shipyards and industrial plants where the eyes are subject to injury from frequent exposure to dust and dirt. No age is known to be immune from keratoconjunctivitis, however, and during outbreaks among industrial employees precautions must be taken in their homes to prevent the spread of the infection to other members of the family.

In addition to inflammation of the eyes and surrounding tissues, a person with this infection has low-grade fever and often headache and malaise. Isolation is considered advisable during the acute stage of the illness. Recovery usually is complete in from two to four weeks, but keratitis with impairment of vision may persist in from 1 to 10 per cent of those affected.

The Middle Coat of the Eyeball. The middle layer, or choroid coat, of the eyeball carries the largest number of blood vessels with which the eye is supplied. These very fine arteries and veins weave in and out to make a dark red tapestry that completely covers the eyeball except for a small peephole in front. This peephole is familiar to us all as the pupil of the eye.

The Shutter of the Eye. The circular band of the choroid coat which surrounds the pupil is also familiar to everyone because it gives the eyes their distinctive color. This colored disk is the iris of the eye. Its color is determined by heredity. Its function is similar to that of a window shade or a camera shutter; that is, it regulates the amount of light entering the interior of the eyes through the pupils. The pupil looks black because the inside of the organ that gives us the power to see is in itself dark. We cannot see the interior of the eyes through the pupils for the same reason that we cannot see the interior of a dark room by looking in through the windows. However, the structures inside the eye can be seen and examined by throwing light into each eye through the pupil by means of an instrument called an ophthalmoscope, much as the interior of a dark room may be seen and examined by throwing light through a window from a flashlight.

It is possible by close observation to see the motions of the iris in regulating the amount of light entering the eye through the pupil. These motions are carried out by means of tiny muscles in the iris which draw it in close to, or away from, the center opening, according to the amount of light striking the eyes. The visible effect is a shrinking or enlarging of the size of the pupil.

Changes in the size of the pupils, according to the amount of light striking the eyes, can readily be demonstrated. One way to do this is to place a child in a darker part of the classroom and cover his eyes with a card. After a minute or so remove the card, turn the child directly toward the light, and observe the shrinking of the pupils. Notice also how small the pupils are when a child is outdoors in the sunlight.

Excitement or fear will cause the pupils to dilate because the tiny muscles moving the iris curtain are controlled by the autonomic nervous system, which responds automatically to emotional stimuli. Also the healthy iris is extremely sensitive to variations in intensity of light. Sluggishness of action as shown by slowness of the pupils to change in size with changes in light intensity, or inequality in the size of the two pupils, should immediately be reported to the nurse or physician.

The iris of the eye is normally clear and of its characteristic color—blue, brown, gray, hazel, black, and so on—and the pupil is normally coal black, regular in outline, and equal in size to its fellow. Dullness or discoloration of the iris, or redness around the iris, or contraction or grayness of the pupil, or unusual sensitivity to light should be called to the attention of the nurse or physician.

The Inner Coat of the Eyeball. The layer of tissue that lines the interior of the eyeball is the retina. It is a highly sensitive film designed to convert the energy of light waves into the nerve impulses that are transmitted to the seeing center of the brain by way of a compact, rounded bundle of nerve fibers called the optic nerve.

Actually, the retina is the terminal in the eye for millions of tiny nerve fibers originating in the brain. The endings of these nerve fibers are the visual receptors. There are two kinds of visual receptors named, according to their shape, rods and cones. The cones, of which there are about seven million, are concerned only with the perception of fine details and colors. The rods, of which there are about 130 million, are concerned only with the perception of light and shade.

Only cones are present in that part of the retina which is capable of acute vision. This region, called the *fovea centralis,* is a tiny pit only about half a millimeter across. It is hard to realize that objects in the outside world cast images so small that they fit upon such a minute spot. The fovea centralis lies in the center of a large yellow area—the yellow spot, or *macula lutea*—located on the outer side of the optic nerve (see Fig. 16-2).

In other parts of the retina the cones are intermingled with the rods. In regions close to the center of acute vision there are more cones than rods. In regions farther away there are more rods than cones.

It takes much less light to stimulate the rods than is needed to stimulate the cones. It is the rods that make it possible to see objects in a dim light. Objects appear gray in twilight because the rods give no sensation of color.

The outer part of the rods contains a pigment known as visual purple, which is bleached by light but is re-formed in darkness. Visual purple can re-form rapidly only when the retina is constantly supplied with vitamin A. Deficiency or a lack of vitamin A in the diet interferes with the renewal of visual purple, thus causing the condition called "night blindness," or inability to see in dim light. People can have night blindness without realizing it, as they can see clearly in daytime. Obviously a person with night blindness is particularly susceptible to twilight accidents. It can be prevented and cured by getting plenty of vitamin A in the diet (see Table 12-4).

SEEING RIGHT

Light, eyes, and brain·—all three—give us the gift of sight. Rays of light reflected, or bounced back, from objects through which they cannot pass enter the eye through the pupil and are focused in rapid succession upon the retina so that tiny inverted images of the objects fall upon the retina. From every point of these tiny upside-down pictures a nerve impulse speeds to the seeing center of the brain by way of the optic nerve. The sum total of the millions of impulses received in the brain produce the sensation, or conscious impression, of seeing what we are looking at.

Through long experience, we have come to know that the pictures cast on the retina do not represent visible objects as they really are. Without any conscious effort on our part the brain enables us to turn the pictures right side up, enlarge them to life size, and interpret them correctly. Destruction of the part of the brain concerned with vision would cause blindness just as complete as if both eyes were destroyed.

Two-eyed Vision

In looking at the eyes one of the first things to catch the attention of the observer is the almost continuous motion of the eyeballs. They can be turned at will in many directions—right, left, up, down, up and right, up and left, down and right, down and left.

The motions of the eyeball are made possible by voluntary muscles attached at one end to the bones of the orbit and at the other end to the eyeball (see Fig. 16-3). These muscles work in antagonistic pairs. One muscle of a pair helps to turn the eyeball to the right, for example, and its fellow helps to turn it to the left. While one "fellow" works, the other relaxes.

Normally the action of the muscles of both eyes is synchronized so that they turn together to focus on the same spot. Even if one eye is covered it turns automatically to look in the same direction as the uncovered eye. That is why both eyes must be bandaged if it is necessary to keep one eye comparatively still.

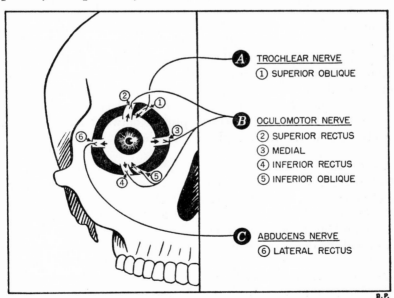

Fig. 16-3. Diagrammatic representation of the muscles that move the eyeball and their controlling nerves.

Binocular, or two-eyed, vision enables us to see things in proper perspective. With one eye we have photographic vision (perception of length and breadth); with two eyes, streoscopic vision (perception of depth, or thickness, as well as length and breadth).

The Focusing Apparatus of the Eyes

The focusing apparatus of the eyes, like that of the camera, is designed to take advantage of the fact that light rays are bent when they pass from one transparent medium, such as air, into another transparent medium of different density, such as glass or water. This bending is called refraction.

In the course of their progress from the air through the window of the eyeball to its back wall, light rays reflected from objects in the outside world pass through several refracting media: (1) the cornea, (2) the watery liquid between the cornea and the crystalline lens, (3) the crystalline lens, and (4) the soft jellylike substance between the lens and the retina. The most important refracting device is the crystalline lens, which is a clear elastic body thicker in the middle than at the edges. Thus its shape is double convex, like that of an ordinary magnifying glass. The first person to describe the shape of the crystalline lens was the great Arab scientist Alhazen (962–1038), who said that it looked like a lentil seed. The English word *lens* comes from the Latin word for "lentil."

The center of the front surface of the crystalline lens coincides with the center of the pupil. The margin of the pupil is in contact with this surface. The lens is enclosed in a highly elastic capsule. Attached to the lens capsule is the suspensory ligament, by which the lens is slung like a hammock from one side to the other of a circular zone of tissue extending from the choroid coat of the eyeball. This zone of tissue is called the ciliary body. It is made up chiefly of the ciliary processes and the ciliary muscle. The ciliary processes project outward like tiny fringes toward the lens, which they completely encircle.

Accommodation

Light rays coming from objects 20 feet or more away are nearly parallel when they reach the eye, and the curvature of the crystalline lens in the normal eye at rest is just right for focusing these parallel rays on the retina. But light rays coming from objects nearer than 20 feet are spread apart, or divergent, when they reach the eye, and in the normal eye at rest are focused behind the retina. How then can we see nearby objects distinctly? This is what happens: The ciliary muscle contracts and in doing so draws the choroid forward. This permits the ciliary processes to move forward and inward, thus reducing the diameter of the ring which they form around the lens. The pressure of the suspensory ligament and lens capsule upon the lens is thus relieved. Consequently, the elastic lens becomes thicker—more convex or spherical—just as the surface of a small rubber ball held tightly between fingers and thumb would round up when the pressure upon it was reduced. The more curved or bulging shape of the crystalline lens increases its focusing power.

The process by which the eye adapts itself to near vision is called accommodation. It happens so smoothly and instantaneously that a person with normal vision is not aware of any change whatever taking place in his eyes when he turns from looking off into the distance to the reading of a book or other close eye work, and vice versa.

SEEING WRONG

Perfect eyes are comparatively rare. Slight imperfections may cause little or no trouble with vision. But according to the most accurate estimates now available, approximately 25 per cent of school-age children have visual difficulties that require correction.

Teachers and school nurses are key persons in the detection of children who may be in need of professional eye care. Even when screening tests for visual acuity are given regularly in school, continuous classroom observation by an alert teacher helps greatly in bringing to professional attention signs and symptoms that may indicate eye trouble. Periodic conferences of teacher and nurse are desirable so that there can be an exchange of information pertinent to the health of the child. Whatever affects general health may affect the eyes. And the constant and excessive fatigue to which the eyes are subjected in trying to overcome visual difficulties may affect not only their own well-being but that of the whole body.

Crossed Eyes

Crossed eyes is the popular name for strabismus, or squint. This condition occurs when the muscles that move the eyeball do not function correctly to focus both eyes simultaneously on the same object. The eye that is directed toward the object looked at is called the fixing eye; the other, the squinting eye. A true image is seen with the fixing eye and a false image with the squinting eye. Hence a person with a squint may have double vision (see Fig. 16-4). However, a child with uncorrected squint usually does not see double by the time he is ready to enter school because he has unconsciously learned to suppress the image from the squinting eye. If the condition is left uncorrected the vision in the squinting eye becomes dim, because progressive loss of function is the penalty nature exacts for disuse of function. This condition, known medically as amblyopia, or lazy-eye blindness, can occur only in a child but, if untreated in childhood, lasts for life.

The Detection of Squint. Squint may be manifest, that is, readily observable; or latent, that is, not readily observable. In the most common forms of manifest squint, the teacher will observe that one of the child's eyes deviates inward toward the nose (esotropia, or convergent squint) or outward away from the nose (exotropia, or divergent squint) while the other eye is fixed on the object being looked at. Sometimes the eyes may take turns in deviating. This is known as alternating strabismus. Convergent squint is the most common form of squint and usually develops between the ages of one and four. Divergent squint usually develops in youth or early adult life.

The squint may be present all the time, or present at some times and absent at others; if intermittent, it may be most noticeable when the child is tired or in poor health. It may be greater for near vision than for distant vision, or vice versa. If vision has been suppressed in the squinting eye, the child may not be able to see with that eye any of the letters or symbols on the vision-testing chart (see Snellen Chart Tests, Fig. 16-10 and Fig. 16-11). Amblyopia, or dimness of vision resulting from long disuse of the squinting eye, means that the child will have to practice using that eye under the supervision of an eye specialist until it has regained its lost function.

In latent squint, one eye may tend to turn in (esophoria) or out (exophoria) because of muscular imbalance. A tendency to vertical deviation (up or down) rarely occurs. A child with latent squint may be able to overcome this tendency by muscular effort because of his

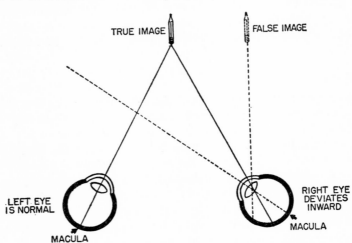

FIG. 16-4. Diagram illustrating double vision in squint. The image seen by the fixing eye (left eye) is distinct because it falls on the macula and hence is called the true image. The image seen by the eye deviating inward (right eye) is less distinct because it falls to the left of the macula and consequently is projected to the right as the false image.

strong desire to maintain binocular vision. In the milder forms, there may be no noticeable signs of squint. In more pronounced forms, there may be some evidence produced by the strain imposed in overcoming the difficulty. Tilting of the head may indicate the child's effort to correct double vision.

Without the aid of special implements or devices, it is difficult for the observer to detect latent squint. However, since both eyes under normal conditions turn in the same direction even when one is covered, a tendency to squint may be detected if an eye that has been covered makes a sudden jump to change its position when the cover is removed. Another simple test may be helpful. The observer holds a pencil or other object in front of the child and asks him to look at it. If the child has a tendency to squint, only the fixing eye will follow the object when it is moved in various directions. A test for muscle balance, that is, the ability of the two eyes to work together, is included in the battery of tests known as the Massachusetts Vision Test (see further on).

In strabismus or in latent squint, careful attention should be given to any difference in the visual acuity of the two eyes. If such difference exists, correctly prescribed and correctly fitted glasses may compensate for it and thus relieve unnecessary muscular effort. It is evident that the sooner any manifest or latent squint is brought to the attention of an eye specialist the greater is the possibility not only of correcting the difficulty, but also of preventing its psychological and social effects. Unthinking playmates may call a cross-eyed child "cockeyed" or give him some offensive nickname that will make him feel different and unwanted.

Eye exercises under the supervision of a specialist in orthoptics are often helpful. It may also be necessary to cover the good eye so that the squinting eye will be forced to work. A child who is obliged to wear a patch or a blacked-out eyeglass lens over one eye should be watched to make sure that he keeps it on. A simple explanation of why Johnny or Jane must wear an eye covering may help to prevent teasing by the other children.

Sometimes a surgical operation may be required to line up the crossed eye with the normal eye. One operation may be all that is needed, but it sometimes takes two or three before the eyes are exactly straight, as several eye muscles may be involved. For older children—and adults too —an operation to correct a cross-eyed appearance will not improve vision, but freedom from the psychological and social handicap of crossed eyes is almost as valuable a reward.

Errors of Refraction

To see nearby and distant objects clearly and distinctly, the light rays reflected from those objects must be focused directly upon the retina of the eye (see Fig. 16-5). If the rays come to a focus in front of, or behind, the retina instead of exactly upon it, blurred vision is the result. Mistakes in vision caused by defects in the structure of the eye are called errors of refraction. Such errors can usually be corrected by placing glass lenses of the required type and strength in front of the eye so as to bring the focal point just enough backward or sufficiently forward to land it squarely on the retina.

Hyperopia (Farsightedness). In hyperopia the vision for distant objects is better than for nearby objects so that the person is said to be farsighted. The most common cause of farsightedness is the possession of an eyeball that is too short from front to back. Consequently, light rays come to a focus behind the retina even when the muscles of accommodation try to be accommodating (Fig. 16-6).

Children are usually farsighted at birth because their eyeballs have not yet reached their full size. As they grow older they may become less farsighted, normal-sighted, or nearsighted. In some children, the eyeball may reach its full development at about the age of nine or ten, but it is not uncommon to find hyperopia, or farsightedness, in older children, even in high school students.

Even to see distant objects distinctly, a farsighted person whose error is uncorrected by glasses requires some accommodation, that is, some alteration in the focus of his eyes. To see nearby objects, he must not only make the alteration required of a person with normal vision, but also an additional adjustment to compensate for his error. The unaided eyes of a farsighted person are never at rest as long as he can see clearly, because to see clearly his eyes must work constantly. No wonder he has eye fatigue!

Very often the testing of a farsighted child's vision does not indicate that anything is wrong with his refracting apparatus. By making an extra effort he may be able to pass the test successfully. Screwing up the eyes when looking at near objects, holding the book far away when reading, and signs and symptoms of eye fatigue observed by the teacher may be the only indications of trouble of this kind.

Myopia (Nearsightedness). In myopia the vision for nearby objects is better than for distant objects so that the person is said to be nearsighted. In nearsightedness the eyeball is too long from front to back so that light rays come to a focus in front of the retina (Fig. 16-8). A child is rarely born with

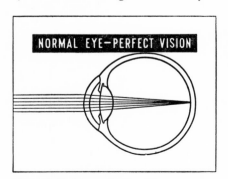

FIG. 16-5. Normal eye. The image is focused directly upon the retina.

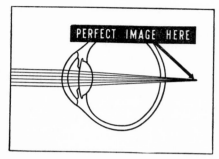

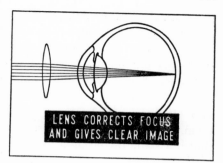

FIG. 16-6. Farsighted eye. The eyeball is too short from front to back, and light rays entering the eye focus the image *behind* the retina. Farsighted eyes cannot see objects near at hand without giving considerable extra work to the muscles of accommodation. This often results in eye fatigue.

FIG. 16-7. Farsighted eyes that have been fitted with convex lenses of suitable power can see nearby objects clearly without overworking the muscles of accommodation.

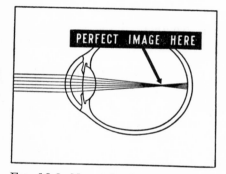

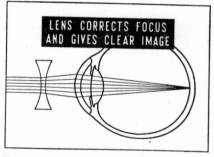

FIG. 16-8. Nearsighted eye. The eyeball is too long from front to back, and light rays entering the eye focus the image in *front* of the retina. Nearsighted people can see objects close at hand, but distant objects appear blurred.

FIG. 16-9. Nearsighted eyes that have been fitted with concave lenses of suitable power will be able to see distant objects clearly.

nearsightedness. However, it usually begins at an early age and nearly always gets worse. Nearsightedness is found in more than 10 per cent of children in the primary grades and increases to 20 per cent or more between the ages of ten and twenty.

Many children who are nearsighted may be able to do close work comfortably and show no symptoms except indistinct vision for distance. Such children can see to read at their desks without difficulty, for example, but may not be able to see clearly what is written on the chalkboard or the details of wall maps or charts. Others may have to hold their books closer to their eyes than the usual 14 inches (Plate 13), look as if they were writing with their noses, and say that their eyes feel tired after doing close work for only a short time.

The pupils of a nearsighted child are likely to be larger than the pupils of a child with normal vision or farsightedness. Hence more light gets into his eyes, and he may complain that strong light or glare hurts them. Also, he may tend to squeeze his eyelids together in an effort to shut out some of the light and so obtain clearer vision. This "squinting" of the eyes in order to see more distinctly is a common sign of near-sightedness.

Whereas farsighted eyes may improve their near vision by making an extra effort to accommodate, or alter their focus, nearsighted eyes cannot improve their focus for distance without the help of lenses of the correct type and strength. In other words, nearsighted eyes are permanently focused for near objects. Hence, eye testing with the Snellen chart at 20 feet will nearly always detect nearsighted children.

Astigmatism. Astigmatism is usually caused by some irregularity in the curvature of the cornea or the lens of the eye. As a result some light rays are bent more sharply than others, so that all the rays are not brought to a sharp focus anywhere on the retina. The astigmatism may be hyperopic, myopic, or mixed.

To persons with astigmatism, details appear blurred and the outlines of objects look hazy as in a photograph out of focus. The image conveyed to the brain resembles that of an object seen through a windowpane which is uneven or wrinkled. The decrease in acuteness of vision caused by astigmatism is present both for distant vision and near vision. Hence, children with astigmatism are subject to constant fatigue, both in using their eyes for close work and in looking at distant objects. A nearsighted child or a farsighted child who is also astigmatic may have all the trouble associated both with farsightedness and nearsightedness.

Efforts to reduce or neutralize the effect of astigmatism are likely to give rise to symptoms of severe continuous eye fatigue and extreme nervousness or irritability in children. A small amount of astigmatism may cause greater eye fatigue than a large amount because the child with severe astigmatism gives up the struggle to see clearly, whereas the child with mild astigmatism continues his straining effort to see clearly.

Color Blindness

Persons who cannot perceive one or more colors are said to be blind to those colors. About nine out of one hundred persons have some form of color blindness. Some persons are blind to red or green or to both. Blindness to blue is rare. Color blindness is usually hereditary and, with few exceptions, affects only boys and men. To a green-blind person, green objects appear grayish. A color mixed with green, such as greenish-blue or greenish-yellow, appears pale blue or yellow. A red-blind person confuses red with green. He may put on bright red socks, for example, thinking that they are dark green or brown. He perceives a color mixed with red, such as purple or orange, as if there were no red present. A purple violet, for example, would appear blue and an orange would appear yellow.

Color blindness is not correctable. It is thought that the retinas of persons with this condition are lacking in the elements sensitive to the colors to which they are blind. As a rule these persons are not aware of their defect.

In occupations such as navigation and railroad operation, in which the ability to distinguish between colored signal lights is essential, color blindness is a dangerous handicap. It is easy to see, also, that color blindness in automobile driving may lead to serious motor accidents because of inability to read traffic lights correctly.

It is recommended that a test for color discrimination be given each child at least once during his school life, as it is important for color-blind students and their parents to become aware of this condition. Vocational counselors also should know whether any of the students who consult them have difficulty in color discrimination so as to prevent the choice of a vocation for which such students are not suited.

VISION SCREENING

The purpose of vision screening in school is to locate children who may be in need of a complete professional eye examination. The National Society for the Prevention of Blindness recommends "as a basic minimum screening procedure for school children an annual test for distance visual acuity using the Snellen chart combined with teacher observation for symptoms that may be related to eye problems." Two other tests may be added if school administrators think it advisable: (1) A test to determine ability to accommodate for close work, which is essentially a test for hyperopia and (2) a test for muscle balance, or the ability of the two eyes to work together, for the detection of latent squint. These two tests together with the Snellen chart test are included in the Massachusetts Vision Test.

Several other screening methods and instruments have been developed for school use. But in carefully controlled comparative studies to evaluate the effectiveness of various screening procedures, the Snellen test combined with teacher observation and the Massachusetts vision test were found to have the highest correlation with the judgment of the eye specialists who examined all children who either passed or failed the screening tests under study. These are the two screening methods recommended by the National Society for the Prevention of Blindness and the

Joint Committee on Health Problems in Education of the National Education Association and the American Medical Association.

In many communities school nurses or public health nurses do vision screening in schools. It has been found, however, that classroom teachers and well-instructed volunteers can screen children for visual acuity with a high degree of accuracy. The National Society for the Prevention of Blindness points out that, "When teachers or volunteers do the screening, the school nurse can devote her attention to coordinating all the services and interpreting the program to parents, teachers, and other professional people in the community. The nurse may screen certain selected children. She usually makes the referrals and does the follow-up to make sure that the children are examined. She may interpret the doctor's findings to the teacher and principal and counsel parents as needed."

The Teacher's Part in Vision Screening

Many signs and symptoms indicating the need for a professional eye examination cannot or may not be detected in periodic vision screening. It sometimes happens that the teacher's close observation is of greater significance than the results of screening tests. Teachers may find the following summary helpful in observing students for indications of possible visual disturbances:

Complaints to Parents or Teachers
    Frequent headaches
    Dizziness
    Nausea
    Blurring of near or distant vision
    Sensitivity to light
Appearance of Eyelids and Eyes
    Crusts on eyelids among lashes
    Frequent sties
    Red or swollen eyelids or reddish conjunctiva
    Watering eyes or discharge from eyes
    Lack of coordination in directing the gaze of both eyes
    Persistent squinting or scowling
Behavior
    Rubs eyes frequently as if to clear away a fog before the eyes
    Acts irritable or cries when using the eyes for close work
    Is inattentive during lessons involving the use of the chalkboard, wall charts, or maps.
    When looking at distant objects:
        Holds body tense
        Screws up face
        Thrusts head forward

When reading:

Blinks continually

Holds book too far from or too close to the face

Frequently moves the book away from or toward the eyes

Stops the effort to read after a brief period

Shuts one eye or covers it with the hand

Tilts the head to one side

Tends to squint at the page

Frequently loses the place on the page

Confuses the following letters in reading or spelling—

o's and a's; e's and c's; n's and m's; h's, n's, and r's; f's and t's

In addition to the signs and symptoms given in this summary, the child's ability to concentrate, to keep up with the class in schoolwork requiring reading, writing, and drawing, to work without tiring easily or acting irritable or inattentive, and to play games requiring both distant and near vision without noticeable awkwardness may also serve as criteria in judging the effectiveness of the child's visual apparatus.

Snellen Chart Test

The Snellen chart test for central distance visual acuity tests the individual's ability to perceive form at 20 feet. It is generally agreed that it is the most important single test of visual ability when properly conducted with correct illumination.

The standard distance from the chart is 20 feet because rays of light reflected from objects at that distance are nearly parallel when they reach the eye and a minimum amount of accommodation is needed to focus them on the retina. In testing the individual's ability to perceive form at 20 feet, the Snellen test can be depended on to screen out the near-sighted children and those with extremes of farsightedness, moderate to severe astigmatism, and other eye conditions that cause a blurred or imperfect visual image.

Snellen Letter Chart. Square-shaped letters are arranged upon a chart, the size of the letters diminishing from above downward. A small numeral at the side of, or above, each row of letters indicates the number of feet away from the chart at which the normal eye should be able to read letters of that size. In the charts ordinarily used in testing the vision of school children, the single top letter is of a size that can be read by the normal eye at a distance from the chart of 200 feet.[1] Then come rows of letters that can normally be read at 100, 70, 50, 40, 30, 20, and 15 feet, respectively (Fig. 16-10).

Acuteness of vision is expressed by a fraction, the numerator of which corresponds to the number of feet separating the child from the chart.

[1] In some schools the top letters of the chart used may be of a size that can be read by the normal eye at 100 feet.

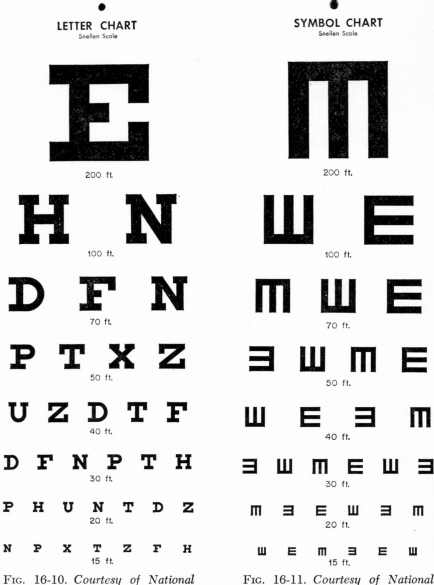

Hence, for testing vision at the standard distance of 20 feet, the numerator is 20. The denominator corresponds to the number indicating the line of smallest letters that the child can read without mistake at that distance. If he can read with one eye the row of letters numbered 20

(that is, letters of a size that the normal eye can read at 20 feet), his sight is considered normal in that eye and is expressed by the fraction 20/20. If he can read only as far down as the fourth row from the top with the other eye (that is, letters that the normal eye can see at 50 feet), the vision of that eye is 20/50. If he cannot read lower than the top letter, it is 20/200. If none of the letters can be read at 20 feet, the child should approach the card until he can read the letter at the top. The distance at which he stands to read that letter will serve as the numerator of the fraction, for example 10/200.

Snellen Symbol Chart. On this second type of chart a series of E's heading downward, upward, to the right and to the left (Fig. 16-11) are printed on numbered lines in sizes corresponding to those of Snellen's test letters. Acuteness of vision is determined by the smallest symbols of which the child, standing at the standard distance of 20 feet from the chart, can correctly tell the direction in which the symbols are open. The Snellen symbol chart is used to test the vision of young children who cannot read and is often preferred to the Snellen letter chart in testing all children. The reasons given for this preference are that the judgment required is simple; the E's of the same size do not vary in visibility as do letters; the symbols are not easy to memorize; fatigue is not produced; and the results can be interpreted by anyone.

In testing with the E chart the child is asked either to tell in which direction the shafts of the E point (up, down, right, or left) or to show with his hand which way the arms of the E point. To make it easier for the child to concentrate on one symbol, a window card, that is, a card with a square hole, should be used to expose only one symbol at a time. The part of the chart not in use should be covered with a cover card.

The Massachusetts Vision Test

The battery of tests that has come to be known as the Massachusetts Vision Test was developed in 1938 by the Massachusetts Department of Public Health. The battery consists of three tests as follows:

1. A test for distance central visual acuity with an illuminated Snellen E chart; the Snellen test is the first test in the battery because it will reveal the majority of students who should be referred for a complete professional eye examination. The test is stopped at the student's first point of failure.

2. A plus-lens test for hyperopia (farsightedness) in which visual acuity is checked while the student is wearing a pair of convex or plus lenses mounted in an inexpensive plastic or metal frame. If the student can see the 20-foot line on the Snellen chart with either eye while wearing these lenses he fails the test because it is assumed that he has as much or more hyperopia as that represented by the lens. Referral for a professional eye examination is therefore indicated.

3. Tests for vertical and horizontal muscle imbalance at 20 feet and for near horizontal muscle imbalance at reading distance. A type of lens known as the Maddox rod is used for these tests. The Maddox rod causes fusion of two images to be disassociated or frustrated, and hence shows the relative position of the eyes without fusion. Two spectacle frames are provided—one with vertical Maddox rods for testing for vertical muscle imbalance and the other with horizontal Maddox rods for testing for inward or outward lateral muscle imbalance (esophoria or exophoria). The unit of measurement used is known as a prism diopter which measures the angle of deviation.

Several companies have produced testing instruments embodying this battery of tests. Instructional manuals on giving the tests are included with each kit. Adequate preparation and thorough understanding of the tests are needed by the persons who conduct them.

The National Society for the Prevention of Blindness suggests that when "the Massachusetts Vision Test battery is introduced it is sometimes practical to start gradually. The plus-lens test may be omitted at first, then added after determination of distance acuity plus teacher observation. Later the test for muscle imbalance can be added. The complete Massachusetts Vision Test might be used every two or three years with Snellen distance testing and teacher observation done annually in the other years."

Eye Testing with the Snellen Charts

The procedure for administering the Snellen test is described here because it identifies nearly as many children in need of eye care as the most elaborate instruments; moreover, it accomplishes this feat with a much lower rate of needless referrals.

Preparation for Eye Testing. In health class the eyes should be the subject for study and discussion in preparation for vision testing. The children should be told what is going to happen and why and be encouraged to ask questions. Also, a demonstration of vision testing may be given so that the children will know exactly what they are to do.

Procedure for Eye Testing. Place the eye-test chart on the wall, which should be light in color. The intensity of illumination on the chart should be equal to from 10 to 30 foot-candles evenly diffused without glare. General illumination should not be less than one-fifth of the illumination of the chart. Too much light on the chart, or spot lighting of the chart, may compensate for some errors of refraction and keep them from being discovered. To avoid contrasts, no bright light should be within the child's field of vision. With daylight illumination the chart should be hung opposite a window and the child placed with his back to the window.

Using a tape measure or yardstick, measure a distance of 20 feet from the wall on which the chart is placed, and mark the 20-foot line on the floor with chalk or adhesive tape. Have each child being tested stand with his heels on the 20-foot line exactly in front of the chart or sit in a chair with the back of the seat directly above the line. The eyes should be at about the level of the 20-foot row of letters or symbols. The chart may be raised or lowered with the varying heights of the children.

Test both eyes together and each eye separately. While one eye is being tested, have the child or a helper hold a card or a folded clean sheet of paper (about 3 by 5 inches when folded) over the eye that is not being tested. Each child should have his own card or paper to avoid the spreading of infection. Show the child how the eye cover should be held. It should be grasped at the edge and placed so that it rests obliquely across the nose. It should not be pressed against the eyeball. Tell the child to keep both eyes open during the test. When the cover is lifted, note whether the eye that has been hidden makes an abrupt movement in order to focus. If so, mention the fact in recording the results of the test.

Test both eyes together first, next the right eye, and then the left eye. If the child wears glasses, have him take the test first with his glasses, and then without. This gives the child a chance to do his best on the first test. Have the child start at the 40-foot line and read downward. If he cannot read this line, have him start again at the 200-foot line. The number of the lowest line of letters on the Snellen letter chart which the child can read without difficulty will be the denominator of the fraction recording the acuity of vision for that eye.

If the symbol E chart is used, expose one vertical and one horizontal symbol on each line with two or more symbols and move down to the next. In the lowest line read correctly, or in the 20-foot line, expose all symbols, one at a time. Reading a majority of the symbols in a line correctly is considered to be satisfactory evidence that the child can see the symbols on that line.

Observe the child carefully while he is taking the test. If he shows signs of straining to see, do not allow him to continue. Record the lowest line correctly read with each eye and any evidences of straining to see. Signs to look for include thrusting the head forward or tilting it to one side, watering of the eyes, scowling or squinting, and rapid blinking of the eyes.

Record results of the test for each eye immediately in the form of a fraction such as, for example, "R. 20/20, L. 20/40." These figures should not be interpreted as representing a fraction of normal vision. They are simply a record of acuteness of vision at a given distance (20 feet). Vision of 20/40 in the left eye, for example, is not one-half of normal vision, but is merely a manner of recording the fact that the best the child can do is to see with his left eye at 20 feet letters or symbols that normally he should be able to see at 40 feet. For children wearing glasses, record the vision for each eye with and without glasses.

Correlating Findings. In order to evaluate the results of the Snellen test, a summary of all the findings for each child should be made. These findings include the visual acuity of each eye as revealed by the test, observations of behavior during the test, a history of recent illness, and any signs and symptoms observed by the classroom teacher that seem to indicate eye trouble.

Criteria for Referral. For children in kindergarten through third grade, a practical criterion for referral for a professional eye examination has been found to be vision of 20/40 or less in one or both eyes. Vision of 20/40 or less means inability to identify accurately letters or symbols on the 30-foot line of the test chart at a distance of 20 feet. For referral of children in the fourth grade and above a practical criterion has been found to be vision of 20/30 or less. This means inability to identify accurately letters or symbols on the 20-foot line of the chart.

Regardless of visual acuity, all children who consistently present any signs and symptoms of visual disturbance also should be referred for a medical eye examination.

Professional Eye Examinations

Long after spectacles first came into use (about A.D. 1300) each individual did his own vision testing. The peddler's pack or hawker's tray was not complete without an array of spectacles, and from it the sufferer picked out the pair that suited him best. The optical errors to which the living eye is subject were not accurately described until the time of the great Dutch ophthalmologist Franz Cornelius Donders (1818–1889). Donders instituted the system of prescribing and fitting eyeglasses which is now in use. Herman Snellen, an ingenious clinician and clever surgeon, who became Donders' "right-hand man" and later his successor to the chair of ophthalmology in the University of Utrecht, invented the Snellen test types.

Specialties Concerned with Eye Care. There are now three different professions concerned with eye care. Each of these professions has high standards for its members.

1. An *ophthalmologist,* or oculist, is a licensed physician who has specialized in the examination of the eye and its related structures, and in the prevention, diagnosis, and treatment of all defects, injuries, and diseases of the eye, including the prescription of eyeglasses when necessary. He is qualified to determine whether the cause of the eye trouble is an error of refraction or some other abnormal condition of the eyes themselves or one of the many diseases in other parts and systems of the body that affect the eyes.

2. An *optometrist* is a nonmedical vision specialist who is qualified by his education and training to examine eyes without the use of drugs. He is licensed to prescribe, fit, and supply eyeglasses and provide visual training for errors of refraction and eye muscle disturbances that are not due to disease. He may not treat eye conditions requiring medicine or surgery, and if his examination of the eyes leads him to suspect a disease or defect requiring such treatment, he will refer the patient to a qualified physician or surgeon.

3. A prescription *optician* is a technician skilled in the grinding of eyeglass lenses. He makes, dispenses, and fits the eyeglasses prescribed by an ophthalmologist or optometrist.

Eye Quacks. As part of their education in the care of the eyes, students should become aware of the fact that in all ages, even to this day, the eye quack has kept many people from consulting professionally trained eye specialists. An eye quack is an unlicensed person who offers to cure dim or failing vision with patent medicines, salves, ointments, or some other remedy. His sole object is to make money out of the natural human fear of blindness and pain. Many a person has had his eyesight ruined or has suffered for years from some correctable defect because he believed the claims of an eye quack instead of going to a qualified specialist.

Methods and Instruments Used in Professional Eye Examinations. The method used for estimating the refraction of the eye with trial lenses and test types is known as the subjective method. The patient must cooperate with the examiner in determining the nature of his optical error, or errors, and say which lens or combination of lenses aids his vision most. Anyone who had had an eye examination knows how difficult it is sometimes to decide this question. For this reason great value is attached to instruments that help the examiner to determine objectively the kind and amount of errors of refraction and accommodation and other eye difficulties.

The first instrument of this kind to be invented was the ophthalmoscope. It is based on the fact that under certain conditions light entering the eye through the pupil is reflected from the fundus, that is, the back part of the eye opposite the pupil, thus making it possible for an observer actually to see the interior of the eye. From earliest times the glowing appearance of the eyes of certain animals (notably the cat) when seen in a dim light had attracted notice. The glow was supposed to be due to the spontaneous development of light within the eye. The famous German scientist Hermann Helmholtz (1821–1894), in his lectures on physiology at the University of Konigsberg, found it necessary to discuss the theory of the emission of light from the eye. The experimental study in which he demonstrated the falsity of this theory resulted in 1851 in the invention of the ophthalmoscope.

This instrument is a device consisting of a perforated mirror or reflector mounted on a handle. The mirror serves to reflect light into the interior of the eye, while the aperture allows a portion of this light, after returning from the patient's eye, to pass into the eye of the observer. A disk containing convex and concave lenses for use in scrutinizing the fundus is set behind the aperture. This disk can be rotated by means of a finger applied to its edge so that any lens on the disk can be placed behind the perforation in the mirror.

It is said that Helmholtz did not at first fully realize the epoch-making character of his invention. It was the brilliant German opthalmologist Albrecht Graefe (1828–1870) who first grasped this. According to a story told in 1886 by Donders, when Graefe, "the greatest of all eye surgeons," used an ophthalmoscope for the first time and saw the background of the eye with its nerve entrance and its blood vessels, his cheeks reddened, and he called out excitely, "Helmholtz has unfolded to us a new world."

The ophthalmoscope has been greatly improved since its invention, and many other instruments have been devised for examining a patient's eyes objectively for evidence of optical errors or disease. The most accurate objective method for determining errors of refraction now in use is retinoscopy, sometimes called the "shadow test." The retinoscope consists of a perforated plane or concave mirror, which can be rotated. The mirror is used to throw light into the patient's eye through the pupil, with the result that the fundus is illuminated. By looking through the sight hole of the mirror, the observer sees the illuminated area and the shadow bounding it. The state of refraction of the patient's eye can be determined by observing the direction of movement of the illuminated area and the shadow when the mirror is rotated.

Before using the ophthalmoscope or retinoscope in examining the eye, the ophthalmologist may use a drug (called a cycloplegic) to paralyze the muscle of accommodation (ciliary muscle). While the effects of the drug last, the eye pupil remains dilated.

Eyeglasses

So many young people wear glasses nowadays that this seeing aid is no longer associated with getting on in years, or excessive studiousness, or old-maidishness, or some other attribute considered undesirable in youth. It would be a very unusual class if none of its members wore glasses.

Information regarding eyeglasses—what they are for and what they mean to the wearer in terms of comfort and clearness of vision—is an important part of the health education of all young people.

Uncorrected errors of refraction not only cause the discomfort of eye fatigue, but also interfere with the clearness and sharpness of vision which contribute so much to enjoyment of life, to efficiency, and to knowledge of the world. Lenses of the proper strength and type correct such errors by placing the focusing power, which should be on the inside of the eyeballs, out in front of the eyes. If the focusing power of lenses is necessary to improve vision or to lessen eye fatigue and discomfort, wearing eyeglasses is the intelligent thing to do. Intelligence may go by the board, however, in the case of some adolescents who have an idea that glasses call attention to the fact that they have a physical disability or who feel that there is something about wearing glasses that makes them less attractive.

It is natural to want to be physically perfect, but perfect eyes are comparatively rare. More glasses are being worn now than in the past not because more eyes are defective—for they are not—but because modern living and working conditions require the use of the eyes for close vision more frequently and over longer periods of time.

Another reason that the popular prejudice against glasses is subsiding among teen-agers is that eyeglass frames are now designed to suit various types of faces. Indeed, becoming glasses improve the appearance of many wearers. This is true especially when they overcome the squinting or bewildered expression that so often accompanies faulty vision.

Younger children who do not wear glasses will not be so likely to tease the wearers if they realize how fortunate they are to have good vision and how wonderful it is that glasses make it possible for others with poor vision to see as well as *they* do.

Safety Glasses. The National Society for the Prevention of Blindness recommends that every child and adult who wears glasses should have the protection of safety lenses mounted in sturdy flame-resistant frames. Safety-glass lenses are made stronger than regular glass lenses by a tempering process similar to the way in which steel is core hardened. As they are shatter-resistant, they serve as a shield for the eyes rather than as an additional hazard in recreational and work activities in which dangers to the eyes are involved.

Safety lenses also are made from optical plastic. These plastic lenses look exactly like glass lenses but weigh only half as much. Plastic lenses are not ground as are glass lenses. Each lens is carefully molded between dies under rising temperature and pressure until it sets. Plastic lenses are shatter-resistant, but they are easily scratched, and the scratches cannot be removed.

Eye specialists often prescribe safety lenses for persons with only one good eye, for workers on jobs hazardous to the eyes, and for athletes as a protective device. Both glass safety lenses and plastic lenses must pass stringent tests for shatter resistance.

Care of Eyeglasses. Young people who wear glasses should be helped to develop a sense of responsibility for wearing their glasses under the circumstances prescribed by the eye specialist and for taking care of their glasses properly. Proper care means keeping the glasses clean and protecting them from bending of the frames and scratching or breaking of the lenses. When not in use glasses should be kept in their case, and when taken off temporarily they should be placed in a safe position on the frames.

Supervision of Children Wearing Glasses. The teacher should have the information that will help her supervise children for whom glasses have been prescribed. She can then cooperate with the eye specialist and the parents in making sure that the child gets the full benefit of his seeing aid. She should know specifically whether a child wearing glasses is supposed to wear them all the time, or only for certain types of visual activity, for example, when he is reading or doing other close work. The teacher may obtain information concerning the wearing of glasses from the child's cumulative health record or, if the record does not give this information, from the child's eye specialist, school physician, nurse, or parents.

EYESIGHT CONSERVATION

The most significant advances in eye care in modern times have been along the lines of sight conservation. Eye health has become an integral part of the school health program. In addition to the early detection of visual errors through adequate vision screening and teacher observation and the correction of such errors by glasses or other means after a complete professional eye examination, the components of the school eye health program include the provision of (1) accurate information about the eyes and their care together with opportunities to establish sound eye health habits and attitudes; (2) a visual environment conducive to eye health, comfort, and efficiency; (3) special adjustments and educational materials designed to help partially seeing children to use the vision they have to best advantage; (4) suitable eye-protective devices for students in school workshops, industrial art classes, and science laboratories; and (5) facilities for the first aid treatment of eye injuries.

Classroom Lighting

For ease, comfort, and efficiency of seeing, proper lighting is essential. Teachers are not responsible for structural elements built into a classroom which affect its illumination, but a knowledge of the principles of good lighting will help them to secure the best possible visual environment for their students.

The purpose of light in a classroom is to produce adequate, evenly distributed illumination of the entire room, without glare and shadow, and adequate intensity of local light for the eye task itself and its immediate surroundings. The intensity, or brightness, of light is measured by a light meter in units known as foot-candles. A foot-candle is the amount of light that reaches a perpendicular screen from a standard candle placed 1 foot away from it.

Teachers will find the standards for proper lighting in classrooms recommended by the Illuminating Engineering Society in a booklet published by the National Society for the Prevention of Blindness entitled *Classroom Lighting*. The local power company will usually make a light meter available to teachers for checking the light in their classrooms.

The brightness pattern in a classroom is a result not only of the amount of light and its distribution but also of the reflecting characteristics of the walls, ceilings, floors, and furniture. Clean pastel-tinted walls and white ceilings reflect the most light and hence improve the level of illumination within the room. Gray-green or blue-green chalkboards are greatly to be preferred to the old-fashioned blackboards. There are paint preparations that can be applied if old blackboards must be used.

Proper classroom lighting plays an important role in health education related to the eyes and their care. It furnishes concrete illustrations of the standards set in the textbooks studied and gives the students opportunities to take an active part in the provision of proper lighting for various eye tasks and in the prevention of direct glare. Consciousness of proper lighting in the classroom will also furnish an incentive for proper lighting conditions in the home.

Avoidance of Glare

The avoidance of glare is one of the most important requirements of good lighting. Glare has been defined as "light in the wrong place." Eyes are likely to become tired or even painful when they are exposed to glare for even short periods of time. The avoidance of direct glare—that is, light shining directly into the eyes from a source of light—depends partly upon the proper placement and shading of windows and lighting fixtures and partly upon proper seating arrangements. The eyes work most accurately in daylight, and the upper portions of windows should be unshaded except when the sun is shining directly on them. Window shades, blinds, or draperies should be adjusted frequently during the day to take maximum advantage of natural light and to control glare. Desks and other work areas should be placed with reference to the source of light so that no student sits where light shines directly into his eyes or works in his own shadow. The teacher should stand or sit in locations in which her students will not have to face a source of light while they are facing her.

Indirect glare is caused indoors by the reflection of light from shiny and glossy surfaces, for example, desks with glass tops or a high polish, varnished floors, glass-covered pictures, and glass doors on cabinets. Books, maps, charts, and posters printed on glossy paper also may produce indirect glare.

The teacher may not be able to take all the measures necessary to prevent indirect glare in her classroom, but she can be a strong advocate for dull finishes on furniture and wall and floor surfaces when finishing jobs are in the making and also for the purchase of textbooks, maps, and other printed materials that have nonglossy surfaces. Also, she can cover glass doors on cabinets and avoid cluttering wall space with glass-covered pictures.

Protection from Sun Damage

When the infrared rays of the sun are focused on the retina of an eye a serious retinal burn results. Fortunately, the sun's light is so blinding that no one normally looks directly at it. Indirect glare from bright sunlight falling upon expanses of snow, ice, water, sand, and other surfaces out of doors also is usually so uncomfortable that most people nowadays wear sunglasses for protection. But there is one time when our eyes may be endangered by the sun without our knowing it. After every eclipse of the sun, there are cases of permanent eye damage, particularly among children.

As the moon partially obscures the sun's intensity, people are able to look directly at the sun. The blinding brilliance is absent, but the damaging infrared rays which we cannot feel are still there. Before an eclipse, students should be warned *not* to look directly at the sun. Eyes can be damaged even by looking through the viewer of a camera.

The safe way to observe the progress of the moon across the sun's face is to punch a pinhole in a sheet of cardboard and allow the sunlight to shine through it onto another cardboard or similar white surface. This will project a clear image of the eclipse and avoid the necessity for looking directly at the sun. A telescope or binoculars can also be used to project an image of the eclipsed sun onto a white screen. The safest way of all is to watch the eclipse on television.

Helping Partially Seeing Children

Partially seeing children are children whose capacity to achieve in school is limited by a vision problem. They are placed in this category if their vision in the better eye is only 20/70 or less after the best possible correction and treatment. Partially seeing children can use vision as their chief channel of learning, and authorities in the field believe that their education should be in the regular schools with their normally seeing companions. They are no different from their classmates except for their handicap and have the same need for school achievement, social acceptance, and opportunities to develop into mature, productive adults within the limits set by their visual capacity.

There are at present three types of educational plans for partially seeing children:

1. *The special classroom.* The visual environment for this classroom is
practically the same as that recommended for all children except that
provisions are made for children with vision problems who need more
than the average amount of illumination and for those who see better in
dim light. The educational materials and equipment usually include such
devices as large-print books, tape recordings and Talking Books, illuminated magnifiers and other low-vision aids, pencils with soft, thick
leads, pens that make thick strokes, and large-type typewriters. Although
the partially seeing child is enrolled in the special classroom, his schedule
is so arranged that he participates to the best of his ability with the
normally seeing children in classroom and play activities.

2. *The resource room.* This room has the same equipment and materials as that provided in special classrooms, but the child is enrolled in a
regular class and goes into the room for special visual help as his need
for it arises. Many educators prefer this plan, as it gives the child more
opportunity to work and play with normally seeing children.

3. *The itinerant program.* This program was developed to provide the
services of qualified teachers of partially seeing children for schools in
rural areas. It has since been extended to include schools in suburban
and urban areas, especially in city schools which previously had not
provided for partially seeing students in the secondary schools. The special teacher makes scheduled visits to schools that have partially seeing
children enrolled in their regular classrooms. Thus the regular classroom teachers have an opportunity to discuss with specialists the particular needs of children with vision problems and plan ways of meeting
them. The visiting teacher also brings necessary educational materials
and equipment and works with individual children according to their
needs.

In spite of the fact that there is an increasing awareness of the importance of providing special educational services for partially seeing
children, there is still a very large number of such children in the school
population who are not receiving special services. This means that the
regular classroom teacher is responsible for meeting the needs of partially
seeing children to the best of her ability. The first step is identification
and, as we have seen, the teacher is an integral part of the vision screening program. From her observation of pupil behavior she may identify
children with visual limitations that are not obvious or that are not
found through screening (see The Teacher's Part in Vision Screening, in
this chapter).

What are some of the vision problems that the teacher may encounter?

In addition to the children with errors of refraction that cannot adequately be compensated for by wearing glasses or by other corrective measures, she must be alert for the child with cataracts (a condition of cloudiness or fogginess of the crystalline lens of the eye, rare in children); the child with albinism (congenital deficiency of pigment in the skin, hair, and eyes, which is often accompanied by astigmatism, sensitivity of the eyes to light, and nystagmus); the child with nystagmus (a condition in which the eye is constantly in rapid motion—sometimes described as "dancing eyeball"); and the child with amblyopia (dimness of vision without detectable organic disease of the eyes). These are only a few examples of the vision problems that a teacher may find among her students.

A booklet published by the National Society for the Prevention of Blindness entitled *Helping the Partially Seeing Child in the Regular Classroom,* describes what the teacher can do to help partially seeing children when no special services are available. It is possible here to highlight only a few of the measures that teachers can take to help children with visual problems.

1. Consult the child's cumulative health record in order to obtain information regarding the child's visual status. Look for any special recommendations made by the child's eye specialist on seating and lighting arrangements and any restrictions on physical activities that may be necessary to safeguard the child's residual sight. The school nurse can be of great help both in interpreting the recommendations of the physician and in putting them into effect.

2. Plan lighting and seating arrangements according to the child's eye condition. The nearsighted child, for example, will need to sit near the chalkboard and demonstration areas in order to have the best view whereas the farsighted child need not necessarily be so close. Some children will need brighter light for various seeing tasks than is adequate for normally seeing children. Others, as in the case of the albino child whose eyes are sensitive to light, will be happy to have less than the normal amount.

3. Obtain information regarding the kinds of educational equipment and materials available for partially seeing children. Many of these children, for example, require books printed in larger than average type. Tape recordings of supplementary materials relieve them of possible fatigue resulting from prolonged reading tasks. Volunteers from the high school may be asked to transcribe material not otherwise available on tape records. In most states there are now full-time directors of special education who can supply information regarding the kinds of special materials available to teachers which the partially seeing child needs to develop his fundamental skills.

4. If a partially seeing child is not restricted in his physical activities by his physician—and few eye conditions require physical restrictions —make sure that he has opportunities to participate successfully in group games. The physical education instructor and other children should know, for safety's sake, that his vision is limited but he should not be made to feel different or unwanted.

5. Make whatever modifications in work arrangements are needed to enable the partially seeing child to keep up with his classmates without making too great an effort to see. Modifying assignments may mean shortening one that is too long, for example, or reducing the amount of drill work in arithmetic, or calling for a report on something heard, such as a radio newscast or play, rather than on something seen, such as a newspaper item or a new book. As the reading load becomes heavier in the upper grades, volunteer readers may be appointed to assist their partially seeing classmates with supplementary reading assignments. Recorded materials also are particularly helpful at the junior and senior high school levels.

6. Remember that most partially seeing children will need help to prepare them to live and work and play in a world that makes itself known to the rest of us so largely through the sense of sight. How the teacher can help most of all has been beautifully summarized in these words written by a junior-senior high school teacher of partially seeing children: [2]

If the teacher can sincerely *feel* that an eye difficulty is offset by real abilities and works on that basis, the class, the parents and the handicapped child will be immeasurably aided in living with the condition. The parents, the oculist, the school nurse and the teacher form a team working for the complete adjustment of most visually-handicapped school children. Each has his own job and each is necessary. But of the team, the teacher is the one who furnishes the clue as to how the child is going to get along in this world. She is the one who can allay fears of anxious parents—often by just failing to lift an eyebrow at a crucial moment or by not getting too disturbed when a chair is bumped or a book is knocked off a desk.

The teacher's *feeling* about a youngster is the most contagious factor in the youngster's life. If the teacher accepts him, his schoolmates accept him—and most important of all—the youngster accepts himself.

FOR REVIEW AND DISCUSSION

1. Match each structure of the eye named in Group A with the condition in Group B which you associate with it.

[2] Amie L. Dennison, "Partially Seeing Children Aren't So Different," *The Sight-Saving Review*, Vol. XXII, No. 4, National Society for the Prevention of Blindness.

Group A   Group B
Eyelid margins   Black eye
Eyelash roots   Pinkeye
Eyelids   Keratitis
Muscles of eyeball   Strabismus
Muscles of accommodation   Errors of refraction
Conjunctiva   Night blindness
Light-focusing apparatus   Sties
  of eye   Eye fatigue
Cornea   Blepharitis
Rods of eye

2. Choose the correct ending for each of the following incomplete sentences:
   a. The only part of the eye that is sensitive to light is the (1) choroid coat, (2) cornea, (3) retina.
   b. Myopia results when (1) the eyeball is too short from front to back, (2) the curvature of the cornea is irregular, (3) the eyeball is too long from front to back.
   c. Vision of 20/40 in one eye means that the child (1) can see only half as well with that eye as he normally should, (2) must be twice as close to an object as he normally should be in order to see it clearly with that eye, (3) must be farsighted in that eye.
   d. A foot-candle is (1) a unit for measuring the intensity of light, (2) a unit of heat, (3) a candle 1 foot tall.

3. Tell the difference between:

   Accommodation and refraction
   Photographic vision and stereoscopic vision
   Amblyopia and hyperopia
   Ophthalmologist and optometrist
   Direct glare and indirect glare

4. Which of the following statements are true and which are false? Rephrase each false statement so as to make it true.
   a. Inability to see distant objects clearly is always noticed by the child affected.
   b. A small amount of astigmatism may cause greater eye fatigue than a large amount.
   c. The teacher's observations are often of greater importance in detecting farsightedness than is vision testing.
   d. A child is likely to outgrow a tendency to squint.
   e. Myopia is nearly always a congenital defect.

5. Have a discussion in class about what a teacher could do to help a child in the class who:

a. Was being teased by other children because he must wear a covering over one eye.

b. Resented having to wear glasses.

c. Did not take proper care of his glasses.

d. Had "something in his eye."

e. Came in from recess with a black eye.

SELECTED REFERENCES

American Medical Association: *The Sense Organs*, Part 8 of *The Wonderful Human Machine* series, The Association, Chicago. (The workings of the human body in words and pictures.)

Best, C. H., and N. B. Taylor: *The Human Body* (first given as reference in Chap. 1). Part X, *The Special Senses*, Chaps. 41–45.

Gregg, James R.: *Parents' Guide to Children's Vision*, Public Affairs Pamphlet No. 339, Public Affairs Committee, Inc., New York.

Hathaway, Winifred: *Education and Health of the Partially Seeing Child*, 4th ed., Columbia University Press, New York, 1959. (A well-written book which clearly outlines the problems of the partially seeing child and delineates methods of identifying these children and meeting their health educational neds.)

Kough, Jack, and Robert F. De Haan: *Teacher's Guidance Handbook* (first given as reference in Chap. 5). Vol. I, *Identifying Children with Special Needs*, Sec. IV, Chap. 20; Vol. II, Sec. IV, Chap. 17.

MacNalty, Arthur S.: *The Preservation of Eyesight*, The Williams & Wilkins Company, Baltimore, 1958. (Simple presentation of anatomy and physiology of the eye, common eye infections, and prevention of eye diseases and injuries in industry.)

National Association for the Prevention of Blindness: *Classroom Lighting*, The Association, New York, 1963.

National Education Association: *Teaching about Light and Sight*, The Association, Washington, D.C.

Perry, John: *Our Wonderful Eyes*, McGraw-Hill Book Company, New York, 1955. (Facts about the eyes presented in an interesting way.)

Sutton-Vane, S.: *The Story of Eyes*, The Viking Press, Inc., New York, 1958. (The evolution of sight from the primitive forms to the complex human eye.)

U.S. Department of Health, Education, and Welfare: *Screening School Children for Visual Defects*, Children's Bureau Publication No. 345, Washington, D.C.

Organizations

Illuminating Engineering Society

National Society for the Prevention of Blindness

Chapter 17   HEARING AND SPEECH

The Organ of Hearing
Middle-ear Infections
Loss of Hearing and Its Detection
Helping Children with Loss of Hearing
Speech and Its Production
Speech Difficulties

So much of learning is associated intimately with the ability of teachers and students to communicate directly with one another that the school is rightly concerned with any condition that interferes with keenness of hearing or clearness of speech. Hearing is the function of the ears. Speech is the production of the vibrating vocal cords modified by a number of other structures. Some knowledge of the structure of these organs and how they work will help teachers to discover and to understand and help children in their classes who have difficulty in hearing or in speaking.

THE ORGAN OF HEARING

As with the sense of sight, so with the sense of hearing, three things are involved. First of all there must be sound waves sent out into the surrounding air by vibrating bodies. Second, there must be an instrument to receive and transmit to the brain the impulses provoked by sound. And third, there must be a center in the brain where sounds are registered and interpreted so that the hearer can recognize them for what they are.

Of these three things, only the instrument—the ears—is to some degree under individual control. A person cannot, of course, fiddle around with his ears as he can with the knobs of a radio or television set in order to change the volume or clearness of the sounds he hears. But there are things the individual can do to protect his ears from the infections and injuries that lessen their efficiency as receivers and transmitters of sound.

The Outer Ear

The part of the ear we see and wash is an appendage of cartilage covered with skin and known as the *pinna,* or wing. Its function is to scoop up sound waves and direct them into the outer ear canal. This winding passageway extends inward and about 1 inch downward to the delicate membrane called the tympanum, or eardrum, which is stretched tightly across its inner end (see Fig. 17-1). The walls of the outer ear canal secrete a thick yellowish wax which acts like flypaper in catching and holding dust and insects that might otherwise injure the eardrum.

"*Something in the Ear.*" The outer ear canal may be temporarily clogged by impacted wax, by water caught in it during swimming, by small objects which children have been known to push into their ears, or by a pimple, boil, or other swelling.

If a child starts to rub or pull at an ear, or to shake the head as if to dislodge something in the ear, or to complain of fullness or stuffiness in the ear, something may be obstructing his outer ear canal. A child usually will confess the details of his ear-plugging experiment, if that is the trouble, when he begins to get a painful or uncomfortable reaction. A live insect usually advertises its presence in the ear canal by its buzzing.

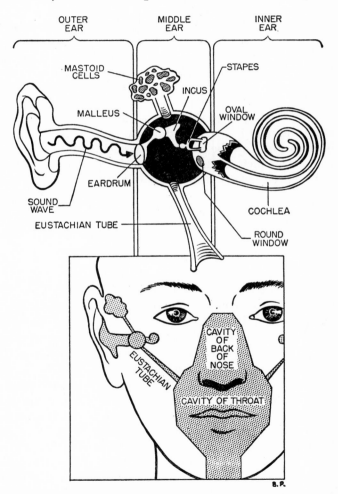

Fig. 17-1. Diagram showing divisions of the ear, with inset showing location with reference to nasopharynx.

Sometimes it is possible to see an obstruction in the outer ear canal by gently pulling the upper part of the ear upward and backward and looking into the opening.

The removal of a foreign body or plug of wax from the outer ear canal can be done safely only by a physician. It is dangerous to poke into the canal with a hairpin, toothpick, match, or other pointed instrument in an effort to get it out. Not only may you push the object further in, but also you may scratch the lining of the ear canal and thereby prepare the ground for an infection. The adage, "Put nothing smaller than your elbow in your ear" is still good advice.

The Middle Ear

The inner end of the outer ear canal is completely sealed by the eardrum. Beyond the eardrum lies the middle ear, a tiny chamber filled with air (see Fig. 17-1). The eardrum cannot vibrate properly under the impact of sound waves unless the pressure of air on each side of it is equal. Hence in evolving the architecture of the ear some method had to be devised to let air into the middle-ear chamber in order to equalize the pressure of air on the two sides of the drum. This was accomplished by connecting the middle ear with the nasopharynx (the meeting place of nose and throat) by a tube called the eustachian tube after its Italian discoverer, Bartolommeo Eustachio, a sixteenth-century anatomist. Before his day, the eustachian tube was unknown in human beings, although some acquaintance with it in animals may have led to the quaint theory that we breathe as well as hear with our ears. Physicians of ancient Egypt believed that "the breath of life enters by the right and that of death by the left ear."

The Eustachian Tube

The eustachian tube is about 1 to 1½ inches wide at its narrowest point. It is lined with mucous membrane which is a continuation of that which lines the nose and throat. It opens into the back of the throat and behind the soft palate. This opening, which flares outward like the mouth of a trumpet, is ordinarily kept closed. However, the mouth of the tube opens in swallowing, yawning, or when high pressure is created in the nasopharynx, as in blowing the nose forcibly or in exhaling forcibly with the mouth and nostrils closed. Practically everyone has had the experience of hearing his ears "pop" when going very far up or down from the place on the earth's surface to which he is accustomed. In going up, as in an elevator or an airplane, the air pressure on the outside of the eardrum decreases and the air in the middle ear drives the eardrum outward. Swallowing or yawning lets air of the same pressure as that on the outside of the drum enter the middle ear via the eustachian tube and the drum snaps or pops back into its original state of tautness. In going suddenly down from a high level to a low one, the pressure of air on the outside of the drum increases and the drum is driven inward until the air pressure on both sides of the drum is equalized by swallowing or yawning.

When the eustachian tube is closed temporarily by the swelling of its mucous membrane lining, as often happens when one has a cold, the pressure of air in the middle ear is below that of atmospheric air. In that event air is gradually absorbed from the middle ear into the bloodstream and the partial vacuum thus created causes the drum membrane to retract or push inward. This is the cause of the stuffy dull feeling in the ears and the dullness of hearing that so often accompany a head cold.

The Auditory Ossicles. The vibrations of the eardrum caused by the beating of sound waves against it are carried across the air-filled middle ear by a bridge of three miniature interlocking bones known as the auditory ossicles. The shapes of the auditory ossicles give them their names—the *malleus,* or hammer; the *incus,* or anvil; and the *stapes,* or stirrup. The handle of the hammer is attached to the eardrum and its club-shaped head articulates with the anvil, which in turn articulates with the base, or footplate, of the stirrup. The base of the stirrup fits tightly against a thin membrane that covers an opening (the oval window) that leads into the inner ear.

The Inner Ear

The inner ear is a small labyrinthine cavity tunneled out of the temporal bone of the skull (see Fig. 17-1). It contains (1) a central chamber, or vestibule, which lies on the inner side of the oval window leading from the middle ear; (2) the cochlea which contains the organ that enables us to hear; and (3) the semicircular canals that enable us to keep our balance (see The Balancing Apparatus, in Chap. 18).

The Cochlea. The cochlea is a spiral-shaped bony canal about as large as a pea. Since it resembles nothing so much as a snail shell, it gets its name from the Latin word for snail shell.

The spiral cochlea makes two and three-quarter turns around a central pillar of bone. A ledge of bone winding around this pillar, like the thread of a screw, divides the spiral canal incompletely throughout its entire length into an upper and a lower compartment or gallery, as shown in Fig. 17-2.

To complete the partition into two compartments, a membrane called the basilar membrane extends from the tip of the spiral bony ledge to the outer wall of the canal (Fig. 17-3). The basilar membrane is built up of a series of parallel fibers, called the auditory strings, of gradually decreasing length like the wires of a piano. However, the standard grand piano has only 240 strings, whereas the human cochlea has 24,000!

A second membrane, called the vestibular membrane, stretches from

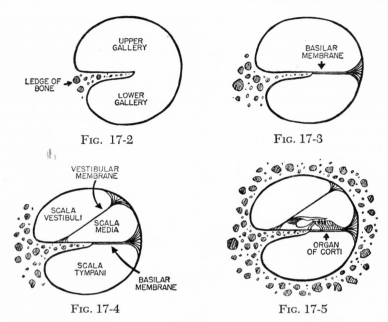

FIG. 17-2   FIG. 17-3

FIG. 17-4   FIG. 17-5

the upper surface of the spiral ledge of bone to a point a short distance above the outer attachment of the basilar membrane.

So we see that the original bony canal is divided throughout its entire length into three spiral compartments or galleries. Giving them their proper names, we now label the cross section as in Fig. 17-4.

The organ of hearing (organ of Corti) lies on the floor (basilar membrane) of the scale media, or middle gallery of the canal, as shown in Fig. 17-5. The organ of Corti consists essentially of rows of sensory sound receptors called hair cells because the surface of each one is equipped with fine hairlike processes. The tips of the hair cells are embedded in the undersurface of a delicate covering (tectorial) membrane, and their bases are connected with the auditory strings of the basilar membrane (Fig. 17-6).

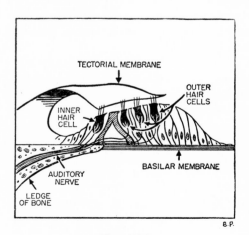

FIG. 17-6

Both the upper gallery (*scala vestibuli*) and the lower gallery (*scala tympani*) are filled with lymph called perilymph (*peri* means "around") to signify that this lymph lies around the middle chamber (*scala media*). The scala media also is filled with lymph called endolymph (*endo-* means "inside of").

The open end of the scala vestibuli is called the oval window, and the open end of the scala tympani is called the round window. Both the windows are covered tightly with curtains of membrane.

A diagrammatic longitudinal section of the cochlear canal as it would appear if straightened out (Fig. 17-7) may at this point help to make its structure clear.

What Happens When We Hear. What happens when we hear is something like what happened in the nursery tale when, given the proper stimulus, the water began to quench the fire, the fire began to burn the stick, the stick began to beat the dog, and so on.

The eardrum vibrates when struck by sound waves set up in air by vibrating bodies, just as a drumhead vibrates when struck with drumsticks. The vibrations of the eardrum are conducted over the bridge of interlocking auditory ossicles spanning the middle ear to the membrane covering the oval window. The rocking of the stapes against this membrane sets up waves in the perilymph in the scala vestibuli. The impact of the miniature "water waves" against the delicate tectorial membrane roofing the organ of hearing sets up similar oscillations in the endolymph. These oscillations cause the basilar membrane, which forms the floor of the scala media, to move up and down. In this way the vibrations of the eardrum are reproduced in the basilar membrane. Thence they are transmitted through the perilymph of the scala tympani to the round window. The membrane of the round window, located between the scala tympani and the middle ear, acts as the shock absorber of the whole system, since it yields readily to pressure.

Each auditory string of the basilar membrane, like each piano string, is tuned to a sound (or note) of a particular wavelength. Hence it vibrates in sympathy when a sound of the corresponding wavelength makes the eardrum vibrate. The frequency of vibration, that is, the number of

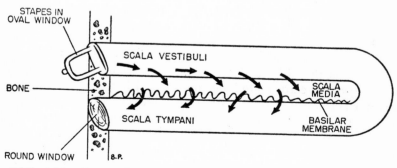

FIG. 17-7. (*After Best and Taylor, "The Human Body; Its Anatomy and Physiology,* 4th ed., *Holt, Rinehart and Winston, Inc., New York, 1963, p. 609.*)

oscillations, or cycles, per second, determines the pitch of the sound we hear.

The auditory cells seated upon the vibrating auditory strings respond to tiny variations in pressure by sending impulses to the brain, via the auditory nerve, where the sound is recognized. A different sensation is received for every sound because the auditory cells seated on each string have their own separate nerve fibers. In the case of complicated sounds a number of auditory strings are thrown into vibration at the same time, the impression conveyed to the brain being the sum total of them all.

The longest and thickest auditory strings are at the top of the cochlea. They vibrate at the rate of about 16 oscillations (cycles) per second. The shortest and most delicate strings are at the base of the cochlea. They vibrate at from 20,000 to 30,000 cps (cycles per second). The ear is most sensitive to pitches ranging from 2,000 to 5,000 cps, that is, for the upper two octaves of the piano.

When a sound is very loud it is felt as well as heard. Feeling is highest for sounds of low frequency, lowest for sounds of high frequency. Hence, a low rumbling sound is felt more than heard, while a high-piched shrill note causes a very painful feeling in the ear.

The faculty of hearing sounds of high frequency is most highly developed in children and declines as persons grow older. A child with normal hearing can detect sounds of 20,000 cps; at thirty years of age the number is decreased to 15,000; and at fifty, to 13,000.

MIDDLE-EAR INFECTIONS

The eustachian tube, as we have seen, is an ingenious device for equalizing air pressure on each side of the eardrum. Its only drawback is the opportunity it permits for the entrance of bacteria into the middle ear from the nose and throat. That is why infection of the middle ear may accompany or follow an acute cold in the head, sinusitis, tonsillitis, influenza, scarlet fever, measles, and other acute infectious diseases involving the upper respiratory tract.

Earache

Severe earache is usually caused by inflammation or abscess of the middle ear (acute otitis media). The pressure set up by pus in the middle ear causes the eardrum to bulge outward. If left to itself, the pressure of the pus perforates or ruptures the eardrum. The ear surgeon prevents this spontaneous rupture, if he sees the child in time, by making an incision near the edge of the drum to allow free drainage. A surgical incision usually heals soon, leaving no loss of hearing. Spontaneous rupture, on the other hand, may result in a large or jagged opening in the eardrum which may heal slowly and in some cases fail to close entirely.

In the latter case the ear may discharge more or less continuously or whenever the child has a cold.

The ears also may ache or feel sore or stuffy during a head cold or at the onset of some other communicable disease affecting the upper respiratory tract. Other possible causes of earache are mumps, a decayed molar tooth, inflammation of the eustachian tube, inflammation or an abscess or boil in the outer ear canal, and inflammation of the mastoid bone back of the ear. Needless to say, medical attention is required for any child who complains of earache. Prompt treatment (with one of the sulfa drugs or antibiotics) can nearly always prevent serious middle-ear infections.

"Runny Ear"

A child whose ear is "running" is quite likely to have a plug of cotton in the affected ear (see Plate 14). In chronic infections, however, the drainage may be indicated only by persistent slight moisture. The teacher should make sure that a child with a discharging ear (acute or chronic) is being looked after by a physician, as this condition may have serious consequences if neglected.

A child with a discharging ear who is free of pain and fever may be permitted by his physician to attend school. In supervising such a child the teacher may find the following information helpful. Usually a physician does not wish to have the ear canal tightly plugged with cotton, as free drainage is important. Cotton may be placed very loosely in the outer portion of the ear canal to absorb the discharge and prevent dripping. The skin area exposed to a persistent discharge tends to become red and raw. Petrolatum or some other bland ointment is often recommended as a help in protecting the skin from an irritating discharge. It is also important to keep the area clean and to encourage the child to keep his fingers away from it.

A severe head injury may result in a watery, blood-tinged discharge from the ears or nose. This is a serious sign, as it may indicate brain damage. A physician should be summoned at once for any child who has been dazed, even momentarily, by an injury to the head.

Chronic Otitis Media

Far more insidious than acute middle-ear infection, which usually makes itself known in accents of severe pain, is chronic inflammation of the middle ear. Sometimes this condition is called chronic catarrh. Repeated or prolonged colds and other long-continued irritations of the nose, the nasal sinuses, the throat, or the passage to the ear may keep the membranes lining the middle ear in a state of constant low-grade inflammation—a sort of mild resentment of the constant nagging which is not provoking enough to cause a full-blown flare-up, but which will result eventually in a thickening of the membranes lining the middle ear and a stiffening of the joints of the three miniature bones bridging it (see further on). The result will be progressive loss of hearing unless the condition is cleared up in time.

Mastoiditis

Nearly always some of the cells in the honeycomb-like mastoid bone which connects with the middle ear are involved in acute middle-ear infection. The mastoid bone may be felt as a hard ridge behind the external ear. Extensive inflammation of the mastoid process results in mastoiditis. In children with a running ear or a recent history of one, complaints of pain and tenderness back of the ear may be symptoms of this infection. Acute or chronic mastoiditis is a serious condition which in the past nearly always required surgical intervention. Now it can usually be prevented or treated successfully with a sulfa drug or one of the antibiotics.

LOSS OF HEARING AND ITS DETECTION

A lack or loss, complete or partial, of the sense of hearing is the medical definition of deafness. It is customary, however, to call a person "deaf" only if he has lost practically all of his sense of hearing.

An estimated million and a half school children have some degree of hearing loss. From one-fourth to one-third of the children have sufficient impairment to handicap them.

Types of Hearing Loss

Loss of hearing may result from a defect or disease in any part of the auditory mechanism. When the trouble is located in the outer ear canal, eardrum, or middle ear—the sound-conducting portions of the ear—the resulting loss of hearing is called transmission, or conduction, deafness. This is by far the most common form of hearing loss.

Loss of hearing due to a lesion of the auditory nerve is called nerve deafness. If the lesion is located along the auditory pathways leading to the auditory center in the brain, or in the auditory center itself, the resulting loss of hearing is called central deafness.

Some cases of deafness are caused by the formation of spongy bone in the inner ear. This condition is called otosclerosis. Hearing may be restored or improved by an operation known as fenestration in which the surgeon cuts a tiny window into the inner ear.

Deaf-mutes are children who are born deaf because of some congenital defect in the hearing mechanism and children who become totally deaf early in infancy. Learning to speak is an imitative process and if a child cannot hear words spoken he has nothing to go by in learning to form words. Deaf-mute children can be trained to read lip movements and to converse with others in sign language. Sometimes they may be taught to talk by imitating lip and throat movements associated with speech.

Observing Children for Loss of Hearing

Loss of hearing, whatever the type or cause, interferes with learning and normal child development. It is often the underlying cause of undesirable behavior or lack of progress in school. If loss of hearing is not recognized, a child may be scolded for seeming stupid, indifferent, or stubborn. As a result of feeling misunderstood at home and in school, he may become emotionally maladjusted—accept the idea of failure and seek compensation in undesirable ways.

As the teacher has no way of observing what is going on in the ears, it is easy to miss indications of loss of hearing. However, she has opportunities to make other observations that will serve as valuable leads when reported to the physician or nurse. Signs indicating chronic nose or throat trouble and early symptoms of chronic middle-ear inflammation should always be brought to the attention of a physician, since trouble of this kind so often leads to progressive loss of hearing.

Early symptoms of chronic middle-ear inflammation of which a child may complain include a persistent feeling of heaviness, dullness, fullness, or stuffiness in the ear; and queer head noises such as buzzing, hissing, or ringing. However, these symptoms may develop so gradually that the child gets used to them before he realizes that he has good grounds for complaint. Hence it is important to watch for the characteristic behavior and appearance that usually accompany some loss of hearing. The teacher may suspect hearing difficulty when any one or more of the following signs are noted:

1. Asking to have words or phrases repeated; cocking an ear toward the speaker when addressed; answering questions incorrectly; seeming to be stupid in understanding instructions or making numerous mistakes in carrying them out; appearing to be inattentive or to take little interest in what is going on about him.

2. Failing to respond when called or failing to locate the source of a sound, as shown by going in the wrong direction when responding to a call.

3. Watching others before beginning to work, or copying from other pupils.

4. Bewildered facial expression showing that the child is not fully aware of what is going on about him; a look of "watchful waiting" (see Plate 14).

5. Faulty articulation out of proportion to age (a child who cannot hear words distinctly will not be able to pronounce them correctly); unnatural pitch of the voice—too high, too low, too loud, or monotonous.

Audiometric Screening Tests for Hearing

Screening tests for hearing are given in most schools in order to find students who should be referred to a hearing specialist (otologist) for professional examination and diagnosis. In several states a hearing test is required by law at or near the beginning of each school year. It is believed, however, that most students with significant hearing loss will be discovered if an audiometric screening test is given (1) to all children entering school for the first time; (2) annually to all children under 10 years of age, except those already known to have a hearing impairment; and (3) possibly to all children just before leaving school, especially to those who terminate their schooling before high school graduation.

In addition to this routine testing program, a screening test should be arranged as soon as possible for children of any age who fall into one of the following special referral categories:

1. A child whose teacher, parents, school nurse, or he himself suspects that his hearing is not normal
2. A child who has frequent or severe respiratory infections or allergic reactions involving the nose, throat, or ears
3. A child who is frequently absent from school
4. A normally intelligent child whose academic work is poor according to the patterns of instruction and grading of the school

Types of Audiometers. Two types of instruments are in general use at the present time for testing the hearing of school children, (1) the phonograph speech audiometer, and (2) the pure-tone audiometer.

The phonograph audiometer was developed to meet the need for a rapid method of testing the hearing acuity of large groups of children. Speech sounds from a phonograph record are led through the instrument and then to a receiver applied to the child's ear. The test sounds in the form of spoken numbers are varied in intensity, or loudness, by means of dials upon the front of the instrument. Groups of up to forty children may be tested at one time. In testing with the phonograph audiometer, the level of intensity at which numbers either are not heard or are heard incorrectly represents a child's degree of hearing acuity.

The pure-tone audiometer provides an instrument for measuring the hearing acuity of individuals for a series of pure tones of a given pitch (intensity) at preselected frequency levels (cycles per second). In performing this test the attenuation dial usually is set or maintained at a predetermined intensity level for each frequency generated by the audiometer in the range of frequencies selected for checking. Variations in the audibility of specific tones in relation to frequency are recorded on a graph known as an audiogram.

The pure-tone audiometer is a more reliable instrument for detecting hearing loss than the phonograph speech audiometer, as it makes possible the detection of high-frequency losses that are not revealed by the phonograph screening method. Early hearing loss often begins in the high-frequency range. High-frequency deficiencies may result in certain types of speech impairment in addition to being medically significant. For those reasons many authorities believe that school testing should be conducted only with the pure-tone audiometer.

Measurement of Sound Intensity. The decibel is the unit by which the intensity, or loudness, of sound is measured. A decibel is one-tenth of a bel, so named after Alexander Graham Bell, the inventor of the telephone. One decibel equals the least intensity or degree of loudness of any given tone at which that tone, or note, can be heard by the normal ear (normal threshold). A whisper is around 10 to 20 decibels in intensity; ordinary conversation, about 50 or 60 decibels. The normal human ear has a range of auditory response up to 120 decibels. Noise is loud enough to be painful to the ear at about 140 decibels.

In the pure-tone audiometer, the intensity of tone is calibrated in intervals of 5 decibels. The standard scale is logarithmic. Therefore, each step of 10 decibels represents ten times the previous step in decibel loss. If the loudness of a sound has to be stepped up to 10 decibels in order to make audible a sound that normally would be heard at 1 decibel (normal threshold), the amount of hearing loss is expressed as 10 decibels. A loss of 20 decibels means that the change in loudness required to hear the sound is 100 times that required at normal threshold; a loss of 30 decibels, 1,000 times; of 40 decibels, 10,000 times; and so on.

Preparation for Audiometric Testing. Many schools have their own audiometers[1] for testing the auditory acuity of children in groups and individually. In some states audiometers may be obtained on loan from the department of health or education, or representatives of the department of health or education may visit schools at stated times to conduct hearing tests.

For accuracy and efficiency it is necessary to have audiometric testing done by adequately trained persons. In many school districts the testing is done by the school nurse. In others, certain teachers or substitute teachers may be designated for special training in conducting the tests and in reading and recording the results.

In preparation for the testing of auditory acuity, the ears and their care should be the subject for study and discussion in health class. As in vision testing, the children should be told what is going to happen and why it is so important to find out how well they can hear.

The room selected for audiometric testing should be the quietest

---

[1] Information concerning various types and models of audiometers can be obtained from the American Hearing Society and from its chapters and affiliates throughout the country.

suitable room in the school building—usually a room on the top floor, or one with no room above, is best. The playgrounds should not be used, and there should be no marching or singing during the periods in which the tests are being given.

Since the hearing of only one child at a time can be tested with the pure-tone audiometer, this test can be conducted in a smaller room than that required for testing with the phonograph audiometer. In many schools the health room is used for this purpose. Considerable time may be saved by having the children brought into the room in groups of four or six at a time. This procedure makes it unnecessary to repeat the instructions to each child, and a minimum of time is lost between tests. As soon as all but one of the children of the small group have been tested they are sent back to their class with orders to send in the next group while the remaining child is being tested.

Results of Audiometric Testing. A child may show some hearing loss in one or both ears at the first or "sweep" test for any of the following reasons:

1. The child may actually have defective hearing.
2. Some extraneous noise may have distracted his attention.
3. He may have been unable to do his best because of nervousness. (Young children unfamiliar with the use of a telephone are especially apt to be nervous.)
4. The receiver may have been improperly adjusted, or some condition, such as an acute cold, may have temporarily impaired his hearing.

Because of the many chances for error in a first test, all children who fail to make a satisfactory score should be retested at least twice. Usually children given a second test after testing with the phonograph audiometer are all those below the seventh grade who fail to hear speech sounds at 9 decibels or better and children in grade seven and above who fail to hear at 6 decibels or better. Children referred for a second test after testing with the pure-tone audiometer are all those who exhibited a loss of 20 decibels or more for two or more tones.

If a child fails the second test his teacher should be informed immediately of the possibility of hearing impairment. He should be tested again approximately three weeks later. This third test, if given with a pure-tone audiometer, should be a threshold test. This test reveals how loud a tone must be to produce the slightest perceptible sensation of sound.

All children who fail to make a satisfactory score on the third test should be given a complete professional examination by an otologist. In making the referral for an otological examination, it will be helpful to the physician making the examination to have the pooled observations of the teacher and school nurse. The record of such observations should include any history of frequent or prolonged upper respiratory tract infection, complaints made by the child of queer noises in the ears or head, and a description of behavior or appearance suggestive of hearing loss. Once a child has been found to have a hearing impairment, prompt and persistent follow-up steps should be taken by the school to ensure adequate care. The child should be removed from the screening program, and thereafter he should be given suitable supervision and his hearing threshold should be tested at appropriate intervals. Frequent threshold retesting may help to motivate the family toward placing the child under the care of a physician as well as to measure the child's progress.

Hearing Tests without the Use of an Audiometer

There are two types of rough-and-ready hearing tests that may be made by teachers in schools where it is impossible to obtain audiometric testing.

The Whisper Test. A whisper can usually be heard in a quiet room by a person with normal hearing at a distance of 20 to 30 feet, depending upon the loudness of the whisper. In making the whisper test, the residual whisper is employed. This is a whisper made with the air remaining in the lungs at the end of an ordinary expiration. It ensures the same degree of loudness of the whisper used in testing all individuals in a group.

In preparation for the whisper test, mark off a distance of 25 feet from the chair in which the child will be seated. At that distance and at intervals of 1 foot inward toward the chair, draw chalk lines parallel to one another. After the child is seated, blindfold him lightly or have him hold a card against the side of his face so that he cannot see your movements. Then instruct him to cover one ear tightly with his hand and to repeat after you each word or number that he can hear. Use either nouns of one syllable or numbers, but do not mix them. If nouns are used, tell the children in advance which ones you are going to whisper. Choose nouns that are familiar to the children. If numbers are used, the ones you are going to whisper should be recited in advance. Such numbers as 5, 19, 25, 26, 27, 33, 66, and 76 test hearing both for low tones and for sibilant sounds.

Be sure that the room is absolutely quiet. Then, standing at the line 1 foot away from the child and facing the ear being tested, whisper a few words or numbers. Enunciate clearly and breathe in and out after each whisper. If he repeats them correctly after you, move back a few feet and whisper different words or numbers. Continue moving back until the point is reached beyond which the child cannot hear. Record the greatest distance at which the child repeats the words or numbers correctly. Test both ears in this way.

The greatest distance at which about three-quarters of the class repeat the words or numbers correctly may be taken as the norm. It is not wise to use a standardized distance, such as 20 feet, as the norm because the "normal distance" will vary according to environmental noise and difference in the loudness of the whisper of the person giving the test.

Record the result for each child as a fraction of the norm. The numerator will be the greatest distance at which the sounds are audible to the child and the denominator the greatest distance at which they are heard by 75 per cent of the children under the same conditions. A hearing distance of even 3 feet less than the norm suggests some loss of hearing, and the child should be referred for medical examination.

The Watch-tick Test. A loud-ticking watch may be substituted for the residual whisper as a rough-and-ready hearing test. In quiet surroundings a loud watch is heard by the normal ear at a distance of about 3 feet. However, it is not safe to use this criterion, and the watch selected should be standardized by repeated trials on children with normal hearing. That is, if the majority of the children tested hear its tick at 3 feet, then 3 feet may be taken as the norm.

Seat the child to be tested, blindfold him, and have him cover one ear with his hand. Place the watch near the uncovered ear and ask him whether he can hear the tick. Move the watch away from his ear until the point is reached at which it ceases to be heard. From this point move the watch back toward the ear and measure and record the distance at which it is just heard. Test both ears in this way.

If a child's hearing distance is much less than the normal distance, the child should be referred for medical examination.

Referral for Otological Examination. It sometimes happens that findings of the whisper test or watch-tick test which seem to indicate some loss of hearing are not confirmed by the ear specialist. For this reason it is considered unwise for the teacher or nurse to tell the parents or guardians the results of the test. The suggestion that an ear examination is advisable, without going into details, should be sufficient.

HELPING CHILDREN WITH LOSS OF HEARING

In many cases of auditory loss, the hearing may be improved or progressive loss of hearing checked by early medical attention. Children whose hearing is irremediably impaired to the point at which the inability to hear constitutes a definite handicap may be helped by training in lipreading or by the wearing of a special hearing aid [2] recommended by the physician or by both. In some school systems provision is made

[2] The American Hearing Society gives information regarding the different hearing aids accepted by the American Medical Association. In some cities a person with impaired hearing may visit the offices of the local chapter or affiliate of this organization, try out hearing aids, and get advice. The Alexander Graham Bell Association for the Deaf provides inquirers with a list of approved hearing-aid clinics throughout the nation where audiometric testing is given and where hearing aids can be tried. (See Addresses of Organizations, at the back of this book.)

for lipreading classes and for special instruction of hard-of-hearing children.

The teacher and school nurse should be informed of the otologist's recommendations in the case of any child whose hearing is impaired so that they can cooperate intelligently with the parents and physician in helping the child to make as good an adjustment as possible.

The child should know that he has hearing loss, but should not be pampered or made to feel self-conscious by too much attention. It is important for him to realize that defective hearing, like defective vision, is nothing to be ashamed of and that it is better to have others know about it than to give a false impression of stupidity or stubbornness. His teacher and his schoolmates can be of great help by looking directly at him and speaking clearly when addressing him. His seat in the classroom should be assigned with a view to making it as easy as possible for him to see and hear the teacher.

Since loss of hearing imposes both a physical and a mental strain, a hard-of-hearing child should be watched carefully for signs of fatigue. Also the teacher should note on the child's health record any signs of change for the better or worse in his ability to hear and her observations as to his behavior and his success or failure in adjusting to the school situation.

SPEECH AND ITS PRODUCTION

A large part of the life and thought we share with our contemporaries is made possible, in Emerson's words, by the fact that "the hearing ear is always found close to the speaking tongue." The ability to send out the sounds of speech, however, is not located in the tongue but rather in the upper part of the larynx directly below the epiglottis (see The Larynx, in Chap. 11).

The Voice Box

The glottis, or "voice box," as it is sometimes called, is an aperture or chink between the vocal cords together with all that part of the larynx concerned with voice production. The two equal sides of the glottis are formed by the vocal cords (see Fig. 17-8), which are strands of yellow elastic tissue that run from the front to the rear of the larynx. They are attached at the rear to two small cartilaginous bodies (the arytenoid cartilages) and are fixed to the wall of the larynx in front. The vocal cords are swung outward against the walls of the larynx or inward toward each other by small muscles which rotate the arytenoid cartilages. Ordinarily the vocal cords lie against the walls of the larynx, leaving the glottis wide open for breathing. In speaking or singing they are brought toward each other until the glottis shrinks to a small chink. The flow of air expelled from the lungs sets the edges of these tautened cords into vibration, thus producing the voice. Slender muscles in the cords themselves make it possible to tighten or slacken them so as to change the frequency of their vibration and thus vary the pitch of the voice. In children and women, the vocal cords are short and high-pitched; in men they are longer and the voice is deeper.

The timbre, or quality, of the voice is produced by numerous resonating spaces, just as the vibrations of violin strings or the reeds of an organ are transformed into a complex tissue of tones by the sounding board of the violin or the pipes of the organ. The resonating spaces of the human vocal instrument include the chest, the throat, the mouth and nose, and the nasal sinuses.

Voice is not speech, but rather a series of musical tones and overtones. To produce the sounds of speech, the sound waves sent forth by the vibrating vocal cords are modified by other structures—the nose, lips, teeth, and tongue. Broadly speaking, there are vowel and consonant sounds. Vowel sounds are formed by the passage of air through the mouth, which assumes characteristic positions for each vowel. Consonants are produced by the blocking or interruption of the passage of expired air in various parts of the vocal pathway by the tongue, teeth, lips, or soft palate.

You can learn a great deal about the production of individual sounds by pronouncing the letters of the alphabet and observing in a mirror the position assumed by the various structures involved.

The voice change from childish soprano to baritone or bass in adolescent boys is caused by the descent of the larynx to a lower position in the

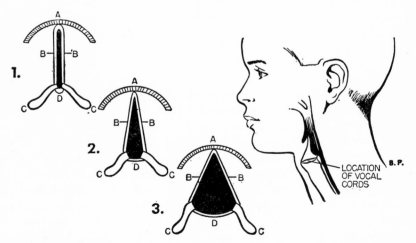

FIG. 17-8. Vocal cords as seen from above. 1, cords brought closely together as in singing a high note. 2, cords brought toward each other as in speaking. 3, cords swung out against wall of larynx as in breathing. A, front of the larynx. B–B, the vocal cords. C–C, the arytenoid cartilages. D, back of larynx.

throat. The cracks or breaks in the voice so characteristic of boys in this transition period are due to the fact that the larynx does not immediately become accustomed to its new position and occasionally moves up to the old.

Falsetto Voice

In some boys the shift in position of the larynx does not take place, with the result that they retain the high soprano of childhood. A soprano voice in a man is called *falsetto* (Italian for false) because of its un-naturalness. The failure of the larynx to descend may be caused by psychic factors, by bad habits of speaking contracted during the change in voice, or by an endocrine disturbance.

An example of a psychic cause is an unconscious fear of assuming the responsibilities of adult life. The resulting anxiety may inhibit the voice change which proclaims to the world that the boy is becoming a man. In that case the muscles that keep the larynx raised (elevator muscles) may retain their dominance over those which lower it (depressor muscles), and the larynx remains high in the throat. If this condition is allowed to persist, the continued psychic blows to the personality may have serious consequences. Fortunately, the larynx may be lowered by manipulation, but this procedure must be reinforced by psychotherapy to remove the basic feeling of inadequacy and by voice training. If the condition is caused by an endocrine disturbance, glandular treatment will be necessary. Whatever the cause, persistent falsetto voice in a boy who in other respects is close to manhood indicates that the assistance of a competent medical specialist is necessary.

SPEECH DIFFICULTIES

It is estimated that there are more than twelve million speech and voice cripples in the United States, upward of one million of whom are in the school population. Generally speaking, speech is considered to be defective or distorted "when it deviates so far from the speech of other people in the group that it calls attention to itself, interferes with communication, or causes its possessor to be maladjusted." [3]

Difficulty in speaking is a serious impediment in social, academic, and work relationships. Even if the difficulty is a physical abnormality, psychological aspects are bound to complicate the picture sooner or later. If young children are permitted to go along with any form of distorted speech, with the idea that they will later outgrow it, not only will the disorder or defect itself be far more difficult to cure but also the child's personality may be warped permanently.

Ideally, children entering school for the first time should have a

[3] C. Van Riper: *Speech Correction—Principles and Methods,* 3d ed., Prentice-Hall, New York, 1954, p. 19.

speech examination by a trained examiner to screen out those with speech difficulties. Not many schools have this service. Authorities agree that the next-best procedure is to have the classroom teachers report speech difficulties to the nurse or physician serving the school. For this reason it is recommended that teachers, as part of their training, learn to recognize speech disorders. The procedure after recognition involves examination by a speech clinician or trained speech correctionist for diagnosis and the planning of treatment. In some cases surgical or psychiatric treatment may be required before voice and speech training are started. In school systems in which speech correctionists or specially trained teachers are not employed, this training may be carried on by the parents or teachers under the supervision of the specialist responsible for the diagnosis and treatment. In some communities speech clinics which offer diagnosis and treatment of speech disorders may be available for the individual or group treatment of children who need it.

Variations of Speech Disorders

Speech disorders differ widely as to cause, kind, and degree of handicapping. Roughly they may be classified as follows:

1. Speech difficulties caused by some structural defect in one or more of the organs involved in speech. Examples of such defects are cleft palate, harelip, protruding upper or lower front teeth and missing front teeth, nasal obstructions, and any abnormality in the larynx.

2. Weakness or sluggishness of the soft palate, tongue, and lips, which results in a distortion of speech because more effort is required in speaking than is normally put forth. Examples are lisping and nasality.

3. Complete or partial loss of the power to speak or to write (motor aphasia) or of the ability to understand spoken or written language (sensory aphasia) because of injury or disease of the speech centers in the brain (see Aphasia, in Chap. 8).

4. A disturbance of the rhythm of speech, usually symptomatic of a personality maladjustment. The outstanding example of such a so-called "emotional disorder of speech" is stuttering or stammering.

5. Poor quality of voice, which may be due to a structural or functional cause. Voices of poor quality may be husky, weak, nasal, shrill, breathy, or monotonous. Excessive loss of hearing or nerve deafness (due to a lesion of the auditory nerve) is quite likely to result in monotonous phonation. Learning to speak is an imitative process. Children cannot learn to speak well if they cannot hear well.

6. Substitution of one speech sound for another beyond the period at which correctness of speech is usually acquired. The popular term for this difficulty is "baby talk." It may be due to a slight temporary interruption of the growth process, or to a home environment in which baby talk is encouraged, or to some emotional blocking.

7. A noticeable unusual accent caused by the influence on English speech of a foreign language, local dialect, or family peculiarities of utterance. Since speech (as we have noted above) is largely imitative, children cannot learn to speak English correctly if they constantly hear English spoken poorly.

In describing speech difficulties that are caused by defects of structure or poor functioning, it will be helpful to have some knowledge of what the organs involved have to do with the production of sounds.

The Tongue in Speech

From time immemorial the tongue has been intimately associated with speech. *Linga*, in Latin, means both "tongue" and "language." In the Old Testament we find Moses complaining to the Lord that he was "slow of speech and of a slow tongue" and Isaiah prophesying that on the day of judgment "the tongue of stammerers shall be ready to speak plainly." At one time it was thought that moistness of the tongue caused stammering, and attempts were made to dry the tongue by blistering it. A more modern version of loosing the "string of the tongue," which is how St. Mark described Christ's cure of a speech sufferer, was the actual cutting of the lingual nerves in attempts to cure stuttering. Thousands of tongues were cut and mutilated until it became evident that operative measures were entirely useless as means of curing stammerers.

The tongue participates in the production of a great variety of speech sounds, although it is not the all-important organ of speech it is popularly supposed to be. It is the only muscle in the body that is attached only at one end. This arrangement makes it especially mobile and flexible. In producing individual sounds it assumes a great many different forms and positions, as you can see for yourself by looking in a mirror while talking.

Tongue-tie. Teachers or parents have often remarked carelessly, "Oh, he is tongue-tied," to explain an otherwise inexplicable speech impediment in a child. As a matter of fact, very few speech difficulties are caused by defects of the tongue, and true tongue-tie is a rare condition.

Normally, the fold of membrane that attaches the undersurface of the tongue to the floor of the mouth is located at some distance back from the tongue tip. You can see this membrane by protruding and lifting your tongue while looking into a mirror. In tongue-tie the membrane is attached close to, or right at, the tip of the tongue. As a result, the tongue literally is tied down.

It is easy for teachers or parents to find out whether a child is truly tongue-tied. If the child can stick out his tongue and curve it upward to touch the groove in the middle of his upper lip; or if he can run the tip of his tongue along the roof of his mouth, with his lips and teeth slightly open, he is not tongue-tied. The operation to correct tongue-tie is a simple one. Of course it should be performed only by a surgeon and only when he says there is need for it.

The Lips in Speech

Several sounds in English speech are primarily lip sounds or lip-teeth sounds. It is impossible, for example, to make the sound of P or B, or to say "which" or "what," without moving the lips. A common fault in speaking is a failure to use the lips enough in forming consonant sounds.

Harelip. Harelip is the defect most commonly involved in speech disorders that are due to structural malformation of the lips. This is a congenital cleft of one or both lips, but usually of the upper lip only. It can be corrected by surgery, the earlier the better for the child born with it. As in cleft palate (see under The Palate in Speech, further on), voice and speech training are required after the defect has been repaired.

The Teeth in Speech

The forcing of air against or between the cutting edges of the front teeth is responsible for several consonant sounds. If the teeth of the upper and lower jaws do not come together (occlude) or if any front teeth are missing, some of these sounds may be made incorrectly.

Lisping. The speech disorder most commonly connected with defective or missing teeth is lisping. In lisping, the sounds for S, Z, Sh, and Zh are made incorrectly or the Th sound is substituted for them. It is easy to understand why a child who is losing his deciduous front teeth may say "ith" for is, "clath" for class, "horth" for horse, "thithers" for scissors, and so on, when we realize that the hissing sound of S and Z is produced by forcing air from behind against the nearly closed cutting edges of the front teeth, whereas in pronouncing Th, the tip of the tongue protrudes from between the teeth.

Sluggishness or wrong manipulation of the tongue may also produce lisping. Some lispers protrude the tongue in pronouncing words in which S or Z sounds are required instead of pointing it at the teeth from behind (lingual lisp); others fail to raise the tongue on both sides, with the result that air slides over the sides instead of through a channel in the middle (lateral lisp). By asking children who lisp for no obvious cause (such as missing teeth or malocclusion) to pronounce such words as sleep, slide, see, shine, wish, show, zoo, zebra, pleasure, and please, and watching their tongues meanwhile, the teacher may be able to observe the trouble in managing the tongue which is responsible. Gymnastic exercises for the tongue which are helpful in efforts to overcome lisp are given in books or manuals on the correction of speech disorders.

The Nose in Speech

The nasal cavities and nasal sinuses are part of the resonating apparatus in the production of voice. Also a few of the sounds of speech normally are produced by blocking the passage of air through the mouth and allowing it to pass out through the nose. These nasal sounds of speech are M, N, and Ng.

The familiar speech distortions often caused by the temporary congestion of the nose during a bad cold in the head illustrate what may happen to the voice as a result of an obstruction due to some structural defect of the nose or throat. The diagnosis and treatment of such defects naturally are the responsibility of the physician.

Nasality. Talking through the nose, or nasal intonation, is one of the most common faults involved in voices that are unpleasant to hear. The nasal voice is a whining voice and the whine, which literally is the low plaintive nasal sound evoked in complaint or distress, is associated with a complaining, nagging personality. Actually a cheerful, happy person may be the unfortunate possessor of a "whining voice."

Nasal intonation is produced by the escape of air into the nose while the person is speaking. The reason that some people talk through their noses can best be explained by describing the structure and functions of the normal palate.

The Palate in Speech

The palate forms the roof of the mouth and the floor of the nose. It has two parts, one hard, one soft (see Fig. 11-2). The function of the palate is to separate the nose from the mouth so that they can work separately.

If you will run your tongue over the roof of your mouth, you will feel a hard bony structure covered with membrane. This is the hard palate. Now look into the back of your mouth in a mirror. You will see a flap of soft muscular tissue which moves as you say "Ah." This is the soft palate. You will also notice that the soft palate hangs down into a finger-like bulge. This is called the uvula.

Between the soft palate and the back of the throat there is a small space called the "postnasal space" which permits air to flow from the throat into the nose in breathing out. During speech this space is closed off by the soft palate and muscles at the top of the throat in much the same manner as a drawstring is used to close a tobacco pouch or old-fashioned purse. The effect is to raise the soft palate and bring it in contact with the back of the throat so as to keep the vocalized air from escaping into the nose, thereby compelling it to flow out through the mouth.

Generally speaking, the larger the postnasal space, the greater the chance of nasality, since a large space is harder to close off than a smaller one. A weakness of the soft palate, requiring more effort than is usually put forth in speaking, also may result in nasality. Functional nasality, that is, nasality without any discoverable defect or weakness of structure may be present in children who have fallen into poor habits of speech.

Voice exercises are of great help in correcting nasality, whether of structural or functional origin. Preferably they should be carried on under the supervision of a speech correctionist. Blowing games are excellent for increasing the mobility of the soft palate and for teaching the child to direct the current of inspired air through the mouth instead of allowing it to escape through the postnasal space into the nose. Such play exercises include blowing bubbles into water through a straw, blowing a small celluloid ball across a flat surface, blowing soap bubbles, and blowing up balloons. For older children, learning to play musical instruments that require blowing, such as the mouth organ or the clarinet, will make the exercises interesting.

Cleft-palate Speech. This term is applied to the speech of a person who has a cleft, or opening, in the roof of the mouth. Although it is comparatively rare, it is one of the most distressing of all speech defects. Cleft palate is a congenital defect; that is, the child is born with it. No matter what may be the size or shape of the cleft, the child has great difficulty in speaking and eating. Speech, as might be expected with a hole through the roof of the mouth, is nasal in character.

Fortunately the cleft can often be closed if the operation is done in time by a surgeon specializing in the repair of such defects. The operation is most successful if it is performed before the child's third or fourth year. Even after a successful operation, however, massage and exercise are needed to make the soft palate move correctly, because a repaired palate is not so flexible and mobile as is a completely normal palate. Postoperative massage, exercises, and speech training are best carried on under the supervision of the trained speech correctionist, but parents or teachers can learn how to give them if a specialist's services are not available.

The Brain in Speech

The mechanics of speech are the functions of the organ of speech and its assistants, the tongue, teeth, nose, lips, and palate. The ability to speak, however, is located in the brain. In learning to speak the little child first associates the sounds (words) he hears with the sensations aroused by the objects he sees, touches, or otherwise apprehends. These associations are stored in his brain as memories. When definite meanings have become attached to certain words, pathways are established between the auditory center of the brain (the area where sounds are recognized and interpreted) and the motor area for speech (the area from which impulses are sent to the muscles involved in speech). The child then tries to form and utter the words that he has heard. As we have seen, this marvelous act of speaking depends upon the coordinated movements of a large group of muscles—the respiratory muscles, and the muscles of the larynx, pharynx, tongue, and lips.

Later on, as the child learns to read, he associates auditory speech with visual symbols of speech, that is, printed words. Finally association is established between the visual symbols of speech and the motor area that directs the movements of the hand. Then the child is able to express in writing both his auditory impressions (what he hears) and his visual impressions (what he sees).

Handedness. In most children the areas involved in speaking, reading, and writing are more highly developed in the left hemisphere of the cerebrum than they are in the right. Since the left half of the brain controls the right half of the body (see Fig. 17-9), most children are right-handed, "right-speaking," and "right-reading."

About 4 per cent of children, however, are left-handed. Babies begin to show their preference for the right or left hand when they are about six

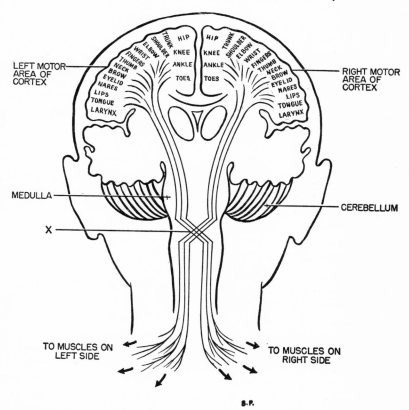

Fig. 17-9. Motor nerves from one half of the brain cross with those descending from the other half at the spot marked X. Hence the left motor area of the brain controls the muscles in the right side of the body and vice versa.

months old. As we live in a right-handed world, parents and teachers may try to correct left-handedness. This is a mistake. There is nothing wrong in being left-handed. Of course the child must put up with the inconvenience of living in a world in which the buttons on his clothes, the knobs on doors, and many other contrivances are designed for right-handed people. However, left-handed children seem to take such inconveniences in their stride. It is only when they are made to feel conscious of their difference from other children by being heckled or ridiculed that speech difficulties or other forms of maladjustment may develop.

Stuttering

Stuttering is a common speech disorder in children. A distinction used to be made between the intermittent blocking of speech called "stammering" and the repetition or prolongation of syllables and words or phrases called "stuttering." Now, "stuttering" is generally used in referring to both conditions.

A distinction should be made between persistent stuttering and the sporadic hesitations and repetitions of which practically all of us are guilty on occasion. We may be speechless, or more or less incoherent, or needlessly repeat certain words or phrases—that is, stutter—when we are nervous or tired or frightened or angry or excited or speak too hurriedly or forget what we started out to say. In children of two or three who are beginning to talk, the speech mechanism often does not work fast enough to allow them to express what they have in mind, and they stutter.

Primary Stuttering. The stuttering of young children is called primary stuttering. Usually it disappears in a few months. In some children, however, normal hesitations in speech are turned into a real speech disorder. Usually the disorder develops so gradually that it is difficult for the parents or speech correctionist to discover exactly why and when a particular child began to show an excessive amount of halting or hesitating in his speech or pronounced repetitions or prolongations of verbal sounds.

It may be found that the child belongs to the small group of children who have difficulty in coordinating the muscles involved in speech. A child with this difficulty will be more susceptible than are most children to emotional conflicts of one kind or another.

Emotional conflicts and frustrations are often expressed in stuttering. At times most of us have been torn between conflicting desires to speak and to remain silent—before making a speech, for example—or in soliciting contributions for a cause, or in asking for a raise. Children are sometimes placed in such situations. We have seen that children may be torn between love and hate. Yet the child who feels deep-seated resentment is required to express his love verbally. The naughty child who doesn't feel sorry at all inside must say "I'm sorry." Frustration may be experienced merely by interruptions or a show of impatience on the part of parents or teachers who do not realize how long it takes for little children to become fluent in expressing themselves. To be commanded in the middle of a sentence to stop and begin over again, or to be ignored or diverted before one is able to get out what one is trying to say, is bound to be frustrating. Occasionally a particular experience may precipitate stuttering. Here are two examples:

By the time Mary was halfway through the fourth grade, her family had moved so many times that she had been in four different schools. Then she began to stutter. When the doctor told her parents that the many school changes were probably the precipitating cause, they pointed out that Mary was a bright child who had never had trouble keeping up in her classwork. They failed to understand that a child who enters a new school from an old one is an outsider who has to be tried and tested by other children before being accepted or rejected. An unusually sensitive child, like Mary, may be able to weather this ordeal once or twice, but cannot go through it repeatedly without ill effects.

Another child—Tom—started to stutter when he tried unsuccessfully to keep up with an older boy who was visiting in his home. The visitor escaped punishment because he was a visitor. All the spankings and scoldings for their misdeeds fell upon Tom. As a result, Tom felt that he was losing his parents' favor and love. He had begun to stutter and was well on the way toward developing deep-seated feelings of inferiority and hostility until the situation was explained to the parents. When the visitor left and peace and harmony were restored, the stuttering disappeared.

Often primary stuttering grows less and less frequent and periods of fluency becomes longer and longer if no attention is paid to it. Eventually the stuttering may disappear altogether. The speech correctionist called in by anxious parents or the nursery school usually explains that the best treatment is no treatment. There must be no interruptions of speech, no rewards or punishment, no expressions of concern that the child can hear. Situations in which fluency in speech is made easy or in which attention is distracted from speech, such as partly verbal games, are suggested. Also adults who are with the child are asked to speak more slowly, more simply, and more calmly. The speech of adults is often too fast or too complicated for children to imitate, and it is imitation that lies at the root of speech development.

Secondary Stuttering. In primary stuttering the child is usually not aware of his difficulty. He prattles along repeating, pausing, prolonging certain syllables without the slightest concern. It is only when he becomes conscious that his speech is unpleasant or funny to others that he is on the way to becoming a secondary or confirmed stutterer.

Although confirmed stuttering is not a disease, it is a very serious affliction because of the social taboo on lack of fluency in speech and on the strange twitches and contortions, especially of the face and lips, which stutterers employ in their effort to force out words.

Many youngsters who stutter form the habit of sidestepping pitfalls in the way of words that are especially difficult for them to pronounce (fear words), with the result that they talk so incoherently that they are looked upon as dumb or silly by their contemporaries. Eventually they may dodge situations in which it is difficult to talk (fear situations) or may greatly limit their conversation. It is easy to see how such "silent stutterers," as they have been called, may grow up to be unhappy, repressed individuals.

When the primary stutterer first notices that his speech is not socially acceptable—perhaps as a result of ridicule from playmates or expressions of concern or even punishment from adults—he first shows signs of bewilderment and then of tension and struggle. Having recognized that the stuttering is an obstacle, he tries to overcome it by force. He attacks words as if they were concrete objects to be forced past his tense tongue or lips by pressing or squeezing harder than usual with his abdominal muscles. Of course, this only makes the tightness worse. Then he may stamp his foot, or beat his side with his fist, or toss his head, or jerk his jaw as if the word could be jarred out with sudden movements. As he does eventually succeed in saying the word, he associates these queer gyrations with his success. Thenceforth whatever forcing device he has employed becomes an established part of his particular stuttering complex until the device no longer works and he has to invent some other trick.

In studying large numbers of stutterers, psychiatric specialists frequently find tension states, anxiety reactions, emotional immaturity, and feelings of insecurity and apprehensiveness. Unfortunately, the stutterer is usually unaware of what is making him stutter until the psychiatrist is able to discover the underlying cause or causes of his anxiety.

Underneath the anxiety and tension the psychiatrist usually finds resentment or hostility toward parents, teachers, or people in general. This is not surprising if we remember that a child begins to be a confirmed stutterer when he realizes that his speech is displeasing to others. It is easy then to take the next step and feel that he himself is displeasing. Without knowing it, the stutterer may project his injured feelings on the world at large. Particular people or perhaps all people are potential enemies lying in wait to take advantage of his weakness. That is why many stutterers are able to talk without difficulty when they believe themselves to be alone. Others will stutter only when in the presence of superiors—parents, teachers, employers—or only when in the classroom surrounded by classmates presumably waiting to laugh. In general, any situations that are anticipated with anxiety—for example, reciting, making a speech, apologizing, explaining a poor report card to parents—will invariably bring on or accentuate the stuttering. On the other hand, situations in which attention is diverted from the stutterer, such as reciting in unison or singing in a group, favor comparatively easy and smooth-flowing speech.

Means of overcoming stuttering have been sought all through history. Engraved on a clay tablet excavated from the ruins of the Biblical town of Beth Shemish was this prayer: "Oh God, cut through the backbone of my stammering. I desire that Thou shalt remove the spring of my impediment." Two of the various cures suggested were running uphill with pebbles in one's mouth reciting as one ran, and chewing pungent substances such as mustard, garlic, and onion. Presumably these practices were designed to take the stutterer's mind off his speech. There have been many modern versions of such distractions, but they have seldom worked a permanent cure because they do nothing to influence the underlying causes.

A stuttering child should have expert attention as early as possible. In some schools, speech correction or speech correction teachers and psychologists and psychiatrists are available for helping children with this form of crippling. In schools without these services, the child should be referred to a speech correctionist, a speech clinician, or a speech clinic for the correction of speech disorders and defects. As there are many so-called "stammering schools" and self-styled "speech experts" who trade on the fear and anxiety associated with stuttering, the teacher or nurse serving the school should get reliable information for the child's parents by consulting the school physician or the local medical society or public health unit.

It is important that a child who is learning to speak correctly, no matter what his defect or disorder, should not be made unduly speech-conscious. In school his teachers should not notice and attempt to correct each mistake as it occurs during ordinary conversations or recitations. It will help the child to realize that he is not the only one who has trouble in speaking—that hesitations and repetitions in speech are not uncommon and that other children in the class may stutter or stammer when called on to recite if they are unprepared or may talk too fast. And it should be explained to the other children, without the stutterer's knowledge, that stuttering is not done on purpose and cannot be overcome at once. They can help their friend to overcome it if they will overlook his handicap and not laugh at or make fun of him.

FOR REVIEW AND DISCUSSION

1. Suppose you were correcting the papers of high school students who had been given a "supply the missing words" test on the organs of

hearing and speech and you found the following mistakes. Make the corrections.

a. Air is let into the middle ear through the *Eustachian tube* ~~outer ear canal~~ in order to equalize the pressure of air on each side of the tympanum.

b. Sound waves are conducted across the middle ear by the vibration of the auditory *~~strings~~*. ossicles

c. The organ of hearing in the inner ear is the *~~cochlea~~*. organ of corti

d. The vocal cords are located in the upper part of the larynx below the *~~glottis~~*. epiglottis

cleft palate *e.* *~~Stuttering~~* is an example of a speech disorder caused by a structural defect.

2. Knowing the derivation of the following words, tell why they are good names for the things they name.

Pinna	Tympanum	Endolymph
Malleus	Incus	Perilymph
Stapes	Cochlea	Scala media
Decibel	Falsetto	

3. Tell the difference between:

a. Conduction deafness and central deafness
b. Otosclerosis and otitis media
c. Phonograph speech audiometer and pure-tone audiometer
d. Sweep test (for hearing) and threshold test
e. Nasopharynx and larynx
f. Glottis and epiglottis
g. Hard palate and soft palate
h. Lisping and nasality
i. Harelip and cleft palate
j. Primary stuttering and secondary stuttering

4. Discuss in class ways of making school life easier:

a. For a child with considerable loss of hearing
b. For a child who has secondary stuttering

SELECTED REFERENCES

Hearing

American Medical Association: *The Sense Organs,* part 8 of *The Wonderful Human Machine* series, The Association, Chicago. (The workings of the human body in words and pictures.)

Best, C. H., and N. B. Taylor: *The Human Body* (first given as reference in Chap. 1). Part X, *The Special Senses,* Chap. 46.

Boyd, G. G.: *Hearing Loss—What Can Be Done about It,* J. B. Lippincott Company, Philadelphia, 1959.

Davis, H., (ed.): *Hearing and Deafness,* Holt, Rinehart and Winston, Inc., New York, 1957. (A guide for laymen.)

Kough, Jack, and Robert F. De Haan: *Teacher's Guidance Handbook* (first given as reference in Chap. 5). Vol. I, *Identifying Children with Special Needs,* Sec. IV, Chaps. 18 and 19; Vol. II, *Helping Children with Special Needs,* Sec. IV, Chaps. 15 and 16.

National Education Association Council for Exceptional Children: *Children with Impaired Hearing—Administration of Special Education in Small School Systems,* 1960. The Association, Washington, D.C.

Speech

Best, C. H., and N. B. Taylor: *The Human Body* (first given as reference in Chap. 1). Part V, Chap. 22, *The Larynx, The Organ of the Voice.*

Johnson, Wendell (ed.): *Speech Problems of Children; A Guide to Care and Correction,* Grune & Stratton, Inc., New York, 1950.

Johnson, Wendell (ed.): *Stuttering and What You Can Do about It,* University of Minnesota Press, Minneapolis, 1961.

Van Riper, Charles: *Your Child's Speech Problems,* Harper & Brothers, New York, 1961.

Van Riper, Charles, and John Irwin: *Voice and Articulation,* Prentice-Hall, Inc., New York, 1959.

Van Riper, Charles, and Katherine Butler: *Speech in the Elementary Classroom,* Harper & Brothers, New York, 1955.

Williams, Jesse Feiring: *Onset of Stuttering; Research Findings and Implications,* University of Minnesota Press, Minneapolis, 1959.

Organizations

Alexander Graham Bell Association for the Deaf
American Hearing Society
American Speech and Hearing Association

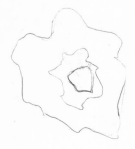

Chapter 18   BODY MECHANICS

The Bones
Bone-moving Muscles
Physical Fitness
Posture and Its Appraisal
Orthopedic Defects in School Children
Identifying and Helping Children with
Orthopedic Defects

The only organs of the body that we can consciously command to do our will are the muscles attached to our bones. Their function is to move bones by furnishing motive power at appropriate points. It is a basic physiologic principle that the use of a function improves the function. The efficiency and ease with which we perform physical tasks are directly related to the amount of work we give our muscles to do.

The physical fitness of American children has become a question of great national concern. Since schools exist everywhere and reach everyone during the years of childhood and youth, teachers, more than most other Americans, have become involved in programs undertaken to improve the physical skills, strength, and endurance of young people. Some knowledge of the bone-muscle system and how its work is integrated with that of other body systems is necessary for an understanding of the part played by physical activity in developing and maintaining physical fitness. This knowledge also will help teachers to recognize and appreciate the difficulties of children who are handicapped by orthopedic defects, that is, defects that occur as a result of disease or injury or faulty habits affecting the bony framework of the body or its operation.

THE BONES

Bones joined together by ligaments form the skeleton or inside framework of the body. The principal mechanical function of this framework is to support the weight of the body above the ground against the pull of gravity, to protect the soft structures of the body, and to act as points of support and leverage for lifting, bending, and other operations.

Bone Architecture

Good framework material combines strength and durability with lightness. Bone is a material of this kind. It consists of a compact ivorylike outer shell with an inner lacelike structure in which innumerable tiny tubes cross and recross each other like miniature beams along the lines of the normal stresses for each particular bone. The walls of these tiny tubes are composed of concentric layers of a complex compound of calcium, phosphorus, and small amounts of other mineral salts. Embedded in the mineral walls in a spiral pattern are fibers of collagen, the chief organic constituent of bone. Collagen is a gelatinous protein substance which can be changed by boiling into glue or gelatin.

Blood vessels and nerves run through the bores of the bony tubes. They are connected by delicate channels with the bone cells which live in tiny hollows in the walls of the tubes. The bone cells build and repair bone with material brought to them by the blood. The work of the bone cells makes possible the repair of a fractured bone. The blood vessels and nerves enter the bone from a thin membrane called the *periosteum* (from the Greek, meaning "around bone") which forms its outer covering.

The long, heavy-duty bones of the arms and legs have very thick outer shells. The shafts of these long bones are hollow and filled with yellow marrow consisting primarily of connective tissue and fat. The ends contain red bone marrow. It is in the red marrow located in the ends of the shafts of the long bones and to a greater extent in the ribs, breastbone, spine, and the loose bony tissue between the inner and outer layers of the bones of the skull that the red cells of the blood are manufactured (see Blood and Its Composition, in Chap. 10).

The shapes of the various bones are adapted to the work they are called upon to do. If protection is the main job of the bone, its form is comparatively flat like that of the shoulder blades, the breastbone, and the bones of the cranium, or brain case. If the bone must act as a lever when moved by the muscles, it is long like those of the arms, legs, and fingers. If flexibility in a group of bones is necessary, the individual bones tend to be short like those of the wrist and ankle, or irregular like those of the spine.

Joints

The meeting places of the various bones that form the skeleton are called joints, or articulations. Some joints are not movable, as in the cranium; some are only slightly movable, as in the spinal column; but the greater number are freely movable, as in the shoulders, elbows, fingers, hips, and knees.

Joints are classified according to the shape of the articulating surfaces. The four most important types of joints in the human body are the ball-and-socket (at the shoulders and hips) which permits movement in all directions; the saddle (between the vertebrae of the spine) which permits movements backward, forward, and sidewise; the hinge (for example, between the bones of the fingers) which permits movement in only one direction; and the rotary (usually combined with a hinge joint, as in the elbow) which allows the bones to rotate at the joint like a corkscrew or a key in turning a lock.

The articulating surfaces of all movable bones are protected with pads of elastic cartilage, and the bones are held in place at the joint by ligaments, that is, bands made up of tough fibers. Nearly all movable joints are enclosed in a capsule of very tough material strengthened by ligaments and lined with a membrane that secretes a thick fluid like white of egg. This fluid acts as a lubricant to reduce friction between the articulating surfaces. In addition the joint capsule is padded with small sacs filled with fluid called bursae. These little "water cushions" are also interposed beneath and between muscles, tendons, or other structures at places where friction with bone would otherwise develop. Chronic irritation of the bursae causes the painful inflammatory condition called bursitis.

The Skeleton

The skeleton is composed of more than 200 separate bones and is divided into two main parts: (1) the axial skeleton, consisting of the spine and its immediate outgrowths, the head, ribs, and sternum (breastbone); and (2) the appendicular skeleton, consisting of the supporting framework for the limbs (the shoulder girdle and the pelvic girdle) and the bones of the arms and legs themselves.

Some knowledge of the way in which the skeleton is put together and moved, and of the functions of its various parts under normal conditions, will be helpful to the teacher in recognizing deviations from normal in posture and gait.

The Axial Skeleton

The Spinal Column. The spinal column is the mainstay of the body. All the rest of the skeleton is directly or indirectly attached to it.

The spine is made up of 33 vertebrae which are piled on top of one another to form a strong hollow column. The vertebrae are bound firmly together by strong ligaments, and between each two is placed a pad of tough elastic cartilage. These pads act as shock absorbers and allow free movement of the neck and trunk.

The vertebrae differ in size and shape, but except for the top two, they are built very much alike. Seen from above, as in *A* in Fig. 18-1, a typical vertebra consists of a solid disk, or body, with an arch of bone extending from it. Spinous processes project sideways and backward from the roof of the arch. The "spines" give the spinal column its name. We see and feel as rounded knobs the "spines" that project backward (*B*, in Fig. 18-1).

The spinal cord passes through the hollow column formed by the arches of the superimposed vertebrae much as the string passes through the hollow centers of spools strung together (C, in Fig. 18-1). Nerve trunks pass out from the spinal cord between each two vertebrae.

The first two vertebrae differ from the rest because they must carry the head. The top vertebra is called the atlas (see Fig. 18-3) because it supports the head as the giant Atlas was fabled to uphold the heavens. Unlike the others, it has no body but consists of a bony ring with cups on the top surface into which knobs of the occipital bone of the skull (see further on) fit. This makes it possible to move the head backward and forward like a rocking chair. A bony peg rising from the second neck vertebra (the axis) forms a pivot around which the atlas rotates like a revolving platform when the head is turned from side to side.

Viewed from the back (Fig. 18-3), the spine is seen to be a column which is narrower at the top than at the base. The vertebrae at the upper levels of the column are small and light because they do not have so much to carry. The vertebrae at the base of the column are large and stout because they must carry the accumulated weight of all parts above them.

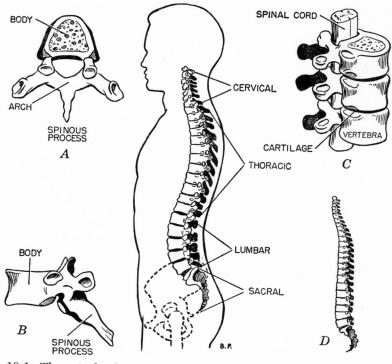

Fig. 18-1. The spinal column of an adult showing normal curves. A, vertebra viewed from above. B, vertebra viewed from left side. C, spinal cord passing through vertebral arches. D, spine of a ten-year-old child.

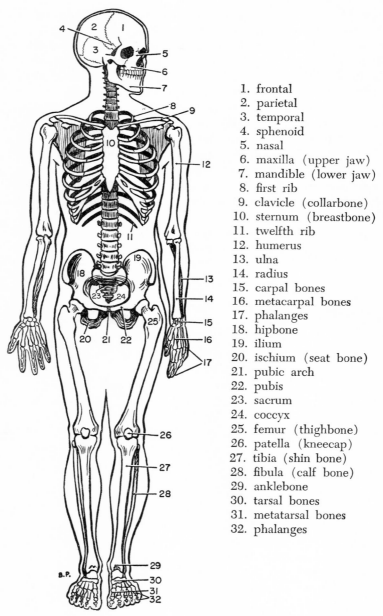

1. frontal
2. parietal
3. temporal
4. sphenoid
5. nasal
6. maxilla (upper jaw)
7. mandible (lower jaw)
8. first rib
9. clavicle (collarbone)
10. sternum (breastbone)
11. twelfth rib
12. humerus
13. ulna
14. radius
15. carpal bones
16. metacarpal bones
17. phalanges
18. hipbone
19. ilium
20. ischium (seat bone)
21. pubic arch
22. pubis
23. sacrum
24. coccyx
25. femur (thighbone)
26. patella (kneecap)
27. tibia (shin bone)
28. fibula (calf bone)
29. anklebone
30. tarsal bones
31. metatarsal bones
32. phalanges

Fig. 18-2. The skeleton of a fifteen-year-old boy, front view.

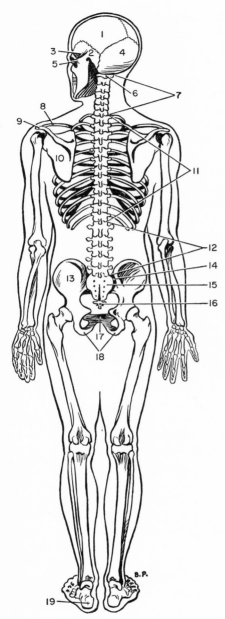

1. parietal
2. temporal
3. sphenoid
4. occipital
5. cheekbone
6. atlas
7. cervical vertebrae (neck)
8. clavicle
9. tip of shoulder
10. scapula (shoulder blade)
11. thoracic vertebrae (chest)
12. lumbar vertebrae
13. hipbone
14. sacroiliac joint
15. sacrum
16. coccyx
17. pubis
18. ischia (seat bones)
19. heel bone

FIG. 18-3. The skeleton of a fifteen-year-old boy, back view.

Viewed from the side, the spinal column curves in and out somewhat like the letter S. The spinal curves help to ease the jolting of the spine in walking, running, jumping, and other body movements. They are so accurately balanced that one curve cannot be increased or decreased without increasing or decreasing the other (see Posture, further on). The four regions of the spinal column (cervical, or neck; thoracic, or chest; lumbar, or lower back; and sacral, or hip) are labeled in Fig. 18-1.

The Sternum (Breastbone) and Ribs. The sternum is a plate of bone about 6 inches long situated in the middle of the front wall of the thorax. It provides points of attachment for the collarbones and ribs (Fig. 18-2).

The ribs are semiflexible arches of bones enclosing the thoracic cavity. At the back the twelve pairs of ribs are attached by strong ligaments to the twelve thoracic vertebrae which form the upper outward curve of the spinal column. In front the first seven pairs of ribs are attached to the sternum by means of elastic cartilages. Each of the next three pairs is attached to the cartilage of the pair immediately above. The front ends of the last two pairs hang free, and so they are called floating ribs.

The cagelike arrangement of bone and cartilage enclosing the chest is an admirable compromise between stability and mobility. The heart and lungs must be protected, yet they cannot be shut up in a rigid box as the brain is, since the lungs must expand in breathing and the heart must beat. The mobile elastic chest cage is more readily influenced by exercise and the deep breathing that goes with it than is any other part of the skeleton. In boys and girls who engage in athletics, the circumference of the chest is larger than in those who have little physical exercise.

The Skull. The skull rests upon the top of the spinal column. It is divided into two parts: the cranium, or brain case, and the face.

The eight immovable interlocking bones of the cranium (Figs. 18-2 and 18-3) form a firm case for the brain. Four of these bones (the occipital, two parietals, and the frontal) are typical flat bones, composed of two dense layers—the outer one thick and tough, the inner one thinner and more brittle—with loose bony material sandwiched between. Hence they are admirably fitted to protect the delicate brain from ordinary bumps and blows.

Blood vessels and nerve trunks pass in and out of the brain through openings at the base of the cranium. The largest opening is an outlet for the constricted part of the brain where it narrows down to join the spinal cord.

The very hard temporal bones, one on each side of the cranium, are hollowed out in a series of small, peculiarly shaped cavities to contain, in addition to the organs of hearing, the organs of equilibrium, which record where we are in space and the direction in which we are moving (see The Balancing Apparatus, further on).

In front of the opening in the occipital bone through which the spinal cord passes downward from the brain, the irregular wedge-shaped sphenoid bone rises steeply. At the top of this declivity, is the tiny saddle-shaped fossa, or ditch, in which the pituitary gland (see The Endocrine System in Action, in Chap. 6) is lodged. The sphenoid bone and the sievelike ethmoid bone in front of it separate the brain cavity from the face.

The olfactory bulbs of the brain rest on a ridge of the ethmoid bone. From these bulbs the olfactory nerves (nerves of smell) pass downward into the nasal cavity through openings in the bone. It was once believed that the mucus, which we know as a secretion of glands in the mucous membrane of the nose lining, was a secretion of the brain. Excessive secretion of mucus, as in a head cold, was considered to be the means by which the brain cleansed itself of noxious "humors."

The face extends from the eyebrows to the chin (Fig. 18-2). The thirteen immovable bones of the face form the bony settings of the eyes, nose, and mouth. The only movable one is the lower jawbone (mandible) which moves up and down and sidewise on sliding hinge joints in speaking and chewing.

Eye Sockets. Above and on either side of the midline of the face are the bony orbits, or sockets, for the eyeballs and their related structures. The promontories represented by the bones of the cheek and upper nose guard the eyes against blows. Lacrimal ducts, through which tears drain into the nose (see Fig. 16-1), pass for part of their distance through canals in the lacrimal bones located in the inner walls of the eye orbits.

Head Sinuses. Above each eye in the frontal bone, on each side of the nose in the maxillae (upper jawbones), and in the sphenoid and ethmoid bones in the floor of the cranium there are air-containing sinuses or cavities. Reference has been made to the troubles caused by the swelling shut of the very narrow openings through which the sinuses lead into the nose (see Sinusitis, in Chap. 11).

The Nose. The upper part of the bridge of the nose is formed by two small bones placed side by side. The lower part of this bridge is made of cartilage. The nasal bones are rather easily broken by a direct blow.

A thin bone shaped somewhat like a plowshare (the vomer) forms part of the septum, or wall, which divides the nose into two corridors. Sometimes it deviates, that is, bends to one side or the other, thus making the nasal corridors of unequal size. The inferior turbinates are thin, scroll-shaped bones situated in the outer wall of each nostril. They overhang the corridors below and help to increase the area over which the air passes as it flows through the nose (see Fig. 11-2). A deviated septum and enlarged inferior turbinates cause some of the more common nose troubles, largely owing to their interference with the ventilation and drainage of the nasal passages and sinuses.

The Jaws. The two maxillae meet in the midline of the face to form the whole of the upper jaw. Together with the palatine bones, they form part of the floor of the eye orbits, the floor and sides of the nose cavities, and the roof of the mouth.

The mandible, or lower jawbone, is shaped like a horseshoe. It is the largest and strongest bone of the face. The curved portion forms the chin, and the two perpendicular portions are joined by sliding hinge joints to the temporal bones of each side of the cranium just in front of the ears. Fractures and dislocations of the lower jawbone are quite common injuries. Sockets in the lower rims of the maxillae and the upper rim of the curved portion of the mandible hold the teeth.

The Hyoid Bone. The base of the tongue is supported by a small U-shaped bone called the hyoid bone (*hyoeides* in Greek means "U-shaped"). This bone also furnishes attachments for some of the tongue's muscles. The hyoid bone may be felt in the neck, just above the Adam's apple.

The Appendicular Skeleton

In human beings a more or less complete division of labor with regard to the two important activities, locomotion and grasping, is reached by the assignment of locomotion to the legs and feet and of grasping to the arms and hands.

Arms and legs are essentially much alike—one long, strong bone nearest to the trunk, then two bones, then several little bones, forming in the arm the wrist and hands, and in the leg the ankle and foot. However, legs are not nearly so flexible as arms. Sturdy support for the body's weight with a reasonable degree of movability is all that is required of legs. The series of bone levers making up the arms and legs are attached to the trunk by a supporting framework consisting of two girdles—the shoulder girdle and the pelvic girdle.

The Shoulder Girdle. This girdle is composed of the two long double-curved collarbones (clavicles) and the two flat triangular shoulder blades (scapulae). Each clavicle is attached at one end to the sternum and at the other end to a scapula (Figs. 18-2 and 18-3). Each scapula is a large, flat triangular bone placed point down over the upper ribs at the back of the thorax. Folded back across its upper portion is a prominent ridge of bone which ends in a projection (the tip of the shoulder) to which the outer end of the clavicle is attached.

The Arm. The bone of the upper arm (the humerus) has a rounded head, or knob, at the top which fits into a shallow, cuplike depression in the scapula, forming a ball-and-socket joint. The shoulder joint is the most freely movable joint in the body and is quite easily dislocated. The curved lower end of the humerus fits into a big notch at the upper end of the large bone of the forearm (the ulna) to form the elbow joint. The lower end of the ulna articulates with a disk of cartilage which separates it from the wrist.

The other bone of the forearm (the radius) is shorter and smaller than the ulna, to which it is attached near both ends. The lower end of the radius articulates with the top row of bones forming the wrist.

The Wrist. The wrist is composed of eight small, irregularly shaped bones (the carpals) united by ligaments. They are arranged in two rows of four bones each and articulate with one another as well as with the bones of the forearm and hand, thus permitting a wide range of motion.

The Hand. The five bones of the palm (metacarpals) articulate at their bases with the lower row of wristbones and at their heads with the first row of finger bones (phalanges). The fourteen finger bones (three in each finger and two in each thumb) give the hand its extraordinary flexibility. The hands are the copartners of the brain in performing all acts of manual dexterity and skill. The thumb is the most important "finger." A good thumb and only one finger make a far more useful hand than four fingers minus a thumb.

The Pelvic Girdle. The two hipbones are joined together in front by a narrow bridge of bone. They form, with the sacrum and coccyx behind, the basin-shaped ring of thick, heavy bones known as the pelvic girdle (Figs. 18-2 and 18-3). This girdle with its attached muscles forms the floor of the abdominal cavity and also serves to attach the lower limbs to the trunk.

The broad, flaring upper portion of each hipbone (the ilium) forms the prominence of the hip. It is joined tightly at the back with the sacrum to form the strong sacroiliac joint. The sacroiliac joints permit little motion in the lower back region but are subjected to very great pressure from the weight of the trunk. One of the common causes of low-back pain is strain of the sacroiliac joints caused by improper lifting of too-heavy objects or by poor distribution of body weight in walking or standing. The ischium is the lowest and strongest portion of the hipbone, and the pubis is the narrow portion which curves around to join its mate on the other side in front to form the pubic arch.

The Thighs. In the outer surface of the hipbone, at the junction of its three portions, there is a deep socket into which the round head of the femur, or thighbone, fits, forming a ball-and-socket joint. The femur is the largest and strongest bone in the skeleton. Its lower end is wider than its upper end and is divided into two large knobs which articulate with the tibia, or shinbone, and the patella, or kneecap, to form the knee joint. The head of the femur is not so easily dislocated as is the less tightly fixed head of the humerus but is much more difficult to put back into its socket.

The Knee. The knee joint is a strong hinged joint which is protected by the patella, or kneecap. The patella is a small lens-shaped bone surrounded by the tendon of a big muscle which is used in kicking.

The Leg. Anatomically speaking, the word leg is used for that portion of the lower limb between the knee and the ankle. It contains two bones, the tibia and the fibula.

The lower end of the tibia, or shinbone, is much smaller than its upper end and is prolonged downward to form the inner rounded prominence of the ankle. The fibula, or calf bone, is attached at the top to the tibia. The lower end is prolonged downward to form the outer pointed prominence of the ankle. The fibula is smaller than the tibia and in proportion to its length is the most slender of all the long bones. It is more often fractured alone than is the tibia, but fracture of both bones is a common injury.

The Ankle, Foot, and Toes. The ankle joint is formed by the junction of the lower ends of the tibia and fibula with the talus (one of the tarsals). The seven tarsals, or anklebones, are firmly bound together by tough ligaments. They are larger and more irregularly shaped than are the wristbones. The heel bone is the largest and strongest, as it must transmit the weight of the body to the ground and form a lever for the muscles of the calf of the leg in walking.

The shape of the foot is roughly like that of a triangle, with the apex at the point where the leg bones fit over the talus. The long arch, or instep, of the foot is formed by five bones (the metatarsals) which extend from the ankle to the base of the toes. The phalanges forming the toes are similar in number and arrangement to the phalanges forming the fingers.

BONE-MOVING MUSCLES

The word muscle comes from the Latin *musculus,* meaning "little mouse," because the spindle shape of the muscles that move bones resembles that of a running mouse. Each skeletal muscle is a bundle of muscle fibers running lengthwise, and its surface is covered with a protecting sheath. The fibers of these bone-moving muscles, which are under the control of the will (voluntary muscles), are striped crosswise or striated, whereas those of the involuntary muscles, which bring about movements in the large organs of the interior (the viscera) are smooth. The action of smooth muscle is slow and rhythmical, like the movements of an earthworm, while that of striped muscle is swift.

Each voluntary muscle is attached by one end to a bone and by the other end to an adjoining bone or to skin or cartilage or some special organ like the eyeball. The ends of muscle fibers that connect muscle with bone have become coarse and hard, forming tough white cords called tendons. Some tendons run through a sheath of dense strong tissue lined with membrane which secretes a lubricating fluid like that which "oils" the joints.

The Mechanics of Muscle Contraction

The special characteristic of muscular tissue which enables it to do its work is the ability to contract—become shorter—and then to relax so that it can be stretched—made longer. Voluntary muscles work in pairs; when one of the pair contracts, its opposite relaxes. The muscles that pull bones toward each other are called flexors. Those that pull bones away from each other are called extensors.

It is easy to see how voluntary muscles bring about movement. When a muscle attached at one end to one part and at the other end to another part becomes shorter and thicker (contracts) it is bound to pull the two parts toward each other in the direction permitted by the joint. This may be demonstrated by lifting the hand to the shoulder. The bulge of the contracting biceps (the flexor) pulling the forearm toward the upper arm is clearly seen. While this contraction is taking place the triceps muscle at the back of the arm (the extensor) is stretched. The tension set up in the stretched muscle produces a tendency to contract and reverse the movement, that is, to extend, or straighten out the arm. The biceps is then stretched and made ready for another contraction (see Fig. 18-4). The continuous alternating contraction and relaxation (stretching) of thousands upon thousands of muscle fibers in paired muscles produce movements of infinite variety in all activities such as walking, running, jumping, climbing, and riding a bicycle.

Muscle Tone. No healthy muscles are ever completely relaxed. Reflex action keeps them always in a state of mild steady contraction like that

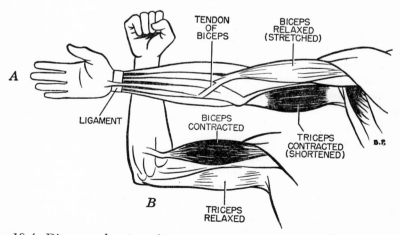

Fig. 18-4. Diagram showing alternate contraction and relaxation in paired voluntary muscles.

of a violin string that is correctly tuned. This state is called muscle tone. Its purpose is to make the muscles springy and ready for instant action when impulses demanding movement come from the brain. If our muscles had to take up slack, so to speak, before starting to pull on the parts to which they are attached, they would use up about a fifth more time and energy in performing their tasks. Muscle tone also has a steadying effect, much as a firm hold on a steering wheel helps to steady a vehicle. When the muscles that work against the pull of gravity are completely relaxed, as in fainting, for example, the body collapses.

Muscle tone varies according to the general condition of the body. This can readily be observed, especially in the face. In healthy rested children the skin of the face is tight and firm. When children are tired or ill, the tone of the facial muscles is decreased and their faces look weary. The slumping or sagging of the body associated with fatigue posture (see further on) is also due partly to a decrease in muscle tone.

The Chemistry of Muscle Contraction

A powerful chemical called acetylcholine, which is liberated from the muscle terminals of motor nerves, serves as a transmitter of the nerve impulses to muscle fibers and so makes them contract. The energy for contraction is obtained through a series of highly complicated chemical reactions, involving the breaking down and rebuilding of various substances present in muscle. Free oxygen is not required in the first stage when the muscle actually contracts. It is necessary only in the recovery stage to rewind the chemical clockwork so that the muscle can contract again.

Toward the end of the contraction stage, the muscle fuel glucose breaks down into lactic acid. Lactic acid is a waste substance in the sense that it must be quickly eliminated or changed. At the beginning of the recovery stage, part of this lactic acid is oxidized, with the result that carbonic acid (CO_2 plus H_2O) is formed. The carbonic acid diffuses into the blood and is carried to the lungs for removal from the body in the form of carbon dioxide and water. The energy obtained from burning a portion of the lactic acid is used to change the remainder back into glucose.

Even when a muscle is completely at rest, glucose is being broken down into lactic acid. This happens so slowly that the lactic acid can be removed as quickly as it is produced. During strenuous muscular activity, however, lactic acid is formed faster than it can be partly oxidized and partly changed back into glucose. The demand for oxygen may increase up to ten or fifteen times the amount required at the resting level. Measures taken to meet this demand are faster, deeper breathing to increase the ventilation of the lungs and faster, more powerful beating of the heart to increase the volume of blood in circulation. Even so, during vigorous exercise it is impossible to take in and deliver enough oxygen to the muscles to dispose of the excess lactic acid they are producing.

Buffering. The mechanism that makes it possible for us to engage in strenuous activities of more than a few moments' duration is that of buffering. The excess lactic acid both in the muscles and in the blood into which it diffuses is rapidly neutralized by alkaline salts, chiefly sodium bicarbonate and alkaline sodium phosphate. These salts, which are dissolved in the body fluids, are called buffer salts because they serve to protect the blood and tissues from any considerable change in the acid direction. So delicate is the acid-alkali balance of the body, which is just on the alkaline side of neutrality, that a change in reaction equal to the difference between distilled water and tap water would make the difference between life and death.

The Oxygen Debt. By the mechanism of buffering we are able to run up an oxygen debt, that is, to keep on working in spite of the fact that lactic acid is being produced in far greater quantities than there is oxygen available to remove it. But as soon as the muscle buffers are exhausted and the reaction of the muscles reaches a certain acidity due to the formation of lactic and other acids, further contraction becomes impossible. This is the condition known as muscular fatigue. Once muscles are fatigued, a rest interval is necessary for their complete recovery.

By puffing and panting we speed up the paying off of the oxygen debt run up during vigorous exercise. The heart also continues to beat rapidly during the recovery period. The time it takes for the heart rate to return to normal values is highly correlated with the level of physical fitness. Unless a person is in good condition it may take him an hour to pay off his oxygen debt after running a half mile and two hours or more after prolonged violent exercise, such as running the marathon.

It has been said that our powers of physical endurance may be no greater than the capacity of our muscle buffers. Improved buffering capacity is one of the desirable results achieved in the process of physical conditioning for athletic competition or for the performance of a certain piece of work. It also explains in part the value of exercise in keeping fit. Any condition that interferes with or improves the nutritive condition of the muscles or the body as a whole also will diminish or increase the efficiency and amount of work that can be obtained from the muscles.

Muscular Coordination

In discussing somatic (body) sensibilities in Chap. 6, reference was made to the sensations that make us aware of the movements of our limbs, trunk, and head. This type of sensory experience is derived from a sense called *kinesthesia,* or muscle sense, whose receptors lie in the muscles, tendons, and joints. These receptors are stimulated by the strains and stresses set up in muscles, tendons, and joints during muscular contraction. As a result of reports received in the central nervous system from these receptors, individual muscles and groups of muscles are guided in working together to produce smooth, finely adjusted, and effective movements. Such coordinated movement would be impossible without this guidance.

The Cerebellum. The cerebellum, or "little brain," also plays an important part in muscular coordination. It lies under the shelter of the back part of the cerebrum and is shaped somewhat like a moth; that is, it has a long narrow body and two wings spread out over the medulla oblongata. The cerebellum is connected with the cerebrum, the brain stem, and the spinal cord by a complicated system of nerve pathways. It receives nonsensory impulses continuously from the muscles and joints of the limbs, neck, trunk, eyes, and from the semicircular canals in the inner ears. These impulses inform the cerebellum of the positions and movements of the various parts. On the basis of information received, the cerebellum sends out messages to the voluntary muscles through its connections with motor nerve centers in the cerebrum and midbrain. These outgoing impulses do not themselves cause the muscles to move. But they do help to keep the muscles in just the right state of tension (tone) and make muscular movements surer and more forceful by reinforcing the voluntary motor impulses sent out by the motor area of the cerebral cortex. These two functions of the cerebellum allow the various muscle groups to make the final delicate adjustments that enable them to work smoothly and harmoniously together as a cooperative whole.

When the cerebellum is damaged by disease or injury, these nice cooperative actions are impossible. As a result voluntary movements become jerky and irregular. This condition is called ataxia. It is thought to be largely due to weakness and loss of tone of the muscles themselves rather than to failure of coordination.

The Balancing Apparatus

The feeling of equilibrium, or balance, is derived from sensations that arise in special organs lodged in three tiny tunnels—the semicircular canals—in the inner ear. These tunnels are no bigger than capillaries. Because of their complicated windings, they are called labyrinths, and keeping our balance is referred to as the labyrinthine function. Lodged in each bony labyrinth is a membranous labyrinth. The membranous labyrinth is filled with fluid, and a similar fluid lies between it and the walls of the bony labyrinth.

The semicircular canals lie in planes that are approximately at right angles to one another (Fig. 18-5). The one toward the outside of the head is the horizontal canal, and the ones toward the front and back are the vertical canals. The planes in which they lie correspond to the three dimensions of space: length (backward and forward), breadth (from side to side), and height (upward and downward).

At one extremity of each canal there is a bulblike arrangement (ampulla) which contains a sense organ consisting of a gelatin-covered mound of delicate hair cells for the reception of messages about body movements. These receptors are supplied with nerve fibers that carry impulses to the medulla oblongata and thence to various parts of the brain including the cerebellum. Now how does this miniature balancing apparatus work?

When the head and body move in one dimension—backward or forward, from side to side, or up and down—the fluid in the corresponding canals flows in the opposite direction. This change of direction stimulates the hair cells to send out the impulses that are interpreted by the brain as changes in the body's position. Because of the shifts in current in the fluid of the semicircular canals and their influence on the hair cells, we can tell when we move forward or backward, when we start or stop, when we slow down or speed up, when we deviate to the right or left, when we are going upward or downward. And with this awareness of the direction and speed of our movements, we automatically make the compensatory movements of the muscles of the neck, trunk, and limbs required to maintain our equilibrium.

The information sent to the cerebellum from the semicircular canals and incoming impulses from the eyes and neck muscles are essential for maintaining the correct position of the head in space. On the basis of this information, the cerebellum dispatches messages to the neck

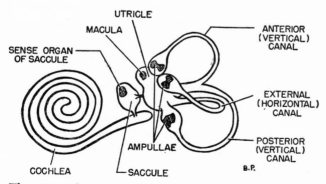

Fig. 18-5. The organ that makes it possible for us to keep our balance (the semicircular canals) is shown at the right; the cochlea, which contains the organ of hearing, at the left.

muscles which keep the head poised at the correct angle no matter what change is made in the body's position. Falling backward or to one side or the other is a common sign of disturbed cerebellar function.

Dizziness. Dizziness is a common sensation. Whatever may be its precipitating cause, the sensation arises immediately as a result of excitation of the semicircular canals or of their connections in the brain or spinal cord.

We may deliberately make ourselves dizzy by spinning around several times, as children do in playing certain games. In rapid rotation the brain becomes confused. It is accustomed to associate a displacement of fluid in the semicircular canals in one direction with a movement in the opposite direction. For example, when we go forward, the fluid in the horizontal canals bends the hair cells backward. This gives the sensation of going forward. When we spin round and round in an erect position, the fluid in the horizontal semicircular canals bends the hair cells backward, just as if we were going forward, but on stopping the fluid in the canals bends the hair cells in the opposite direction. This gives us the feeling of revolving in the opposite direction. However, our legs and our common sense tell us that we are standing still. We solve that problem by assuming that it is the world and not ourselves that is spinning about us in the reverse direction. This sensation is called vertigo. To keep from falling, we sway to one side or the other, or backward or forward, depending upon the position of the head during rotation.

Dizziness arises from many other causes besides rotation, for example, alcoholic intoxication, gastrointestinal upsets, infections, and high blood pressure. Often people complain of feeling dizzy when they are nauseated or very tired or about to faint. Unusual or abnormal actions of the eye muscles also produce dizziness. Just as the semicircular canals influence eye movements, so eye movements influence the semicircular canals. Dizziness is therefore a common effect of eye fatigue or of watching the landscape from a rapidly moving vehicle, such as an automobile or train.

Motion Sickness. Motions that involve repeated rapid changes of direction create strong disturbances in the semicircular canals which make some persons feel dizzy and sick. This sickness is known as motion sickness. It may be caused by the motions of an airplane (airsickness), of a boat (seasickness), or of a train, streetcar, bus, or automobile (car sickness). Swinging may make some children feel sick until they become accustomed to the motions. Indeed, frequent repetition of the motions that cause motion sickness may educate the semicircular canals so the persons suffering from it may get over it. Certain drugs are very effective in the prevention of motion sickness. Dramamine was the first drug of this kind to be developed.

PHYSICAL FITNESS

The physical fitness of young Americans has become a matter of national concern at several periods in the twentieth century. Theodore Roosevelt started the first one early in the century with his advocacy of the "strenuous life" as a way of making our nation strong. The second and third periods coincided with the two world wars when medical examinations given to determine fitness for military service revealed that a large fraction of American boys were disqualified because of inadequate levels of physical and mental or emotional fitness.

The fourth surge of interest began in the 1950s with the wide publicity given to the results of tests of muscular strength, flexibility, and agility applied to American boys and girls and to children of comparable ages in several European and Far Eastern countries. The fact that the performances of children of other countries were superior to those of our own youngsters was wounding to national pride, if nothing else. At best they focused attention on the need for promoting a higher level of physical fitness in American youth.

The President's Council on Youth Fitness at Cabinet level was formed, and great efforts continue to be made to improve the fitness of American youth by strong programs of health education and physical education, including a daily fifteen-minute period of vigorous exercise for all school children and the administration of standardized tests for identifying physically underdeveloped children.[1]

What Is Fitness?

The spotlighting of physical fitness led to the definition of a much broader concept of fitness than that confined to its physical aspects alone. In this definition fitness is described as that state in which a person is able to develop most effectively *all* his potentialities—mental, moral, social, and emotional, as well as physical.

Although physical fitness is not the whole of health, it is certainly an inseparable part of it. It has been defined in several different ways depending upon the special interests of those defining it.

In physiologic terms physical fitness is the capability of the body to respond to the demands of physical work and exercise with minimum evidence of strain. The question that immediately arises is why be physically fit? Nowadays much of the work done to earn a living is sitting-down work. Automobiles, motorboats, television, and spectator sports dominate the recreational scene. It is not surprising that motivation is the most important factor in physical fitness programs when one

---

[1] These tests are included in the government publication entitled *Youth Physical Fitness: Suggested Elements of a School-centered Program*, President's Council on Youth Fitness, July, 1961.

considers that contemporary society has taken away so many of the incentives and the opportunities for becoming physically fit.

The crux of the problem seems to be that of obtaining evidence for beneficial results that will motivate people—young and old alike—to include a larger amount of physical work or exercise in their daily lives. A good deal of research is going on in this field. But there is much that can be said right now for the value of exercise.

Physiological Effects of Exercise

Exercise makes muscles stronger and more efficient not, as we have seen, by increasing the number of muscle fibers but by increasing the size and strength of each fiber. The circulation of blood within muscular tissue improves, possibly through an increase of the capillary bed. Motor skills are increased by practicing the moves called for in games, sports, and other forms of physical activity. But it is not so much the effect of exercise on muscle strength and coordination as its effect upon the body as a whole that makes exercise as essential for the best health at every age as are good nutrition, adequate rest and relaxation, good medical care, satisfying work, and peace of mind.

During vigorous exercise physiologic mechanisms are brought into play which greatly increase the ventilation of the lungs and the output of blood from the heart. These increases, accompanied by the buffering capacity of the blood, enable the body to meet the high metabolic demands placed on it by vigorous exercise. Repeated exercise leads to an increase in the capability of the body to maintain a given level of activity at lower cost and consequently to increase endurance.

It is well known that some people can drive their muscles harder and longer without fatigue than others can. All-round physical fitness and special conditioning for a particular activity—running or rowing, for example—make a tremendous difference in strength and endurance. Comparatively few of us, however, are born athletes headed for exceptional proficiency in sports and games or for record-breaking performances in events calling for a high degree of muscular strength, agility, and skill. What most of us are interested in is what regular daily exercise can do for us in terms of ordinary everyday living. Doctors tell us that what it can do is to allow us to engage in our usual round of activities with the least possible fatigue and the greatest possible ease. Everyone— young and old alike—unless prevented by serious disease or crippling handicaps can improve his stamina and strength by establishing the habit of getting enough exercise every day and keeping it up through thick and thin.

The form exercise takes does not matter to muscles. They need work and do not care whether they get it from climbing a tree or making a touchdown or walking to school or work. The form exercise takes does matter to people, however. Either one does, or one does not, enjoy a game or a sport or a work activity. The habit of daily exercise is much more likely to be established in youth if boys and girls are given opportunities to try out several different activities and to acquire enough skill to enjoy the ones that suit them.

Meeting the Challenge of Stress

Enjoyable physical activities help to relieve the stresses and tensions to which most people, including children, are subjected today. Furthermore, very few persons escape periods of abnormal stress which demand a fully efficient body, not a sluggish one that is adequate only for sitting around and not doing much. Being fit, with reserves of stamina to draw on, makes a big difference in the capacity to respond to stress; it may even mean the difference between life and death. The margin of safety necessary to bounce back from abnormal stress can be built up only through the regular use of all our physical and mental capacities.

Keeping Weight Down

Besides the part it plays in helping to build up and maintain a high level of fitness, daily vigorous exercise taken either in the form of recreation or as part of one's job (including getting to and returning from work) tends to prevent overweight and obesity with all their medical complications (see Overweight and Underweight, in Chap. 12). Many individuals get soft and flabby from too little exercise as they get older. Young people, except those who are already overweight, are not likely to be concerned with what's going to happen to their waistlines in middle age, but they can be encouraged to choose one or more recreational activities that they can keep on enjoying in later life. If they get to be good enough at swimming, skating, bowling, badminton, dancing, or golf, for example, the chances are they will keep on with it as an adult. An interest in one or more sports or games that a young person can continue to enjoy after he is through school will pay big dividends in helping to curb any tendency to put on weight in the years ahead.

Physical Activity and Heart Disease

There is as yet no evidence that physical activity helps to prevent any specific disease. Several interesting observations have been made, however, on the possible association of coronary heart disease with levels of exercise. In one study, the risk of death from coronary heart disease among London bus drivers (who sit at work) was compared with that of London bus conductors who spend much of their time running up and down between the lower and upper decks. In another more recent study, made in Washington, the subjects were sedentary post office clerks and physically active post office carriers. The findings of these and other studies tend to indicate that there is a relationship between physical activity of work and heart disease. No hard and fast conclusions can be drawn, however, until all the many other factors that may be involved have been investigated. This will be a complex and difficult task.

POSTURE AND ITS APPRAISAL

It is customary to think of posture as meaning the general impression of body carriage conveyed to the beholder when one is stationary. The familiar command "straighten up" is associated with this conception. To "straighten up" somehow implies ramrod stiffness—the disciplining of a body that has fallen into bad habits.

Actually, good posture means much more than "standing straight." It is the use of all parts of the body to maintain balance with ease and grace. It involves constant shifts in position of various parts of the body in relation to other parts at all times and under all circumstances. These shifts are the reactions of the muscles within to physical forces acting upon the body from without. The primary force is gravity. Like all other objects on the earth's surface, the body is continuously subject to a pull toward the earth's center and must incessantly meet it.

The center of gravity of any body is the center of its mass or weight. In the upright human body, this is located in the back wall of the pelvis in line with the spinal column. When the center of gravity is "supported" —that is, when a line dropped from it passes through the base of any body—that body is in equilibrium and will not fall. The base of the upright human body is represented by the feet and the area between them.

When body weights are distributed too far to one side or the other, or too far to the front or back of the spinal column, the center of gravity is thrown off center. In that case, the body is off balance and compensating shifts of weight must be made to withstand the pull of gravity. The muscles are called upon to bear the burden of these off-center weights. Yet the bones properly are the weight bearers, and the main job of the muscles is to move the bones. They should not be called upon unnecessarily for the support of off-center weights in order to maintain equilibrium. Not only does an unbalanced adjustment of weights strain the muscles, which must contract against the pull of gravity, but also the bones themselves must suffer.

The three principal segments of body weight are the head, the thorax, and the pelvis. The weight of the head rests on top of the spinal column and the combined weights of the head, thorax, and pelvis are supported on the heads of the powerful thighbones. Gravity pulls perpendicularly on the erect body, that is, down through the vertical axis represented by the spinal column. Body balance in the erect position, or good posture, as we are accustomed to call it, means simply that body weights are so adjusted that they stay up by themselves on the two leg props with the least possible effort on the part of the muscles to hold them in line.

The curves of the spinal column are of great assistance in this adjustment of weights. If the spinal column were straight up and down, like the pole of a clothes tree, for example, the weight of the organs of the chest and abdomen would pull the body forward out of balance, just as several heavy overcoats suspended on the hooks at the front of a clothes tree would topple it over. As it is, the four spinal curves, alternately convex and concave, not only balance each other but also divide up the weight of the three loads supported by the spinal column—the head, the chest, and the pelvis—and balance these loads as they accumulate toward the base represented by the heads of the thighbones.

It would be a mistake to think that balance is brought about in the body by opposing weight for weight at equal distances from the center line as can be done in draping clothes on a clothes tree or in building a tower of blocks or a snowman. The weights are there to be supported in the positions assigned to them. And the weight bearers—the bones— have muscular attachments which can shift such burdens within limits as the need arises.

It sometimes happens, however, that for one cause or another—weak muscles, chronic fatigue, poor posture sense, or bone deformities, for example—these weights must be held out of balance more or less constantly. The essential supporting mechanism—the spinal column—must then adapt itself to these off-balance weights. It can do this because its flexibility enables it to accent or even to distort the normal curves so as to compensate for poor weight distribution. This throws extra work on the muscles and ligaments attached to the individual vertebrae. Also, other muscles, those in the neck, for example, may be called upon to bear more weight than is their proper task.

Postural Characteristics According to Age

As children grow from babyhood into childhood and on into adolescence, their posture tends to change (see Fig. 18-6). That is why an indispensable factor in observing children for postural characteristics is the age of the child observed. It is important not to confuse real defects with conditions that children normally outgrow.

The characteristic changes in posture come about through skeletal growth and development and the strengthening of the child's muscles as he learns to sit up, creep, stand, and finally to walk, run, climb, and take part in active play. When the child enters school the abdomen normally protrudes because of the relative weakness of the abdominal muscles. In proportion to the prominence of the abdomen the lower spinal curve (lumbar curve) normally is exaggerated (lumbar lordosis).

The muscles of the shoulders, neck, and upper trunk all help to hold the head, shoulders, and chest in position. It is normal for young children to hold their heads slightly forward and to have chests deeper in proportion to their breadth. The chest gradually becomes broader and flatter and the shoulder blades closer together during the years immediately before and after entering school. Good muscular and skeletal development makes it possible for the child of school age to carry his head, neck, chest, and shoulders in good balance.

With the increase in strength of the muscles of the abdomen and buttocks in the adolescent period, the abdomen flattens and the lumbar curve straightens out so that the lower back becomes less "hollow." In this period types of body build (see Chap. 3) become apparent, and the posture reveals trends that become definite characteristics in adult life (see Fig. 18-7 for characteristics of good posture).

It is at this time also that posture faults are most likely to develop. However, it may be difficult to distinguish between real defects and temporary maladjustments or retarded development of the mature spinal curves. For example, girls, becoming aware of their maturing breasts, may try to conceal them by letting their shoulders droop forward, and tall weedy boys may slouch to make their height conform more nearly to that of their associates. Also, as has been pointed out (see Chap. 3), rapid growth during adolescence may result in awkwardness in body movements. On the other hand, adolescent youngsters learn that an attractive physical appearance contributes to social success. This idea furnishes a strong incentive for efforts to correct postural defects and to develop the strong muscles that help to maintain good body balance.

Although various postural characteristics considered undesirable in

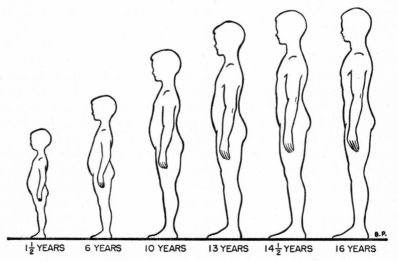

FIG. 18-6. Postural characteristics of a boy according to age.

General Appearance	A well-poised body giving the effect of good physical and emotional health and enthusiasm for life.		
Head	Head erect, or inclined slightly forward, with chin in.		
Shoulders	Level and down in back with flat shoulder blades. Upper outer tips curved slightly forward in front.	**Back** Normal spinal curves. Neck curves slightly inward (toward front); upper back curves outward ("dorsal prominence"); lower back curves inward ("lumbar curve"). † Buttocks curve outward.	
Chest	Moderately elevated and symmetrical.		
Abdomen	Flat from the hips to the breastbone.*		
Thighs	Curved slightly backward.		
Knees	Straight, barely touching each other.		
Feet	Toes pointed straight forward, inner sides parallel, body weight carried on balls and outer sides of the feet.		

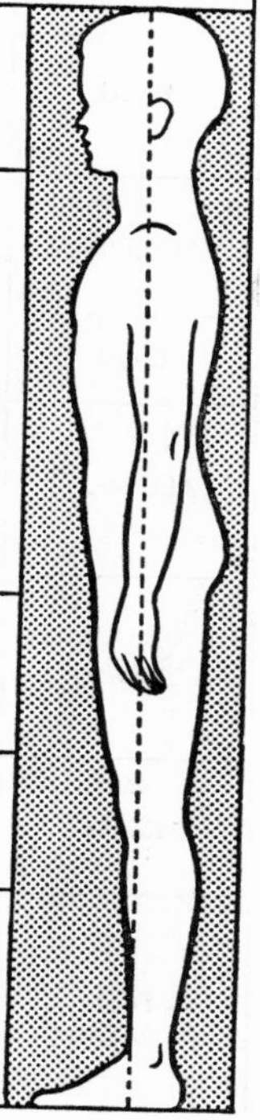

* A protruding abdomen is normal in pre-adolescent children.
† A straight upper back and an exaggerated lumbar curve are normal in childhood.

B.P.

FIG. 18-7. Good posture.

physically mature individuals are normal in earlier stages of development, it is important to be on the lookout for conditions that persist beyond the time at which they should be outgrown (see Fig. 18-8). Conditions that should be referred for attention at all ages are exaggerated front-to-back (natural) spinal curves, lateral (unnatural) spinal curves (see Spinal Curvature, further on), chest deformities, flat feet (see further on), cramped toes, hips out of line, round shoulders and forward head, and generally poor body balance due to lowered muscle tone.

Every person who is healthy and who has no defects or deformities that interfere with body mechanics can have good posture. Why is it then that so many young people develop poor posture? Partly it's because they have fallen into careless habits of standing, walking, and sitting. Partly it's because they have not had enough exercise to strengthen

General Appearance	A slumping body giving the effect of substandard health, fatigue, inadequacy for life.	
Head	Markedly inclined forward.	
Shoulders	One shoulder higher than other. In back, shoulder blades stick out.* In front, shoulders sag forward.	**Back** Exaggerated curvature of dorsal prominence (kyphosis, or "humpback"); extreme curvature in lumbar region (lordosis); deviation of spinal column to right or left (scoliosis, or lateral spinal curvature).
Chest	Markedly depressed or deformed ("funnel breast" or "chicken breast").†	
Abdomen	Markedly protruding and sagging.	
Thighs	Curved slightly forward.	
Knees	Slightly bent, close together.	
Feet	Toes pointed outward, ankles turned inward, body weight carried on inner sides of feet.	

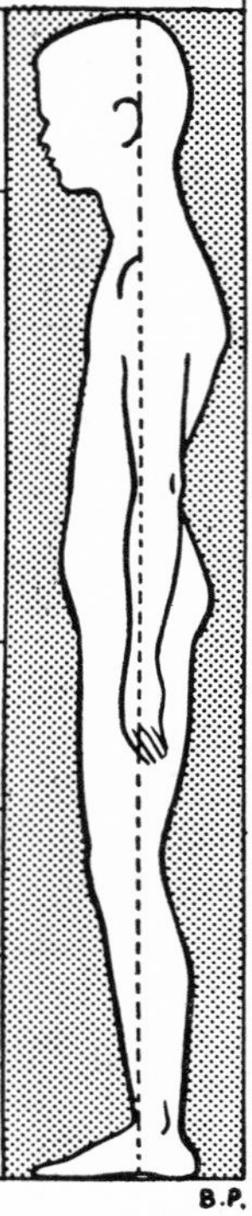

B.P.

* Slight pressure only required to place the fingers definitely under the inner border or tips of the shoulder blade.

† Funnel-like depression at the end of the breastbone or a forward bulging of the breastbone with the ribs sloping away to the sides.

FIG. 18-8. Poor posture.

the muscles used in posture—particularly those of the abdomen and back. And partly it's because no one has ever shown them how to stand, walk, and sit correctly.

Getting the "Feel" of Balance

Long before the child enters school, he has succeeded in his early efforts to cope with the forces of gravity and has developed skill in maintaining the equilibrium of his erect jointed body over a small base of support. His spine has been changed from a horizontal beam for the suspension of weights, as in the all-fours, or quadruped, position, to a vertical column for the support of weights in the two-footed, or biped, position. By mechanical necessity his spine curves forward at the small of his back; his shoulders fall back and down of their own weight; his chest is lifted, giving room for lung expansion; and by a series of shelf-like and basketlike arrangements, the organs of his trunk are being supported and given maximum space for full and vigorous function.

Cultivation of the child's posture sense, or overall feeling for balance, is more important than the singling out for correction of separate portions of his anatomy which, from an adult point of view, are held incorrectly. Such commands as "Push your head up," "Hold your chin in," "Stick your chest out and up," and "Throw your shoulders back" suggest effort and tension and, in effect, are futile. The teacher may, however, make suggestions that will help the child to get the feel of the proper position. Good posture is relaxed and comfortable, graceful, attractive, and efficient. When the various segments of body weight are well poised one above the other, total weight is carried directly to the seat or ground by the bones with a minimum of effort on the part of the muscles.

In getting the feel of balance in oneself and in observing children, it is helpful to think of the weights at the front of the body as passing upward toward the shoulders and head and the weights at the back of the body as passing downward from the top of the spine to the base. In thinking "up in front and down in back" it is useful to visualize a belt conveyor traveling upward with loaded cups and dumping the load as it travels downward. In this up-in-front-down-in-back picture of erect posture, the head, shoulders, chest, abdomen, and back have the appearance noted in Fig. 18-7.

Standing and Walking

No one ever stands completely still. Standing, even when the body weights are perfectly balanced, requires delicately graded alternations of muscle tension which may be as tiring as walking. The entire weight of the body in standing is borne by the feet. It is the arched formation of the feet that gives them the power to absorb and distribute the crushing weight of the body. The heel bone gives one point of contact of the foot with the ground, and the heads of the metatarsal bones give the other points of contact. The five metatarsal bones bound together by ligaments and covered with flesh give the effect of a single long arch. The back part of this arch is the instep. The heads of the metatarsal bones form the transverse, or cross, arch. The rounded part of the sole, right under this arch, is the ball of the foot. In proper standing the weight of the body is distributed evenly on both feet with weight felt as falling mostly on the balls and slightly to the outside of the feet.

In walking, the motion of the ankles, feet, and toes is produced largely by the action of muscles located in the legs. These muscles are connected with the bones they move by long tendons. The muscles of the leg act as shock absorbers in walking and running. They also are largely responsible for holding the feet in proper position (see further on). These muscles are strengthened as the child learns to stand and walk. As he becomes increasingly active, they help to keep his whole body in good balance.

When the feet are used correctly in walking, the toes point straight ahead, the inner sides of the feet are parallel with each other, and the knees just miss each other. In stepping forward, the heel and the ball of the foot strike the ground at nearly the same time, with the heel touching first. The weight of the body falls toward the outer edge. To get the most good out of walking, the arms should swing forward and backward from the shoulders as the legs swing forward and backwards from the hips.

Feet and Their Troubles. Babies who are learning to stand and walk are very unsteady on their feet. All toddlers have knock-knees (knees together with ankles far apart) and some degree of toeing out of the feet. At about the age of six, the knees normally become straight and the toeing out is greatly decreased. In some children, however, knock-knees and toeing out remain to become the defect known as "pronated feet."

A child with pronated feet walks with the toes pointed outward and the ankles turned inward. This position increases the strain on the ligaments and fatigues the muscles on the inner side of the foot. As a result the foot sags on the inner side below and in front of the ankle. The long arch of the foot is weakened and in severe cases "flatfoot" or "fallen arches" develop. In children with pronated feet the heels of the shoes are usually worn over on the inside (Plate 15). Often faulty weight bearing and weak or flattened arches can be corrected by special exercises for the feet.

There are flat feet of many varieties. One common variety is congenital flatfoot. That is, the arch of the instep is flat from birth. As a result, the entire sole of the foot rests flat on the ground. Congenital flatfoot runs in certain families and usually causes little trouble.

Sitting

In sitting, the weight of the head and trunk properly falls on the rockerlike lower portions (ischia) of the hipbones (see above). For this reason the ischia are sometimes called the seat bones. It is easy to fall into bad habits of sitting because the very fact of having a seat permits almost any slumps or contortions of the body. Standing would be impossible with the spinal sag in which many people sit for much of the time. Children sit in school for a large part of the school day. It is inevitable that habits in sitting will be formed. To make possible natural, comfortable sitting positions so that such positions will become habitual is the object of adjusting chairs and desks or tables to the individual child in school.

What the seat must accomplish is to ensure that when the child relaxes in it his posture will be erect and comfortable (see Fig. 18-9). This means that the pelvis must sit vertically with the forward lumbar curve preserved and the shoulders hanging back freely. The points of the seat bones, the crests of the hipbones, and the shoulder tips should be in the same plane, and in this position there should be no uncomfortable pressures, strains, pushes, or pulls.

A bad habit that is easy to fall into in the seated position is that of sliding forward so that one sits on the end of the spine instead of upon the seat bones. In the typical stoop or slump characteristic of a tendency to slide forward on the

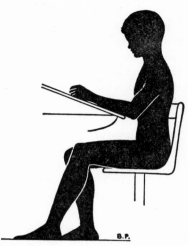

FIG. 18-9. Good sitting posture in school is made possible by an adjustable desk top and an adjustable seat that gives proper support to the lower back and thighs.

seat or to pitch forward at the shoulders, the pelvis tips backward so that a plane passing through the seat bones and the crests of the hips would pass far behind the shoulders. Then the forward curve in the small of the back disappears and there is a single continuous outward curve from seat to neck, with consequent displacement and crowding of the organs of the chest, abdomen, and pelvis.

To prevent any forward-sliding tendency, the seat should slope slightly backward. It should also provide support under the thighs when the feet are extended forward but should not be so high or so deep, front to back, as to cause pressure under the knees when the child sits as far back as the back support permits. The seat should be just high enough above the ground to allow the feet to rest comfortably on the floor while the lower part of the back is supported by the chair back. The desk or table at which a child sits at work should be just high enough to allow him to rest his forearms on the top surface at right angles to the upper arms with the shoulders relaxed.

Influences on Posture

A naturally easy graceful carriage can be maintained only by strong muscles and well-shaped bones working efficiently together. Several factors influence posture by their favorable or unfavorable effect on the bone-muscle team itself or the conditions under which this team does its work.

Nutrition. Good nutrition, without which good health is impossible, is a most important contributor to good posture. A well-balanced diet provides liberal amounts of the materials the body uses in building and repairing muscles and bones. The composite picture of a well-nourished child and a malnourished child described in Chap. 12 (under Observing the Nutritional Status of School Children) indicates other postural differences between the two which the teacher may observe.

Physical Defects. Physical defects of various kinds are often reflected in poor posture. Poor eyesight or hearing tends to make a child lean forward or sideways or cock his head or take other unnatural positions in order to see or hear better. More serious are the crippling defects with which some children are born or which develop as a result of disease or injury (see further on).

Exercise. Exercise, as we have seen, strengthens muscles and gives them practice in moving the bones with speed and ease. One of the principal causes of poor posture is soft, lazy muscles—particularly those of the abdomen and back—that lack the strength and agility for good body mechanics. Another contribution to poor posture is a lack of symmetry in muscular development brought about by lack of variety in exercise. It is easy to see that muscular development may be unsymmetrical, or uneven, if one part of the body is exercised much more than other parts. Children can attain symmetrical muscular development by taking part in vigorous outdoor games and sports that make them use many muscles.

Fatigue. The fatigue caused by poor posture is due to the muscular and nervous strains required to balance the body when the weight masses are out of line. The fatigue associated with malnutrition, the effects of illness, a focal infection, skeletal or muscular defects, nervous strain, or emotional instability is usually reflected in poor posture. Fatigue posture in a sitting position is illustrated in Plate 16.

The tendency of the body to slump is the chief characteristic of fatigue posture. Practically all of us have experienced loss of muscle tone after a hard day's work or a period of prolonged or strenuous physical exercise. We start out feeling fresh and rested, with erect body and springy step. At the end of the day or after a long hike, for example, we have actually become smaller with rounded shoulders, perhaps, and forward-drooping head, because the tone of the muscles is decreased.

A period of rest or a good night's sleep is all that is needed to cure temporary fatigue. Even if children tend to droop at the end of the day, there is nothing to worry about if they come to school in the morning looking rested and glowing with vitality. It is only when a child seems to tire more easily than most children do or habitually slumps in his seat or moves in a listless manner that medical attention is needed to determine the cause.

Emotional Factors. Posture very often gives feelings away. It is difficult to stand up straight when one is weighted down with a load on one's mind. A young person's posture alone may show that he is suffering from hurt feelings, worries, fears, shyness, a grudge, a notion of not being understood, or lack of interest in life.

Clothing. Clothes that are so tight that they interfere with freedom of movement obviously have an unfavorable effect on posture. Fortunately, today's styles in children's play and school clothes allow plenty of room for action. Girdles or other foundation garments worn by adolescent girls, however, may be so tight that they do the work of supporting the body that the abdominal muscles should be doing. These muscles may get flabby if they are braced up all the time.

Shoes. No one can be happy on his feet, let alone have good posture, unless his shoes fit properly. Most parents realize the importance of frequent changes in their children's shoes. Youngsters often have a great deal to say about shoe purchases because being in style—"being like everybody else"—is of great importance to them. Pointers on shoe selection are often included in health courses. The points usually emphasized are (1) snug fit around the heel so that the heel does not slide up and down when walking; (2) a relatively straight inner border; (3) enough width in front to accommodate the toes with room to spare; and (4) the allowance of at least ½ inch between the tip of the shoe and the end of the big toe.

The question of the height of the heels is of great concern to girls. There is no doubt that high heels throw more weight on the balls of the feet than they would normally be called on to support. The muscles of the legs can take care of the necessary adjustments without too much difficulty over short periods of time. But if a girl wears high-heeled shoes constantly, the wear and tear on her legs and feet may become so great that she is in for real trouble.

Among the more familiar miseries are aching arches, sore calves, painful calluses under the balls of the feet, headaches, and backaches. It may be possible to persuade girls that they can avoid troubles of this kind by making a sensible compromise—that is, by reserving their spike heels and other less-than-ideal shoes in style at the moment for dances and other social occasions—and shoeing their feet sensibly and comfortably for school and work. Many shoe manufacturers now combine correct shape with attractive styling in designing shoes for daytime wear.

Furniture. Seating arrangements that make possible good sitting positions at work have already been described. Sitting at leisure seems to encourage the strange contortions of the body so common among adolescent youngsters. Learning to sit correctly when reading, watching television, talking on the telephone, or just lounging is a matter of learning the correct positions and then forming the habit of taking them. These positions, rather than the incorrect ones, will then be comfortable. A good comfortable position to take while sitting in an easy chair is to sit well back or to slide the lower part of the body forward and place a cushion under the lower part of the back for support.

Strained sleeping positions may be caused by sagging bedsprings and a too-soft mattress that lets the heavy parts of the body sink down. A mattress that makes good sleeping posture possible is firm and flat but not so rigid that it doesn't allow for natural body curves. Bedclothes should be light in weight and not so tightly tucked in that they interfere with changes of position during sleep. The pillow should not be so large that it bends the neck forward.

ORTHOPEDIC DEFECTS IN SCHOOL CHILDREN

Radical changes have occurred in recent years in the types of orthopedic defects that are found in school-age children. These changes reflect the advances made by medical science in the prevention and treatment of infections that often have crippling aftereffects and the great strides that have been made in orthopedic surgery.

By far the leading cause of orthopedic impairments among school children was once poliomyelitis (see Poliomyelitis, in Chap. 8). With the advent of successful vaccines for preventing this disease, there has been a sharp decline in the number of polio cripples. It has been confidently predicted that there will be none at all in years to come. The incidence of other orthopedic defects caused by infection or by nutritional deficiency also has been greatly reduced—in some cases almost to the vanishing point—largely because of the advances made in chemotherapy and in the science of nutrition. (See Osteomyelitis, Tuberculosis of the Bones and Joints, and Rickets, further on.)

The decline in orthopedic defects caused by infections or nutritional deficiencies has been counterbalanced by rises in crippling conditions caused by cerebral palsy (see Cerebral Palsy, in Chap. 8), muscular dystrophy, congenital defects and birth injuries, and childhood accidents.

Crippled Children in School

There are two main reasons why crippled children may appear in the school population in increasing numbers. The first reason is related to the improved surgical and treatment methods that are making it possible for more children malformed at birth to survive. It is conjectured "that the percentage of children in special classes with cerebral palsy, congenital anomalies, and other neurological conditions due to birth injury will continue to grow as a result of this decrease in infant mortality. . . . Many of those surviving will be more severely handicapped than in the past and will present more diverse educational problems resulting from central nervous system disorders." [2]

The second reason is the change that is taking place in the educational planning for crippled children. Formerly children suffering from crippling conditions and other special health problems were required to undergo long-term treatment and care away from home. Instructional programs for these children were instituted in hospitals and in convalescent and rehabilitation homes. At present, advances made in medicine, greater accessibility of medical care, and the progress made in the rehabilitation of the handicapped have materially reduced the confinement away from home of most children with crippling conditions. As a result many of these children are attending regular classes or special classes in the public schools.

Congenital and Prenatal Conditions

As one would expect, congenital defects and birth injuries are responsible for the majority of orthopedic handicaps in the early years of life. Since many of these defects can be corrected or their effects greatly minimized by early treatment, they become numerically less important in the later years of childhood, and acquired defects become numerically more important. Orthopedic surgery is now undertaken much more frequently than in the past for the correction of conditions that cannot be remedied in other ways. In some cases, of course, it is impossible to correct a crippling defect. But the orthopedist can do a great deal to help his patient to adjust to it.

When uncorrected, deformities due to congenital conditions or birth injuries cause various abnormalities in posture or gait. Some of the more common are briefly described here.

Some foot deformities are the result of congenital conditions. One of the most common is *talipes* (Latin for "clubfoot"). In this condition the foot is twisted out of shape or position. Some forms of clubfoot may be acquired after birth by disease or injury. A child with clubfoot may walk on the heel with the toes elevated, or on the toes or forepart of one or both feet, or on the inner borders of the feet with the feet turned outward (pronated), or on the outer borders with the feet turned upward (supinated).

In uncorrected congenital dislocation of the hips, the child may walk with a waddling gait ("duck walk") but usually he can get about with relative freedom.

In wryneck (*torticollis*), caused by the contraction of the muscles on

[2] Joseph Fenton and Frances P. Connor, "The Changing Picture in the Education of Children with Crippling Conditions and Special Health Problems," reprinted from *Exceptional Children*, February, 1959.

one side of the neck as the result of a birth injury, the head is tilted to one side and the child looks as if he were "listening to his shoulder."

There are several other forms of wryneck other than congenital torticollis, some of which are temporary in character. Most of us are familiar with the tendency to screw the neck into the least painful position when the neck muscles feel sore and tight as a result of a cold or "a touch of rheumatism." Uncorrected hearing and visual defects, as we have seen, often affect the position of the head. Habitually cocking one side of the head toward the speaker is a common indication of loss of hearing in one ear. A high degree of astigmatism is so closely associated with wryneck that ocular torticollis is a well-recognized condition.

Wryneck also may be a sign of hysteria or a form of tic or habit spasm in which there is spasmodic contraction of the neck muscles, producing deviations of the head.

In _Erb's palsy_, caused by injury at birth to the network of nerves supplying the muscles of the arms (brachial plexus), there is paralysis of one or both arms. The affected arm hangs limply at the side and is turned inward toward the body. The child, when asked to bring the palm of his hand to his mouth, will "kiss the back of the hand" instead.

Muscular dystrophy is a disease of the voluntary muscles which is growing in importance as a cause of crippling and premature death. Its cause is the inheritance of one or two abnormal genes, according to the type of muscular dystrophy inherited. It may, however, be caused by the conversion in the egg or sperm of a normal gene into an abnormal one. This is the process known as mutation. In this disease there is progressive loss of muscle fibers resulting in progressive wasting and hence weakening of the voluntary muscles.

There are several different kinds of muscular dystrophy, but the three most common types are known as the childhood type, the juvenile type, and the adult type. The childhood type begins typically in the first few years of life and rarely as late as puberty. It starts in the hip region and progresses rapidly. Death often occurs in the teens or early twenties. Its victims are boys; girls are rarely if ever affected but may act as carriers. It was announced in 1964 that a method involving several tests has been worked out for identifying women carriers of the childhood type.

The juvenile type begins usually in early adolescence in both the shoulder and hip regions. The adult type seldom appears before puberty and is slowly progressive. The muscles of the face and shoulder girdle are typically affected first. The usual course in all three types is one of gradually increasing disability.

There is as yet no cure for muscular dystrophy although treatment may be helpful in maintaining muscular activity for as long as possible. The Muscular Dystrophy Association of America provides year-round services to patients and their parents and sponsors educational and recreational programs for the victims. The main emphasis, however, is on the establishment of a nationwide network of clinics and on the support of research on the care and cure of the disease.

Acquired Orthopedic Impairments

The infections, other than poliomyelitis, that are responsible for an appreciable number of orthopedic impairments among children are osteomyelitis and tuberculosis.

Osteomyelitis. Osteomyelitis is an infection of the bone which is usually caused by staphylococci, although other bacteria—notably the streptococcus and the pneumococcus—may be responsible. This infection occurs most frequently before the age of ten. It may be acute or chronic. Destruction of the bone takes place in both forms but is less active in chronic osteomyelitis. The long bones, especially the large bone of the leg (tibia), are most often affected.

Following a compound fracture, osteomyelitis may develop as a result of infection with staphylococci introduced from the skin. It may develop, however, without apparent injury.

The infection may remain localized at one spot or spread to the marrow and thence throughout the bone. In acute osteomyelitis there is, in addition, general poisoning by the staphylococcal toxin, and in about half the cases the staphylococci invade the bloodstream.

The onset of acute osteomyelitis is usually abrupt with signs of severe illness, accompanied by pain, swelling, and redness at the site of the infection. It is extremely important to get the child under a doctor's care at once, because the use of sulfadiazine or penicillin in the early stages of osteomyelitis may avert a serious illness and extensive bone destruction with severe crippling.

Tuberculosis of the Bones and Joints. Tuberculous infection of the bones and joints was a prominent cause of disability only a generation ago. Since then it has decreased markedly in frequency and now accounts for only a small fraction of all orthopedic defects among children under twenty-one. The hipbones, the knee joints, and the spinal vertebrae are the most common sites of tuberculosis of the joints and bones in the young. Tuberculosis of the spine is known as Pott's disease. With adequate treatment it may be arrested, but it frequently leaves the child with a permanent deformity.

Rickets. The fundamental feature of rickets is a disturbance of calcium-phosphorus metabolism, which results in the defective formation of bones. Vitamin D is essential for the absorption and proper utilization of calcium and phosphorus to form normal bone. Hence Vitamin D deficiency is a prime factor in the cause of rickets.

Since the bones are relatively soft and pliable in rickets, they are easily bent and twisted by muscular action, and the natural curvatures of the long bones become exaggerated. The various bone deformities that develop include knock-knees, bowlegs, lateral spinal curvature (scoliosis), malformation of the chest (pigeon breast, chicken breast, funnel breast), narrow pelvis, soft depressible areas in the skull, and bosses or beadings on the sides and ends of bone (for example, "beading of the ribs").

Rickets is essentially a disease of the first two years of life, when bone formation and growth are most active. Infantile rickets seldom commences after the second year nor does it usually progress beyond that time. However, the deformities caused by it persist. Owing to the great strides made in orthopedic surgery, it is now possible in many cases to correct the crippling aftereffects of infantile rickets.

In the days before the antirachitic properties of Vitamin D were discovered, rickets was a very common cause of crippling. It is now rarely encountered in our country, largely because of the widespread use of Vitamin D milk instead of ordinary milk in the feeding of infants and children.

Spinal Curvature. Curvature of the spine, especially lateral curvature (scoliosis), is among the leading causes of orthopedic impairment among children. There are few individuals with ideally curved spines. In observing children we are concerned only with pronounced degrees of deviation from the technically ideal form. A distinction is usually made between structural scoliosis, in which there is a true spinal deformity, and postural or functional scoliosis.

Congenital weakness of the ligamentary apparatus or muscular attachments of the spine accounts for some cases of structural scoliosis. In others, disease of the vertebrae or the supporting muscles may be to blame.

Postural or functional scoliosis in children is rare. It may result from habitually assuming poor body positions. This poor posture is usually caused by weak musculature. Postural scoliosis can be overcome voluntarily when contributing causes, such as poor nutrition, too little rest, or improper seating, have been eliminated and the child's cooperation in correcting his faulty posture, through corrective exercises, has been secured.

Other Crippling Conditions. There is a large group of miscellaneous conditions that cause crippling but are of relatively infrequent occurrence. Of these the most common are disturbances of the normal process of bone growth at the epiphyses (see How Bones Grow, in Chap. 3). The cause of such disturbances is unknown; in some cases it may be congenital. The bones most frequently affected are the upper end of the thighbone (femur) and less commonly the upper end of the large leg bone (tibia). Children from five to ten are most likely to be affected. The onset is gradual. The early sign is a limp, which may be associated with pain and tenderness.

IDENTIFYING AND HELPING CHILDREN WITH ORTHOPEDIC DEFECTS

Many children with orthopedic disabilities come to orthopedic specialists or clinics too late to have the condition corrected by the simpler forms of treatment. Defects found during the early years of life are more amenable to treatment because the body framework is then more plastic. It is believed by many persons doing orthopedic work that teachers should be just as much on the lookout for signs indicating orthopedic defects as they are for defects of vision and hearing.

In observing children for orthopedic defects it is not the function of the teacher to say why the pupil limps, or why the posture is poor or the spine curved, but to refer children who have these conditions for an orthopedic examination.

If a child obviously needs orthopedic care and is not getting it, the school should assume the responsibility for giving his family the necessary information as to the location of clinics or other facilities in the community for diagnosis and treatment.

Observing Children for Orthopedic Defects

To give screening examinations for orthopedic defects it is necessary to remove the greater part of the clothing. Very few school systems have teachers or nurses who have been trained to give such an examination. However, any teacher can make valuable observations even when the child is fully clothed if she is alerted to the importance of noticing deviations from normal in gait and posture. In junior and senior high schools, where the children wear gymnasium suits while participating in physical education activities, the physical education teacher occupies a strategic position for observing abnormal spinal curvatures, winged scapulae, and other defects not easily detected in the fully clothed child.

In Table 18-1 are listed deviations from normal which teachers can observe in children dressed in ordinary clothes or which children may report to her.

Educational Procedures for Orthopedically Handicapped Children

In practically every school there are children who need special attention because of orthopedic difficulties. These children may be classed in three groups according to the severity of the condition.

In the first group are children who have no definite orthopedic defects but who show signs of poor body mechanics, poor coordination, and the like. These children need careful watching and more frequent medical examinations than are given to the rest of the school population. The postural difficulties of these borderline cases may be met by a program of physical education and participation in physical activities suited to individual needs.

Table 18-1

INDICATIONS OF ORTHOPEDIC DEFECTS*

Point of observation	Deviations from normal
Gait..................	Limping
	Dragging of foot
	Spastic gait (each leg swings forward as a solid piece in a narrow arc with the feet turned inward and toes scraping along the floor; called the "scissors gait," as the legs tend to cross each other in walking)
	Waddling gait (called the "duck walk")
	Walking on the toes or heels
	Walking on the inner or outer borders of feet
Feet and toes..........	Habitually standing with toes pointed in (pigeon toes) or out
	Standing with ankles rolled inward (weak ankle posture)
	Heels of shoes worn down on the inside or outside in a short time
	Complaints of pains in the feet or legs
	Reporting of corns, bunions, blisters, calluses on balls of feet
Legs.................	Bowlegs
	Knock-knees
Back and shoulders......	Upper back humped (kyphosis)
	Lower back hollow (lordosis)
	Round shoulders
	One shoulder considerably higher than the other
	Complaints of backache
Chest.................	Abnormally high
	Hollow-chested
	Narrow-chested
Arms and hands.........	Limp, or flaccid
	Deformities of fingers
Head and neck..........	Head abnormally large
	Wryneck (head tilted to side)

* See also Figures 18-7 and 18-8.

In the second group are children with crippling conditions so severe that they require special educational procedures. These children are usually enrolled in special classes, and their classrooms are equipped with ramps and other facilities that enable them to participate successfully in class activities.

The third group is made up of crippled children who can adjust to regular class programs. Practically all those who work with orthopedically handicapped children agree that such children should attend regular classes if it is at all possible for them to do so. The effects of isolation in special classes may tend to accentuate feelings of difference and inadequacy in some children. In regular classes handicapped children have an opportunity to make normal social adjustments as well as to benefit from general school activities, such as assembly and extracurricular programs. In several states local school systems are reimbursed for the cost of salaries of approved special teachers to assist regular classroom teachers in providing educational services for physically handicapped children in regular classes.

It has already been pointed out that the teacher who has a crippled child in her class can do that child the greatest service by unobtrusively making it possible for him to become as independent as possible. Physically handicapped children have the same sort of feelings as normal children. They want to be as much like the others as possible, to have fun and companionship and a chance to excel—to amount to something in their own eyes and those of their peers. It is the teacher's privilege to set the stage for the making of good social adjustments and for successful participation in school activities.

The special needs of physically handicapped children are usually taken care of by professional workers in the field or fields involved. It is considered highly desirable that students in training for regular classroom teaching should become familiar with the functions of the professional workers who work with handicapped children in the schools.

The "team" approach, with the teacher, speech correctionist, physician, physical therapist, occupational therapist, school psychologist, social worker and vocational rehabilitation counselor joining hands in behalf of the "whole" child has become a standard operating procedural goal in almost all instances. Admission to special class facilities, for example, long a prerogative of the physician only, is to a growing extent no longer based upon medical recommendations alone. The physical findings and recommendations comprise one aspect for consideration in balance with the social, psychological, and educational needs of the child with the ultimate decisions being made by the "team." [3]

[3] Ibid., p. 7.

FOR REVIEW AND DISCUSSION

1. Match each group of words in column A with the word or term in column B that you associate with it.

A	B
The outer covering of bones	Mandible
Topmost vertebra	Kinesthesia
A ball-and-socket joint	Triceps
A hinge joint	Shoulder joint
The spinal column	Femur
Chief organic constituent of bone	Clavicles
The only movable bone of the face	Lactic acid
Shoulder girdle	Phalanges
Bones of the fingers and toes	Semicircular canals
Largest and strongest bone in the skeleton	Periosteum
A flexor	The knee
An extensor	Atlas
Waste product of muscle contraction	Biceps
Sense of balance	Vertebrae
Muscle sense	Collagen

2. Tell the difference between

   a. Smooth muscle fibers and striped muscle fibers
   b. Red bone marrow and yellow bone marrow
   c. Ilium and ischium
   d. The instep and the ball of the foot
   e. Muscle tone and muscle buffering
   f. Cerebellum and cerebrum
   g. Congenital orthopedic defects and acquired orthopedic defects

3. In the following groupings of diseases and conditions, one does not belong in the group. Select the one that is out of place and tell why.

   a. Kyphosis, lordosis, tuberculosis, scoliosis
   b. Osteomyelitis, poliomyelitis, rickets, Pott's disease
   c. Erb's palsy, ataxia, muscular dystrophy, congenital torticollis

4. Select the word or phrase which applies to the key word or term.

   a. Posture: (1) standing straight and tall, (2) the position in which you hold your body in everything you do, (3) having good muscle tone.
   b. Center of gravity of the body: (1) back wall of the pelvis, (2) the feet and the area between, (3) the semicircular canals.
   c. Pronated feet: (1) fallen arches, (2) pigeon toes, (3) feet with the toes pointed outward and the ankles turned inward in walking.

d. Congenital flatfoot: (1) flat feet caused by wearing high-heeled shoes, (2) flat feet caused by wearing shoes with heels worn down in the inside, (3) feet in which the arch of the instep is flat from birth.

e. Physical fitness: (1) that state in which the body can respond to physical work and exercise with a minimum amount of strain, (2) that state in which the muscles have become strong and agile as a result of daily exercise, (3) that state in which a person has become fit in all ways for life as he must live it.

5. Discuss in class ways in which a teacher can help (*a*) a child who is orthopedically handicapped, (*b*) a child whose posture is poor because of a poorly balanced program of rest and exercise, (*c*) a physically lazy high school boy or girl who doesn't see much point in exercise.

SELECTED REFERENCES

American Association for Health, Physical Education, and Recreation: *Physical Education for High School Students,* The Association, Washington, D.C. (A complete handbook of sports, games, dances, recreational activities, and athletics.)

American Association for Health, Physical Education, and Recreation: *Outdoor Recreation for American Youth,* (an illustrated text for teaching teen-agers to enjoy the outdoors.)

American Medical Association, Chicago:
ABC's of Posture
Exercise and Fitness
Seven Paths to Fitness

Andrews, Gladys, and others: *Physical Education for Today's Boys and Girls,* Allyn and Bacon, Inc., Boston, 1960.

Best, C. H., and N. B. Taylor: *The Human Body* (first given as reference in Chap. 1). Part II, *The Skeleton and the Muscular System,* Part V, Chap. 23, *Muscular Exercise and Physical Training.*

Davies, Evelyn A.: *The Elementary School Child and His Posture Patterns,* Appleton-Century-Crofts, Inc., New York, 1959.

Frohse, Franz, Max Brodel, and Leon Schlossberg: *Atlas of Human Anatomy,* 6th ed., Barnes & Noble, Inc., New York, 1961. (A series of colored anatomical charts with explanatory text.)

Johnson, David G., and Oscar Heidenstam: *Modern Bodybuilding: a Complete Guide to the Promotion of Fitness, Strength, and Physique,* Emerson Books, Inc., New York, 1958.

Kauth, Benjamin: *Walk and Be Happy—A Specialist's Guide to Healthy Feet,* The John Day Company, Inc., New York, 1960.

Kough, Jack, and Robert F. De Haan: *Teacher's Guidance Handbook* (first given as reference in Chap. 5). Vol. I, *Identifying Children with Special Needs,* Sec. IV, Chap. 21; Vol. II, *Helping Children with Special Needs,* Sec. IV, Chap. 18.

Methany, Eleanor: *Body Dynamics,* McGraw-Hill Book Company, New York, 1952. (The essentials of body mechanics and physical education. Contains suggestions for teaching about posture.)

Meredith, Florence: *Health and Fitness,* 4th ed., McGraw-Hill Book Company, New York, 1962.

Morehouse, L. E., and A. T. Miller: *Physiology of Exercise,* 3d ed., The C. V. Mosby Company, St. Louis, 1959. (A text for the nonmedical physiology or physical education student. It examines the role during exercise of the neuromuscular system and presents an overall account of the body's responses to physical exertion.)

National Education Association: *Your Child's Health and Fitness,* The Association, Washington, D.C., 1962.

National Education Association: *Youth and Fitness,* The Association, Washington, D.C., 1959.

Prudden, Bonnie, and Dorothy Stull: *Bonnie Prudden's Fitness Book,* The Ronald Press Company, New York, 1959.

Tucker, W. E.: *Active Alerted Posture,* The Williams & Wilkins Company, Baltimore, 1960.

Williams, Jesse Feiring: *Administration of Health Education and Physical Education,* 5th ed., W. B. Saunders Company, Philadelphia, 1958.

Youth Physical Fitness: Suggested Elements of a School-centered Program, President's Council on Youth Fitness, Washington, D.C., 1961.

Organizations

American Association for Health, Physical Education, and Recreation
Institute for the Crippled and Disabled
The National Foundation
National Society for Crippled Children and Adults

Appendix A IMMUNIZATION TIMETABLE*

Diseases	*Ages and special times*
Diphtheria Tetanus Whooping cough	At 1½ to 2 months of age—the first of a series of 3 injections with combined toxoid (diphtheria toxoid, tetanus toxoid, and whooping cough vaccine). At 3 months of age and again at 4 months of age injections are repeated to complete the series. One year after the first, or primary, immunization has been completed—a reinforcing, or booster, injection of combined toxoid. At 4 years of age and at 8 years of age the booster injection of combined toxoid should be repeated.
Diphtheria..........	At 12 years of age—a booster injection of diphtheria toxoid. After exposure and during epidemics—a booster injection of diphtheria toxoid may be given to increase the protection of previously immunized children. An antibiotic can be used to give temporary protection to children not previously immunized. In some cases diphtheria antitoxin also may be given. In older children and adults the physician may make tests for susceptibility to diphtheria as well as sensitivity to the injection material before deciding what treatment to give.
Tetanus.............	At 12 years of age and every 5 years throughout life—booster injections of tetanus toxoid. Following an injury from which there is danger of tetanus infection—a booster injection of tetanus toxoid may be given to those previously immunized. Tetanus antitoxin can be used to give temporary protection (lasting about 10 days) to those not previously immunized, provided precautions are taken to avoid unfavorable reactions in persons sensitive to the immunizing material.
Whooping cough.....	After exposure and during epidemics—a booster injection of whooping cough vaccine may be given to previously immunized children. Several substances are available to give temporary protection to children not previously immunized.
Poliomyelitis........	If the oral (Sabin) type polio vaccine (OPV) is used, first immunization at 2 months of age; second at 3 months of age; and third at 4 months of age. A booster dose is given at 15 months of age. If the Salk type polio vaccine (IPV) is used, the same schedule as for OPV; in addition, booster injection at 2 years of age and every two years thereafter.
Smallpox...........	At 12 months of age—the first vaccination with smallpox vaccine. At 6 years of age—revaccination. Every 5 years and in epidemics or after exposure—revaccination. A successful vaccination usually protects from 5 to 7 years.
Typhoid fever........	Periodically or when going on a vacation trip where there is danger of exposure to typhoid fever—an injection of typhoid vaccine (protection lasts for about 1 year).
Measles.............	At 9 months of age or as soon as possible thereafter—innoculation with attenuated live measles virus vaccine plus gamma globulin.

* Adapted from recommendations of the American Academy of Pediatrics and the American Public Health Association.

Appendix B COMMUNICABLE DISEASES

	Chicken pox (varicella)	German measles (rubella)	Measles (rubeola)
Cause	A virus; present in discharges from the mouth and nose and in discharges from vesicles on the skin.	A virus; present in discharges from the nose and throat.	A virus; present in discharges from the mouth and nose.
How spread	By direct and indirect contact.* Very contagious	By direct and indirect contact.* Very contagious.	By direct and indirect contact.* Very contagious.
Incubation period	From 14 to 16 days (occasionally as long as 21 days).	From 14 to 25 days; usually about 18 days.	About 10 days to onset of fever, 13 to 15 days to appearance of rash.
Onset	Mild constitutional symptoms, slight fever, loss of appetite.	Symptoms of mild cold; slight fever; sore throat.	Slight fever; red, watery, puffy eyes; signs of cold with tight hacking cough.
Site of eruption	Scalp and trunk; less abundant on arms and legs.	Scalp, sides of face, arms and hands, spreading rapidly over entire body.	Behind ears, on forehead or cheeks, then downward over body and limbs.
Character of eruption	Begins to appear about 24 hours after early signs. Successive crops of rose-pink spots which change into vesicles and finally to crusts. Each crop completes its course in from 2 to 4 days.	Minute, rosy, itching papules giving appearance of rose-colored rash. Lasts for about 1 to 3 days.	Begins to appear 3 or 4 days after onset. Red spots which collect in large red blotches and usually itch. Ordinarily lasts about 5 days. Peeling in the form of fine, branlike flakes.
Period of communicability	From 1 day before onset to about 6 days after appearance of first crop of blisters.	From onset of symptoms of a cold to from 4 to 7 days. Exact period uncertain	About 9 days (from 4 days before rash appears to 5 days afterwards).
Ages and seasons of greatest prevalence	Most common among children less than 15 years. Winter and spring.	Most common among children but fairly frequent in adults. Winter and spring.	Chiefly children from 5 to 14 years but common also in those less than 5. Winter and spring.
Methods of control	No specific preventive. Exclusion from school during period of communicability. Immunity usual after one attack.	No specific preventive. Immunity usual after one attack.	Active immunization with measles virus vaccine (see Appendix A, Immunization Timetable). Isolation during period of communicability. Immunity usual after one attack.

Source: *Control of Communicable Diseases in Man*, 9th ed., American Public Health Association, 1960; and *Report of the Committee on the Control of Infectious Diseases*, American Academy of Pediatrics, 1964.

* Direct contact means directly from person to person. Indirect contact means indirectly through handling, eating, or drinking anything soiled by discharges from the sick person or carrier.

Meningococcal meningitis	Scarlet fever (scarlatina)	Smallpox (variola)
The meningococcus (*Neisseria meningitidis*); present in discharges from the mouth and nose.	Group A hemolytic streptococci of several strains;† present in discharges from the mouth and nose and from ears, lymph nodes, etc., if affected.	A virus; present in the sores (pocks) on the skin and mucous membranes lining body openings (and so in discharges from the mouth, nose, bowels, and bladder).
By direct and indirect contact.* Carriers are important sources of infection during epidemics. Attack rate very low in those exposed.	By direct and indirect contact.* Floor dust, lint from bedding or clothing, and contaminated milk or other food may be important sources of infection.	By direct and indirect contact.* (Except for short distances, transmission through the air unlikely.) Very contagious.
From 2 to 10 days; usually 3 to 7 days.	From 2 to 5 days.	From 7 to 16 days, commonly 12, rarely 21.
Usually sudden in severe cases with chills, fever, malaise, muscle pains, intense headache, and often vomiting.	Lassitude, restlessness, followed by sore throat and fever.	Chills, intense headache, severe pains in back, vomiting, rapid pulse, quick rise in temperature.
When present, scattered over body.	Neck and chest, then over most of the body.	Face and limbs; less abundant on trunk.
Purpuric spots on skin in a small percentage of sporadic cases and in the majority of cases during epidemics. The purpuric spots are followed by small, bright red spots, which in 12 to 24 hours become successively dark red, purple, and finally blue black.	Little flat red points, close together. Under white coating on tongue red spots appear, and gradually tongue assumes a bright red color (strawberry tongue). Usually peeling begins in second week and lasts 2 or 3 weeks.	Begins to appear from 1 to 5 days after early signs. Red spots on skin which change first to blisters and then to typical smallpox pustules. Crusts form over the pustules and fall off in 10 to 40 days. In severe cases, pitted scars, or pock marks, are left after the crusts fall off.
For as long as meningococci are present in the nasopharynx.	Uncertain. Usually from first symptoms to complete recovery (about 14 days) or until all discharges have ceased.	From first symptoms until all scabs and crusts have disappeared. Most contagious in early stages.
Between epidemics, cases most common in children; during epidemics, severe cases most common in young adults.	Children and adults; children less than 10 years, especially less than 5, most susceptible.	Children and adults, especially adult males. Occurs in epidemics where vaccination is not enforced.
Winter and spring.	Late winter and spring.	Winter.
Administration of sulfadiazine eliminates meningococci from nasopharynx of convalescents and carriers.	Under certain conditions, penicillin to protect exposed persons (see Scarlet Scarlet Fever, in Chap. 11).	Active immunization with smallpox vaccine (see Appendix A, Immunization Timetable).
Isolation for 14 days or until nasopharynx is free of meningococci.	Penicillin may be used to shorten the attack and reduce the period of communicability.	Isolation during period of communicability.
Duration of immunity after an attack, unknown.	Isolation during period of communicability (usually 2 weeks). Boiling or pasteurization of milk. Immunity to rash-producing toxin usually after one attack.‡	Immunity usual after one attack.

† Some of these strains produce a toxin which causes scarlet fever *with* a rash. Other strains produce only infections of the nose and throat (streptococcal sore throat—scarlet fever *without* a rash). See Scarlet Fever and Streptococcal Sore Throat, in Chap. 11 and Sec. 2, Appendix B.

‡ In some cases rheumatic fever or acute glomerular nephritis develops after recovery from the acute attack.

Appendix B Communicable Diseases (continued)

Section 2. DISEASES SPREAD BY RESPIRATORY TRACT DISCHARGES BUT NOT CHARACTERIZED BY A SKIN ERUPTION

	Diphtheria	Mumps (infectious parotitis)	Streptococcal sore throat †	Whooping cough (pertussis)
Cause	The diphtheria bacillus (Corynebacterium diphtheriae) present in discharges from the nose and throat, open wounds, etc.	A virus; present in the saliva of an infected person.	Several strains of Group A hemolytic streptococci; present in discharges from the nose and throat, and from ears, lymph nodes, etc., if affected.	Pertussis bacillus; present in discharges from the nose and mouth.
How spread	By direct and indirect contact.* Contaminated milk or milk products and healthy carriers of the bacillus are important sources of infection.	By direct and indirect contact.* Less contagious than other common communicable diseases of childhood.	By direct and indirect contact.* Explosive milk-borne epidemics are usually called "septic sore throat." Carriers are important sources of infection.	By direct and indirect contact.*
Incubation period	Usually from 2 to 6 days, but occasionally longer.	From 12 to 26 days; average 18 days.	From 2 to 5 days.	From 5 to 10 days; not more than 21 days.
Onset	Sore throat and slight fever; possibly mild constitutional symptoms.	Moderate fever and congestion of upper respiratory tract followed by swelling of the salivary glands.	Sudden, with sore throat and fever, accompanied by muscle soreness, headache, and nausea.	Slow with catarrhal symptoms and tight dry cough. Cough becomes paroxysmal within 1 to 2 weeks after onset.
Period of communicability	For as long as the bacilli are present in the throat; usually for 2 weeks or less, rarely for more than 4 weeks.	Uncertain. Probably from 1 or 2 days before onset of symptoms until swelling of affected salivary glands subsides.	Uncertain. Usually from first symptoms to complete recovery (about 14 days) or until all discharges have ceased.	From early catarrhal stage to about 3 weeks after onset of typical spasmodic cough.
Character of the infection	The bacilli grow on the mucous membranes of the nose and throat and produce a powerful toxin which is absorbed by the	The virus attacks the salivary glands, especially the parotids, causing swelling and tenderness of the glands and mild constitu-	The streptococci grow on the mucous membranes of the tonsils and pharynx and produce a toxin which is absorbed by the	The bacilli grow on the mucous membranes of the respiratory tract and produce thick, ropy, sticky bronchial secretions which

body, resulting in systemic poisoning. Often a dirty white false membrane is formed locally by the action of the bacilli; this may block the breathing passages and cause suffocation.	tional symptoms. After puberty the testes (in boys) and the ovaries (in girls) may become involved.	body and causes constitutional symptoms.	are expelled with great difficulty. The violent repetitive coughing is characterized by a sudden inspiratory "crow" or "whoop."
Ages and seasons of greatest prevalence			
Most common among children less than 10 years of age.	Chiefly children and young adults; less prevalent than other common childhood diseases.	Children and adults.	Chiefly children less than 7 years of age.
Fall and winter.	Winter and spring.	Late winter and spring.	Variable but mostly in spring.
Methods of control			
Active immunization with diphtheria toxoid (see Appendix A, Immunization Timetable).	Hyperimmune gamma globulin from mumps convalescent serum may be administered to give temporary protection to boys exposed after puberty so as to reduce chances of sex-gland involvement.	Antibiotics may be used to shorten the attack and reduce the period of communicability.	Active immunization with whooping cough vaccine (see Appendix A, Immunization Timetable).
Penicillin, plus diphtheria antitoxin in certain cases, for exposed susceptible children followed by active immunization with diphtheria toxoid.		Isolation required during period of communicability (usually 2 weeks).	Immune serums are available for giving passive (temporary) immunity to exposed susceptible children and for making cases lighter.
Isolation required until 2 cultures obtained from nose and throat at intervals of 24 hours show that no diphtheria bacilli are present.	Isolation until the swelling of the salivary glands has disappeared.	Boiling or pasteurization of milk.	Separation of infected child from other children (especially those under 5), and exclusion from school and public places.
Immunity often, but not always, develops after one attack.	Immunity usual after one attack, but second attacks are not rare.	Immunity from infecting strain of streptococcus may develop but not from other strains.	Immunity usual after one attack.

Source: Control of Communicable Diseases in Man, 9th ed., American Public Health Association, New York, 1960; and Report of the Committee on the Control of Infectious Diseases, American Academy of Pediatrics, 1964.

* Direct contact means directly from person to person. Indirect contact means indirectly through handling, eating, or drinking anything soiled by discharges from the sick person or carrier.

† See also footnotes under scarlet fever, Sec. 1, Appendix B, and Scarlet Fever and Streptococcal Sore Throat, in Chap. 11.

Appendix B Communicable Diseases (continued)

	Bacillary dysentery (shigellosis)	Food infections (salmonellosis)	Food poisoning (staphylococcal intoxication)
Cause	Bacilli of the *Shigella* group; present in intestinal discharges.	Bacteria of the *Samonella* group; present in feces of infected persons or carriers and in feces of infected fowl, rodents, and domestic animals; in eggs of infected ducks and hens.	The toxin of certain strains of staphylococci present in contaminated foods.
How spread	By consuming milk and milk products, other foods, and water contaminated with bowel discharges of infected persons or carriers; by hand-to-mouth transfer of such discharges by objects soiled with them. (Flies may carry bacilli on their feet.)	By consuming food or milk contaminated by feces of infected rodents or other infected animals; by feces—soiled hands of infected food handlers; also by eating insufficiently cooked foods containing dried duck eggs or hen eggs.	By consuming milk from infected cows and foods in which staphylococci have been deposited by infected food handlers. Starchy foods, such as custard-filled pastry and salad dressings, when kept at room temperature, are especially good culture media for the staphylococci.
Incubation period	From 1 to 7 days; usually less than 4.	From 6 to 48 hours; usually about 12.	From $\frac{1}{2}$ hour to 4 hours; usually 2 to 4 hours.
Onset	Usually sudden with fever, irritability or drowsiness, loss of appetite, vomiting or nausea, diarrhea, and abdominal pain.	Sudden with diarrhea, abdominal cramps, fever; occasionally nausea and vomiting.	Sudden with severe nausea, vomiting, prostration; in some cases, severe diarrhea.
Period of communicability	From onset until bowel discharges are free of bacilli.	For duration of illness; usually 3 days to 3 weeks or as long as carrier state persists.	None.
Character of the infection	The bacilli grow in the intestinal mucosa and excrete a toxin. Mild cases are characterized by abdominal discomfort, slight fever, and a few loose stools; in severe cases there are fever, nausea, vomiting, stools containing blood and pus, and colicky pains.	Salmonella grow rapidly in the intestinal tract and produce a toxin which causes the diarrhea and other signs and symptoms. Recovery is usually complete in from 2 to 4 days. Explosive outbreaks occur among large numbers of individuals who have consumed the offending food.	The toxin produced by the staphylococci in food *before it is eaten* is responsible for the signs and symptoms of acute gastrointestinal poisoning. Staphylococcal toxin is probably the principal cause of acute food poisoning.
Methods of control*	No specific preventive.	No specific preventive.	No specific preventive.
	Adequate treatment with sulfa drugs or antibiotics brings freedom from infection within 7 days.	Isolation not required, but adults excluded from food handling and care of children until recovery.	Exclusion from food handing of individuals suffering from boils and other skin infections until infection has cleared up.
	Isolation during acute illness.	No lasting immunity after attack.	No immunity after attack.
	Relative temporary immunity after attack.		

Source: *Control of Communicable Diseases in Man,* 9th ed. American Public Health Association, 1960; and *Report of. the Committee on the Control of Infectious Diseases,* American Academy of Pediatrics, 1964.

* General preventive measures for the control of water-borne, milk-borne, and food-borne diseases include protection and purification of water supplies; pasteurization of milk supplies; sanitary disposal of excreta; prevention of fly breeding; elimination of rodents and other vermin; protection of food from flies, rodents, and other vermin; methods of refrigeration and cooking which inhibit bacterial growth or destroy bacteria or other pathogens in possibly contaminated foods; detection and elimination of infected persons and carriers in eating establishments; sanitary dishwashing; and thorough washing of the hands with soap and water after toilet and before handling or eating food.

† Direct contact means directly from person to person. Indirect contact means indirectly through handling, eating, or drinking anything soiled by discharges from the sick person or carrier.

Hepatitis, infectious	Typhoid fever	Undulant fever (brucellosis)
Infectious hepatitis (IH) virus; present in intestinal discharges, in blood, and possibly in nose and throat discharges of infected persons	The typhoid bacillus (Salmonella typhosa); present in intestinal discharges and in urine.	Bacilli of the type species Brucella; present in the tissues, blood, milk, and urine of infected goats, cattle, sheep, and swine.
Uncertain; probably by direct and indirect contact;† epidemics occur most commonly in groups of children or young adults living closely together, as in camps or institutions. See also Serum Hepatitis, in Chap. 13.	By direct and indirect contact † with sick persons and carriers. Contaminated food, milk, water, and shellfish important sources of infection. Flies may spread the bacilli from feces to food under some conditions.	By consuming raw milk or milk products from infected cows and goats and by direct contact with infected animals and the tissues of slaughtered infected animals.
Variable; 10 to 40 days; commonly 25 days.	From 1 to 3 weeks; average 2 weeks.	Variable; usually 5 to 21 days; occasionally several months.
Slow or abrupt, with fever, loss of appetite, nausea, vomiting, and abdominal distress.	Slow with headache, malaise, loss of appetite, and congestion of upper respiratory passages; slight fever which steadily rises day by day.	Slow with irregular fever, sweating, chills or chilliness, and muscle and joint pains.
Unknown; virus persists in stools for as long as 1 month after onset; may persist in blood for as long as a year.	For as long as typhoid bacilli appear in the excreta. Usually from onset throughout illness until all symptoms cease.	Practically not communicable from person to person, but bacilli may be present in the urine or other discharges.
The virus causes inflammation of the liver; as a result jaundice develops in from 5 to 7 days after onset. Recovery usually takes place in 2 or more weeks. In some cases convalescence is slow, with lassitude, weakness, mental depression, and loss of appetite.	The bacilli penetrate the intestinal mucosa, thereby gaining entrance to the bloodstream and causing a systemic infection. Rose spots (small hemorrhages into the skin) may appear over the chest and abdomen between the tenth and fifteenth day. Illness is protracted, convalescence slow, and relapses are common.	The bacilli enter the bloodstream from the intestinal tract or skin and cause a systemic infection. Acute cases usually recover in from 1 to 3 months. Periods of apparent recovery and relapses alternate in a characteristic pattern. If allergy to the bacillus develops, subacute or chronic brucellosis (lasting for from 1 to 20 years) may follow the acute attack.
Gamma globulin obtained from pooled human blood plasma injected promptly after exposure gives passive protection lasting 6 to 8 weeks.	Typhoid vaccine gives active immunization for about 1 year. Chloramphenicol (an antibiotic) is effective in treatment.	Avoidance of unpasteurized milk and milk products is the best preventive for the general population.
Isolation during the first week of illness is recommended. Persons who have had the infection should not act as blood donors.	Isolation required in flyproof room until repeated negative cultures of stool and urine specimens, taken at 24-hour intervals, have been obtained.	Combined therapy consisting of certain antibiotics and sulfadiazine is effective. Isolation not required.
Immunity usual after attack.	Immunity usual after attack.	Duration of immunity uncertain.

493

Section 4. THREE DISEASES SPREAD BY BLOOD-SUCKING INSECTS

	Ma'aria	Endemic typhus	Spotted fever
Cause	Any one of four species of malarial parasites (Sporozoa) of the genus Plasmodium.	Rickettsia prowazekii.	Rickettsia rickettsii.
How spread	By the bite of infected anopheline mosquitoes. The mosquito is infected by biting someone who has malaria when the sexual forms of the malarial parasites are present in the blood. After going through certain changes in the mosquito's body for 10 to 14 days (21 days for the quartan type) the parasites appear in the mosquito's salivary glands ready to be injected into the bloodstream of every person bitten thereafter.	By the bite of infected rat fleas commonly of the species Xenopsylla cheopis. The fleas are infected by biting rats suffering from the disease. Infected black rats (Rattus rattus) and infected brown rats (Rattus norvegicus) are the chief reservoirs of infection.	By the bite of infected ticks or contact of the unbroken skin with crushed infected ticks. In the East and South, the tick carrier of spotted fever is the dog tick (Dermacentor variabilis); in the Northwest, the wood tick (Dermacentor andersoni); in the Southwest, occasionally the lone-star tick (Amblyomma americanum). Even in highly endemic areas only about one out of every 200 to 300 ticks is infected.
Incubation period	Varies with the species of infecting plasmodium; 14 days for the most common variety.	From 6 to 14 days; usually 12 days.	From 3 to about 10 days.
Character of the attack	Abrupt onset, with a shaking chill followed by a burning fever accompanied by severe aching, thirst, and nausea. A few hours later a drenching sweat sets in and the fever goes down. Then there is a fever-free interval before the next episode. The variety of malarial parasite present in the blood determines whether the chills and fever recur every day, every other day, every third day, or at irregular intervals. Treatment with the appropriate antimalarial drug usually reduces the number of episodes of chills and fever. Without treatment the episodes may continue for some time before the attack runs its course.	Abrupt onset, with fever, chills, headache, and prostration. The fever rises rather rapidly for three or four days and then continues for 14 days, rarely for more than 16 days. On about the fifth day a skin eruption of small, pink or bright red spots develops. It usually begins with a few spots on the abdomen or on the inner surfaces of the forearms and within 24 hours becomes scattered. It seldom involves the face. Early treatment with the appropriate antibiotic usually shortens the course of the disease.	Abrupt onset, with fever, headache, and reddened eyes. About 3 or 4 days after the fever begins, a pinkish skin rash appears. The individual spots which give the disease its name are small and distinct and characteristically break out first on the ankles and wrists, whence they spread rapidly over the entire body. Early treatment with the proper antibiotic usually shortens the course of the disease.
Occurrence	Endemic malaria has been virtually eradicated or its incidence greatly reduced by modern control measures in countries where it was once a major health problem; still a major cause of illness in many tropical and subtropical regions.	Worldwide in areas where man and rats occupy the same buildings. Most prevalent during summer months.	Occurs widely throughout the United States in the spring and early summer when the adult ticks become active.
Resistance	Susceptibility to malaria is universal but may be lessened by previous infection. In highly malarious areas, suppressive drugs have great value in preventing attacks in susceptible and semi-immune persons.	No one is naturally resistant. Immunity (which is not always lasting) follows an attack.	No one is naturally resistant. Immunity (which may or may not be lasting) follows an attack.

Addresses of Organizations

Alexander Graham Bell Association for the Deaf
1537 35th Street, N.W., Washington, D.C. 20007

Allergy Foundation of America
801 Second Avenue, New York, N.Y. 10017

American Association for Gifted Children
15 Gramercy Park, New York, N.Y. 10003

American Association for Health, Physical Education, and Recreation
1201 16th Street, N.W., Washington, D.C. 20006

American Cancer Society
219 East 42d Street, New York, N.Y. 10017

American Council on Education
1785 Massachusetts Avenue, N.W., Washington, D.C. 20006

American Dental Association
222 East Superior Street, Chicago, Ill. 60611

American Diabetes Association
18 East 48th Street, New York, N.Y. 10017

American Hearing Society
919 18th Street, N.W., Washington, D.C. 20006

American Heart Association
44 East 23d Street, New York, N.Y. 10010

American Home Economics Association
1600 20th Street, N.W., Washington, D.C. 20009

American Medical Association
535 North Dearborn Street, Chicago, Ill. 60610

American National Red Cross
17th and D Streets, N.W., Washington, D.C. 20006

American Public Health Association
1790 Broadway, New York, N.Y. 10019

American Social Health Association
1790 Broadway, New York, N.Y. 10019

American Speech and Hearing Association
1001 Connecticut Avenue, N.W., Washington, D.C. 20006

Association for Childhood Education
3615 Wisconsin Avenue, N.W., Washington, D.C. 20006

Child Study Association of America
9 East 89th Street, New York, N.Y. 10028

Council for Exceptional Children (National Education Association)
1201 16th Street, N.W., Washington, D.C. 20006

Equitable Life Assurance Society
1285 Avenue of Americas, New York, N.Y. 10019

Food and Nutrition Board of the National Research Council
Washington, D.C. 20025

Illuminating Engineering Society
United Nations Plaza, 47th Street, New York, N.Y. 10017

Institute for the Crippled and Disabled
400 First Avenue, New York, N.Y. 10010

John Hancock Mutual Life Insurance Company
200 Berkeley St., Boston, Mass. 02117

Metropolitan Life Insurance Company
1 Madison Avenue, New York, N.Y. 10010

National Association for Mental Health
10 Columbus Circle, New York, N.Y. 10019

National Association for Retarded Children
386 Park Avenue South, New York, N.Y. 10016

National Commission on Safety Education
1201 16th Street, N.W., Washington, D.C. 20006

National Education Association
1201 16th Street, N.W., Washington, D.C. 20006

National Epilepsy League
203 N. Wabash Street, Chicago, Ill. 60606

National Foundation, The
800 Second Avenue, New York, N.Y. 10017

National Health Council
1790 Broadway, New York, N.Y. 10019

National League for Nursing
10 Columbus Circle, New York, N.Y. 10019

National Public Relations Council of Health and Welfare Services, Inc.
257 Park Avenue South, New York, N.Y. 10010

National Safety Council
425 North Michigan Avenue, Chicago, Ill. 60611

National Society for Crippled Children and Adults
2023 West Ogden Avenue, Chicago, Ill. 60640

National Society for the Prevention of Blindness
16 East 40th Street, New York, N.Y. 10017

National Tuberculosis Association
1790 Broadway, New York, N.Y. 10019

New York Association for Brain-Injured Children
305 Broadway, New York, N.Y. 10007

Public Affairs Committee, Inc.
381 Park Ave. South, New York, N.Y. 10016

Science Research Associates, Inc.
259 E. Erie, Chicago, Ill. 60610

Science Service
1719 N Street, N.W., Washington, D.C. 20006

U.S. Department of Health, Education, and Welfare
Washington, D.C. 20025

> Children's Bureau
> Office of Education
> Public Health Service

INDEX

Hemoglobin, breakdown of, 321
  deficiency of, in anemias, 230
  as oxygen carrier, 226, 275, 353
Hemolysins, 130
Hemophilia, 225
Hemorrhage (bleeding), 225, 230
  from external wound, first aid for, 222–223
  intracranial, 163, 423
  from nose (nosebleed), first aid for, 223
  subcutaneous, in bruises, 351, 382
  in scurvy, 291
Hepatitis, infectious, 327, 493
  gamma globulin in control of, 225, 327, 493
  jaundice in, 322
  serum, 327
Heredity, 13–15
  constitution and, 78
  dental caries and, 339
  in determination, of eye color, 13–14, 387
    of hair color, 356
    of shape of jaw, 344
  in development, of diabetes, 170
    of epilepsy, 160–161
    of familial allergy, 138–139
    of rheumatic fever, 217
  emotional stability and, 78
  environment and, 16–17
  hemophilia and, 225
  influence of, on growth pattern, 50, 51
    on intelligence, 78, 100
    on skeletal growth, 51
  mental defectiveness and, 166–167
  personality and, 13–14
Heroin addiction in adolescence, 201–202
Herpes simplex (cold sores), 334–335
Hinge joints, 447–448, 454
Hipbones, 450, 451, 455
  in sitting, 472, 473
Hips, congenital dislocation of, 477
  joints of, 447
Histamine, in allergic reactions, 140–141
  in sunburn, 350
Hives (urticaria), 138, 141, 363–364
Hoarseness, 255
Hookworm (ancylostomiasis), 330–331
Hormones, 121–124
  of adrenal cortex, 53, 123–124, 169
  of adrenal medulla (epinephrine), 123–125
  amino acids in manufacture of, 285
  of anterior pituitary, 53, 123, 168
  female (estrogens), 123, 124
  gonadal, 53, 123, 124, 169
  influence of, on growth, 53, 123, 168–169
  of islands of Langerhans (insulin), 123, 124, 170–173
  of parathyroids, 124
  of thyroid (thyroxine), 53, 124, 166, 168–169, 286
Hostility, 178
  behavior reactions to, 179, 196

Hostility, behavior reactions to, in adolescence, 197–203
  psychogenic, 126
  in stuttering, 442–443
  and guilt, 178
Humerus, 450, 455
Hunger, 320
  in diabetes, 170
  in insulin reaction, 172
Hydraulic pressure of blood, 236
Hydrochloric acid in gastric juice, 317
Hyoid bone, 454
Hyperopia (see Farsightedness)
Hypersensitivity in allergy, 139
Hypertension, 214
Hyperthyroidism, 168, 183
Hypoproteinemia, 225
Hypothyroidism, 168–169
Hysteria, anxiety, 183
  wryneck and, 478

Ileum, 304
Ilium (hipbone), 450, 455
Immunity, active, artificially acquired, 137
  naturally acquired, 135–136, 150, 265–266
  passive, 137
Immunization, 136–137
  in adenovirus infections, 256
  in colds, 253
  in communicable disease control, 40–41, 137
  in influenza, 257–258
  in measles, 44, 165, 263–264
  in mumps, 337
  in poliomyelitis, 41, 151–153
  schools and, 270
  in tetanus, 157
  in tuberculosis, 269–270
Immunization timetable, 487
Impetigo contagiosa, 366–367, 377
Impulse, nerve, 119–120
Inadequacy, feelings of, 180–181, 197
Inattentiveness, in hearing loss, 7, 425
  in petit mal, 161
Incisors, 337–338
Incus, 417, 419
Indigestion, 316–317
  acid, 317
  nervous, 146, 309
  as symptom, 183, 328, 331
Infection, causes of, 130–133
  definition of, 374–375
  inapparent (mild), in bacillary dysentery, 324
  in meningococcal meningitis, 155–156
  in poliomyelitis, 148
  in undulant fever, 326
  observing children for signs of, 270–271
  reactions of body to, 130–135
  resistance to, 250–252, 285–286
Infestations, skin, 374–377
Inflammation, 133–135